PSYCHIATRIC/MENTAL HEALTH NURSING CONTEMPORARY READINGS

PSYCHIATRIC/MENTAL HEALTH NURSING: CONTEMPORARY READINGS

Barbara A. Backer, M.S., M.A., R.N.

Patricia M. Dubbert, M.A., R.N.,

Elaine J. P. Eisenman, M.S., R.N.

Department of Nursing,
Herbert H. Lehman College of
The City University of New York.

D. VAN NOSTRAND COMPANY, INC.
New York • Cincinnati • Toronto • London • Melbourne

D. Van Nostrand Company Regional Offices:
New York   Cincinnati

D. Van Nostrand Company International Offices:
London   Toronto   Melbourne

Copyright © 1978 by Litton Educational Publishing, Inc.
Library of Congress Catalog Card Number: 77–86704
ISBN: 0–442–20479–5

Published by D. Van Nostrand Company
135 West 50th Street, New York, N.Y. 10020

10 9 8 7 6 5 4 3 2

Forword

IN THE PAST THIRTY YEARS WE HAVE SEEN the field of psychiatric nursing develop from its almost unlettered infancy into a highly sophisticated entity. That psychiatric nursing has come a long way in these three decades is well exemplified in this excellent anthology whose contents, for the most part, are derived from nursing literature and describe nursing practice. The progress made by psychiatric nurses in this period has changed the image of the psychiatric nurse from one who worked with psychiatric patients as custodian and carer for physical ills to that of a therapist—intervening on the basis of psychosocial and physiological assessments.

Rather than repeat what is readily available in other books, the editors have focused on the "how to" of psychiatric nursing. In selecting papers which apply theoretical concepts to actual clinical situations the editors have deliberately focused on the set of observations necessary before the nurse can put theory into action. To this end they have included an excellent section on the gathering of data—the first step in the solution of any problem, including problems in relationships. In this section, as in the others, the selection of articles is both comprehensive and finite and suggests that the book's contents will stimulate one's thinking to answer such questions as—who is the patient, what does the nurse need to know, and what is the scope of the nurse's practice. These themes are present throughout the book as a variety of modes of intervention are discussed by each author.

The articles in this book should provide a needed resource for nursing students and practitioners. They will also serve to provide information to other professionals about the nature of psychiatric nursing.

Claire M. Fagin Ph.D., R.N.

Preface

THIS ANTHOLOGY HAS BEEN COMPILED WITH THE PRIMARY purpose of bringing together in one volume a selection of materials illustrating the practice of contemporary psychiatric mental health nursing. The need for such a book became evident to us in our roles as instructors supervising senior students working with families, agencies, and institutions in the community and as clinical instructors supervising students in a psychiatric nursing course. For the most part, psychiatric nursing texts present only the most universally accepted and therefore general explanations of human emotional and behavioral problems. This approach is sometimes successful in its avoidance of favoring one theoretical position over another, but it tends to reduce to a minimum specific, theory-based recommendations for nursing intervention. Yet it is precisely these specific suggestions which students and generalist-prepared practitioners need if they are to advance their clinical nursing practice. No book can substitute for individual supervision as a method of teaching safe and effective nursing management of psychiatric/mental health problems, but we believe that a book of readings describing some specific views and approaches can help bridge the gap between general theoretical concepts and application of knowledge and skills to actual clinical situations.

In this collection, the reader has a source of materials drawn from a variety of professional journals. The content has been selected for its relevance to interventions and issues of importance for the generalist-prepared nurse. Readings are arranged by content area, with each section preceded by a brief introduction. Most readings were selected from the nursing literature of the last decade and particularly the last five years. In our review of the recent nursing literature, several themes emerged: the influence of the women's movement, a shift from predominance of analytic and intrapsychic approaches toward eclecticism, the independent practitioner role of the nurse, and the community mental health movement. It is exciting to follow the evolution from a position of dependence on other disciplines to a more colleague-oriented, self-directive nursing practice.

In our selections, we tried to avoid duplication of content. We also decided not to include articles whose content is important primarily for the historical development of psychiatric nursing.

Content related to child psychiatric nursing was not included because of our belief that this is a specialty area and this book was designed for the generalist practitioner.

Our primary themes reflect the many issues confronting practitioners, both in their practices and in the settings in which their practices occur. As will be apparent from the selections, psychiatric nurses are functioning in a variety of settings-inpatient wards, out-patient clinics, emergency rooms, homes, and community agencies.

Unit One is devoted to an assessment of the individual and the family, indicating the significance we attach to careful data collection and problem definition. Units two-four review the process of nursing intervention in therapeutic relationships with individuals, groups, and families—both designated psychiatric clients and others who may be undergoing extreme emotional stress. Unit five on psychopharmacology is a two-part article which we feel represents one of the most comprehensive discussions of this treatment modality. Unit six presents the nurse as a change-agent and nurses' participation in milieu therapy. Last, in order to enable the reader to begin to consider philosophical and moral issues concerning care of those labelled mentally ill, Unit seven is devoted to articles which both question traditional processes and present a variety of goals and methods of psychiatric treatment.

Acknowledgements

MANY PEOPLE HAVE HELPED AND ENCOURAGED US IN the development of this book. We especially wish to mention:

—Our students, who through their enthusiasm and questions provided us with the motivation to search out articles to assist them in planning care for their clients.

—Our friends and colleagues who helped us to retain our sense of humor.

—Noreen Garvey, without whose typing skills and high tolerance for ambiguity, the manuscript might never have been completed.

—Steven Eisenman, for his encouragement, assistance, and encyclopedic knowledge of trivia.

CONTENTS

1. Mental Health Assessment of Individuals and Families

2. Management

3. Crisis Intervention

4. Working with Groups and Families

5. Psychotropic Medications

read! (handwritten annotation)

6. Change In The Social System and Use of Therapeutic Milieu

7. Issues, Controversies, and Some Alternative Approaches

MENTAL HEALTH ASSESSMENT OF INDIVIDUALS AND FAMILIES

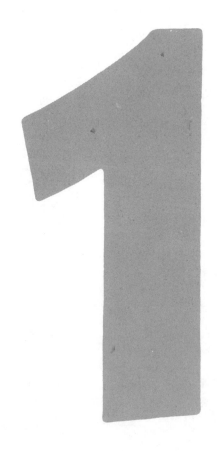

Introduction

The basis for therapeutic intervention is, first and foremost, comprehensive assessment, for only with adequate assessment is evaluation and case formulation possible. A deficit in any component of the data base prevents client-centered intervention from occurring. For this reason, a determination of the past and present functional levels and abilities of the individual and his family is essential in order to make decisions regarding health care. The ability to perform comprehensive evaluations, then, is a critical skill for nurses to possess. This skill may also be considered an art, as it involves the ability to help the client depict, perhaps for the first time, how he feels in his present situation. Similarily, the family may be helped to look at their own roles and sources of pain in a non-judgemental atmosphere.

Ideally, a thorough assessment of any individual would include a complete mental and emotional status assessment, a home visit and interview with the family (or if no family at least a home visit to determine where this person is coming from and returning to), and a problem-oriented physical examination or referral for a physical exam in order to rule out any physical etiology. The omission of any of these base-line components, as well as the depth and extent of the initial interview, is determined both by the needs of the individual and, often, by the treatment setting.

Regardless of the setting, this initial opportunity to elicit primary data lays the foundation for the therapeutic relationship as well as providing the data base for a care plan. Because the focus of nursing is on health promotion and maintenance, the assessment focuses on the client and his family's present reality and strengths. This primary contact and planned interaction helps to convey to the client and his family the nurse's role on the health care team, and serves to legitimize future contacts.

This unit is comprised of five articles, four of which speak to the initiation and enactment of mental health assessment of individuals and families; the fifth presents one method for presentation of data. Discussion of the interpretation and evaluation of data falls within the realm of textbooks on psychiatric nursing and psychiatry, and, as such, is not included here.

First, Eisenman and Dubbert present the structure and content of a comprehensive mental health interview. They include both a brief discussion of essential interview techniques specific to this type of interview and an in-depth discussion of the content areas to be assessed with suggested means for eliciting information. Also included is a detailed outline of the entire content focus for assessment and a sample case report and problem list.

Since the individual client is often but one member of a larger family unit, it is important to understand the interactional dynamics of that unit as well. Sedgewick discusses the family as a system of relationships, and, in doing so, provides five indices by which to examine these relationships. A more detailed means for family assessment is provided by Ackerman in an excerpt from *The Psychodynamics of Family Life*, a classic in the field of family therapy. Ackerman was one of the first clinician/theoreticians to consider the home visit as a critical component in the assessment process; he emphasized the value of family observation during mealtime as an essential insight into the dynamic structure. This guide provides a framework for an evaluation of interactional patterns, relationship components, and alliances both in terms of the family's internal environment and their explorations in the outside world.

One of the most overtly lethal forms of family dysfunction is that of child abuse and neglect. It is often possible to intervene in this crisis situation on a primary intervention level through early and adequate assessment of abuse potential. Kohrt's article addresses the problem of assessment and presents specific techniques for success at it.

The final article by Smith, Hawley, and Grant describes an innovative and highly efficient means for recording one's findings. The problem-oriented Weed system is one which is becoming incorporated into the charting system of many health care facilities because of its simplicity, logic, and readily understandable application to all settings. The four components of the problem-oriented record: data base, problem list, initial plan, and progress notes are discussed through a presentation of key questions and answers about this system, and through examples of charting identified health and behavioral problems.

The papers in this unit provide a foundation for the mental health assessment of individuals and families as well as a means for recording the data. Understanding the format and rationale for mental health assessment and evaluation of family functioning permits the nurse to gather data in a logical and systematic manner. Such an approach allows for a holistic view of the individual; this view is essential to nursing practice, as it clarifies the close interplay between physical and emotional problems and allows for a plan of care tailored specifically to the whole person in his place in society.

1 THE MENTAL HEALTH ASSESSMENT INTERVIEW

Elaine J. P. Eisenman, M.S., R.N.;
Patricia M. Dubbert, M.A., R.N.

NURSES IN MANY SETTINGS ARE ASSUMING MORE RESPONSIBILITY for health assessment. This trend is reflected in nursing literature by the number of recent publications describing physical examination techniques and use of the problem-oriented record system for recording health care data. Although nurses have traditionally recognized the interrelationships between a person's behavior, emotions, and physical health, this recent interest in physical assessment has apparently not been matched by corresponding attention to mental health assessment. We believe that a psychiatric assessment should be part of the nursing evaluation of every client's health status. Its purpose should be to provide specific information about a client's behavior, thoughts, and feelings and how these are related to environmental stimuli, including the immediate interview situation and any unusual or severe stresses in the client's current experience. It may explain behavior which cannot be accounted for by physical examination and serves as the baseline against which any alterations in behavior or emotions can be evaluated.

The techniques of mental health assessment which we describe can help nurses accomplish a more comprehensive assessment of their

Some of the content of this paper has been adapted from a series of three videotape programs, "Mental and Emotional Assessment of the Psychiatric Patient," by Elaine J.P. Eisenman, Patricia M. Dubbert (Larkin) and Madeline Nagle McGowan, Distributed by Blue Hill Educational Systems, Spring Valley, New York, 1975.
This article was written specifically for inclusion in this book. Copyright 1977 Elaine J.P. Eisenman and Patricia M. Dubbert.

clients. We discuss the evaluation as completed in a single, initial interview, as it would usually be carried out in psychiatric treatment settings. The data base and interviewing methods remain essentially the same (however, the structure and depth may be considerably altered) when the evaluation is part of the assessment of a client whose primary problem is physical illness or when the data is collected through a series of brief contacts, perhaps while the nurse is performing physical care. What is essential for skilled assessment is accurate, systematic observation of the client's behavior as well as communication of genuine concern so that the client can begin to gain confidence in the nurse as a helping and trustworthy person.

The Data Base

The assessment interview allows the client the opportunity to define himself as a unique individual. He is helped to share, in his own words, how he views himself and why he has come for help at this time. Here, as in any initial assessment, the nurse's goal is to obtain sufficient information to identify immediate problems in order to formulate beginning plans for intervention. The subjective data (history) is obtained through elicitation of the client's perceptions and recollections in three broad content areas: present problem and its development; descriptions of client's current functioning and lifestyle; and a brief biographical sketch of the client's family, education, social relationships, and work experience. The emphasis in history-taking is on what the client says, not the style of presentation. The completeness of the data is also important, with attention paid to what is omitted as well as what is included. In the event that the client is unable or unwilling to provide a historical overview, secondary sources are acceptable, and should be sought with the client's permission.

The direct mental status examination is considered objective data, and, as such, parallels the physical examination. This segment of the interview consists of skilled observations of the client's level of cognitive and emotional functioning as demonstrated throughout the interview. To this end, physical appearance, motor behavior and other non-verbal cues, speech patterns, and emotionality seen through mood and affect are observed and noted. Evaluation and interpretations of these observations coupled with the historical data enable the nurse to make further inferences about other areas of mental function such as thought processes, thought content, intellectual abilities, memory, degree of orientation and reality testing, insight, and judgement.

Interviewing Techniques for Mental Health Assessment

Since many clients are hesitant to reveal information which they fear will be considered socially unacceptable or "crazy", the establishment of a basis for a trusting relationship is a primary goal. The interview must be managed in such a way as to obtain sensitive information and to convey the interviewer as a skilled listener and caring person. In general, the techniques used to elicit information for physical health histories are also applicable in psychiatric assessment. There are, however, several distinctive differences between these two types of interviews as noted by Mathews and Stevens (cited in Menninger, 1952), and these are reviewed below.

First, in a psychiatric history, past medical illnesses and treatments used for symptom relief are of concern, but the focus changes to the client's emotional and behavioral responses to the illness or other stress. If a woman reports that she discovered a breast lump, but waited six months before visiting a health practitioner, the medical history would be most concerned about what was found and the subsequent treatment. In psychiatric assessment, the most pertinent data is how and why the woman reacted in that way to the experience and how she copes with comparable stresses.

Next, the client rarely knows what to expect from a psychiatric interview. He feels quite threatened about the potential responses to his feelings, thoughts, and perceptions. Many times he will have come to talk about these changes only because of pressure from his family, friends, employer, or family physician. In these situations, clients are likely to be resentful and defensive. The nurse must recognize that, at best, our society's relatively negative attitudes toward the person with emotional problems may make even a voluntary decision to seek psychiatric help a difficult and painful one.

A third difference concerns the client's accuracy as a historian. Clients can usually remember dates and events regarding physical illnesses, but the details and chronology of emotional difficulties are often blurred, forgotten or denied. Similarly, while abdominal pain can often easily be described in terms of precipitating causes, location, duration and severity, depression or a similar affective disorder can rarely be described with such precision.

Although specific interview techniques should always be tailored to the client's presenting behavior as well as the interviewer's own individual style, there are general recommendations which apply to all situations. Psychiatric assessment requires a less directive, more open-ended type of interviewing than that utilized in a medical history. The goal of the interview is to gain as full a picture of the client as possible and this is best accomplished when the client is encouraged to spontaneously expand his answers. Closed-ended, strictly worded questions will not achieve this goal. Ideally, questions which result in "yes" or "no" answers should be avoided, just as questions which ask "why" something occurred should not be asked. Far more data will be elicited through questions which consider the "who", "what", "where", and "when" of events and perceptions. Sullivan (1970) suggests that the interviewer attempt to

---

imagine what it would be like to undergo the events described . . to be where the client claims he was . . . to have a strong sense of its being possible to really follow what is being said, and if not, to say you don't understand—when you can't follow, ask questions—It's that simple—competence in language is essential. Remember that it is hard enough to describe something that one is clearly aware of, but how much more difficult it is to describe something which one is not clearly aware of but is disturbed by and then to put this in a form that a second party will understand.

Since the majority of clients will be highly anxious at the initiation of the interview, beginning with neutral topics may assist in decreasing the client's anxiety to an optimum level. It is important that the client not feel rushed or pressured into discussing something which he is not yet able to discuss. The nurse will be far more successful if she does not follow an outline too closely or require a strict chronology of presentation. The more freedom and support that a client feels in the interview situation, the more likely he is to talk about what is truly upsetting to him. While the client should be helped to do most of the talking, setting limits is also important. If the client rambles or is tangential, it is necessary to help him focus through specific questions and identification of his behavior. In this way, the client learns that the nurse is attempting to find meaning in his descriptions. When the reverse occurs, and the client says very little, he can often be helped to expand on his answers when the interviewer restates the questions and identifies the difficulty the client appears to be experiencing. Also, reassurance that his thoughts are important so that he can best be helped is useful. A flexible and supportive approach is most likely to engage the client in the interview. The more subtle, non-verbal cues are of equal importance in understanding the presenting problem. The process of the interview, that is, the covert response and interchange between the client and the nurse, tell a great deal more about the client's ability to respond to his environment.

Content and Process of the Interview

Interview content—words spoken, facial expressions, body movements, and other observable behavior—is always related to the interview process—what is happening in the relationship between the interviewer and client. What a person says and does can very often have more than one meaning and must be interpreted in the context of simultaneous messages that may conflict with one another. When a person calls a suicide "hotline" to say, "I just wanted to let you know I'm going to kill myself—everybody will be better off without me", the content of that message cannot be taken at face value. Consider the process of the interaction: the person initiated contact with a helping agency, an action certain to evoke vigorous efforts to preserve the caller's life. With this in mind, the total meaning of the client's communication can be interpreted as more on the order of, "I'm desperate, I'm planning to end my life, but maybe you can change my mind." The nurse who really listens is one who "hears" and responds to the total meaning of such communication.

In order to be aware of the process of an interview, it is necessary that the nurse assume the role of participant-observer. Through this role, the nurse is able to maintain an awareness of her own participation in the session as well as the client's participation. An important clue to the process is one's own emotional response to what is occurring. In the process of establishing rapport, for example, it is not possible to directly observe its development, but one can develop the ability to infer it from the flow of verbal content, the client's non-verbal conduct, and one's own increasing comfort. The timing and frequency of communications also provide important clues to the process of the interview. Changes in or repeated return to topics, constant or infrequent alterations in body positioning, emotional expression, and the occurrence of silences are signals which reflect discomfort or increasing anxiety on the part of the client as well as on the part of the interviewer; the message is the same regardless of who is sending it. When, for example, the nurse changes the topic whenever sexual problems are brought up, the client quickly learns that sex cannot be discussed in this relationship, that sex is a negatively-valued topic. If the nurse remains unaware of her covert communications, she may be puzzled as to what is truly happening with her client, and the client may hesitate to share information about other parts of his life as well.

In the role of participant-observer, the nurse can utilize her own feelings as a mirror for the client's feelings and experience. It is not unusual for the nurse to find herself reacting with specific emotional responses to what the client is communicating before either she or the client is aware of the total meaning of the communication. A commonly cited example of this phenomenon is the "masked" depression of a client who presents himself only with somatic complaints, but whose underlying depression is picked up by the empathic response of the nurse. Awareness of one's own emotional responses does not decrease one's objectivity; it results in developing one's self as a listening instrument far more sensitive than the finest stethoscope. The danger occurs when emotional responses go unrecognized or unacknowledged, clouding one's objectivity and making professional distance impossible.

Awareness of the process as well as the content of an interview results in a more in-depth understanding of what is being communicated. When a client responds with thinly veiled hostility or appears overly eager to please, it is necessary to understand the several levels of messages. It is not always appropriate, however, to immediately verbalize interpretations and connections between events, as the purpose of an evaluation interview is data collection, not instant analysis. This is not to say that specific feeling tones cannot be identified to facilitate the client's comfort by accepting his expression of personal feelings. For the most part, however, process and content observations are noted as part of the growing data base; further information will be needed to validate initial impressions.

Conducting the Evaluation Interview

In this section, an overview of the format of the psychiatric interview will be presented, as well as a discussion of some areas of information gathering which are usually most difficult. A detailed outline of the specific content areas to be assessed is presented at the end of this paper, followed by a brief example of a mental health assessment write-up and problem list. The outline is merely a guide to assessment and should be used with discrimination as to its appropriateness in specific situations and with sensitivity to the needs of the client. As noted earlier, the interview should not be closely structured around the outline, nor should the outline be used as a checklist as in a physical assessment review of systems. Such a presentation would be counter-productive, as it would prevent the client from spontaneously sharing his feelings, concerns, and ideas. Detail in the outline is given only to indicate the many areas of the pertinent information which might be reviewed in ideal circumstances, which, however, rarely exist. If they did, it would take several hours to cover all this data, which would also be inappropriate. Ideally, an initial interview lasts 1-1½ hours, but this can vary and depends on the needs and tolerance of the client. The critical factor is the determination of which areas of data are essential to the particular client and his particular problem. The depth and breadth of the interview is based on this determination.

In beginning the interview, it is important that the nurse introduce herself and explain her role to the client, e.g. "I'm Ms. Adams, the nurse from the clinic." If this is a referral, the client should be told by whom he was referred, and, briefly, why. The client might then be asked if he agrees that there is a problem. If he responds "yes" he should be encouraged to expand his story. If he does not agree, it is helpful to ask him about what he disagrees with and why he believes that the referring person identified an erroneous problem. He is then encouraged to present "his side". In this way, the client's initial anxieties over what the nurse knows about him are decreased, and he can begin to view the interviewer as someone who is honest and trustworthy. The interview is then seen as a shared experience in which the client's views and feelings are important (Sullivan, 1954).

When no background or referring data are available, the nurse might begin by asking the client how he has been feeling lately and/or if he has noticed any changes from the way he usually feels. If the client is unable to relate to this type of general question, a more concrete and specific introduction can be helpful. By asking the client to provide purely statistical or demographic data such as age, occupations, address, living situation and so on, the client is allowed time to relax and orient himself to the interview. By gently posing questions without pressuring for answers, the nurse continually reinforces that this is the client time and that his information and feelings are all that is important.

The importance of assisting the client to present his own ideas in his own words cannot be overemphasized. The data collected will be valid only if it is truly reflective of the client in his own words with his own priorities; if this data is filtered through the nurse's perception and depiction of the events, it is her story and not the client's. Therefore, reactions such as "You must have been angry" are inappropriate and do not provide the confirming data that "How did you feel when that happened?" provides.

It is most reassuring and least threatening if all questions build from fairly simple and general topics up to potentially emotionally-laden questions, all based, of course, on the client's statements. An example of such a sequence is as follows: the general question of "Have you had any troubling experiences lately?" could build into "Are you bothered by crowds?" which may then lead into "Do you feel that people stare at you for no reason?" and on to "Do you hear people that you don't know talk about you?" and "Does this happen when you are alone as well as when you're with others?" to "Do they hear it also?" and so on (Bellack, 1973). These questions should be asked slowly in response to the client's answers. He should not be made to feel that he is being "machine-gunned" by questions.

Often asking such questions in a concerned but matter-of-fact manner, puts the client at ease. Projection of calm acceptance is important as it may provide the client with a frame of reference different from that which he has previously received. Friends or relatives may have expressed shock, disbelief, or anger at his feelings or fears, with the result that he may have become highly defensive and convinced that he is totally alone or insane. Lack of surprise at his feelings will indicate that he is not the only person who has ever felt this way. The nurse's acceptance is essential to the client's ultimate acceptance of himself and recognition that his symptoms do not mean that he is without hope.

An additional factor which is both essential to the comprehensive nursing assessment and a way of decreasing the client's discomfort in the interview is the emphasis the interviewer places on the client's strengths and successful past coping efforts. Questions such as, "What kind of things do you enjoy doing?" and "What do you like best about yourself?" or comments like, "When you feel good, you've been able to handle some difficult situations very well" imply the client is seen as a responsible, competent person, with assets as well as problems. Assessment of strengths serves also as beginning intervention in such areas as helping a despairing client see himself and his situation more realistically.

The client may be unable to discuss various issues about his present or past life which are most emotionally charged. It cannot be emphasized enough that one should not push too hard for the client to produce. While anxiety is necessary in working through conflicts, the purpose of the initial interview is to decrease anxiety and assess its possible origins, while offering the possibility of help. Therefore, when it beomes apparent that a topic is too threatening because the client begins to retreat or defend, the topic should be left. The nurse can verbally identify this as an area which causes anxiety, and note that while it is important that it be discussed, it can be returned to later on when the client is better able to discuss it.

Assessment of the presenting problem necessitates an exploration of the client's perception of his current mental health status and a description of any changes in his usual mode of functioning. Here it is important for the nurse to keep in mind that a consideration of changes in one's relationships, thoughts, and feelings can be extremely threatening. The client should not be pressured into admitting changes. If the client is highly defensive or resistant, the nurse can acknowledge the difficulty that he is having in discussing such matters, and may remark that other people also have similar feelings. If the client still resists or denies problems and his anxiety continues to increase, the nurse should note this response, and continue on with less threatening matters. In this first interview it is inappropriate to confront the client with his resistances. As noted earlier, the task is simply to gather a data base for planning interventions, and resistance to sharing information simply becomes part of that data base.

Some clients deny emotional alterations by focusing entirely on somatic changes. If this occurs, the nurse should communicate to the client that she recognizes that these problems concern him, but to fully understand them, she must have other information to consider other possibilities. When a client begins to focus in on only one area of experience, he needs assistance in beginning to widen his self-perception and level of insight.

The assessment of integrative patterns consists of evaluating how well the client sees himself as fitting into the world. His description of himself and his personal and occupational responsibilities and ability to meet these responsibilities as well as his depiction of his lifestyle and social relationships provide the data for assessment. The nurse must also elicit data regarding changes in these varied but overlapping spheres of functioning. Does he see himself changing while others remain the same or vice versa? Is it only his feelings which are changing or is it his perception of his body as well? Does he feel out of step with the world or only an observer? Does it ever seem that there is a filter between him and everyone else? Can he influence people and/or situations or is he a helpless victim? Does he feel as though he is in a dream? and so on. (Bellack, 1973). When the nurse elicits and clarifies positive findings in these areas, she may be assisting the client in articulating what he has experienced but been unable or afraid to express to others.

Another content area for assessment is historical data. The importance of this area has been subject to controversy, as many nurses believe that obtaining the history is irrelevant to the client's present life experience. The question is often raised as to how one can even begin to consider, for example, a woman's relationship with her mother, when presently she cannot leave her apartment. Such an attitude is naive and counterproductive. While one should not attempt to take a complete history from an extremely agitated, actively suicidal, or obviously hallucinating client, this omission would be due to an assessment of priorities, just as a complete health history would be inappropriate for a hemmorrhaging accident victim. Under routine circumstances, however, a relevant, closely circumscribed personal and familial history which focuses on coping patterns and psychiatric antecedants to present behaviors is essential for planning.

Thus, the nurse is not concerned (unless the client is) with the very specific and esoteric data such as age of toilet training, early perceptions of parents and such, but rather with the general data which comprise the developmental background. A fuller picture will emerge if the client is asked to describe what he was like during the different periods of his life rather than what he did i.e., school record, jobs held. With this data, the nurse can begin to assess the client's functioning in terms of those developmental tasks he has mastered and those which were associated with high levels of stress. The questions that the nurse seeks to answer include the following: Is his present pattern of functioning part of a clearly recognizable life pattern? How does he usually cope with stress? Which coping methods are successful, which are not? Has he had close relationships in the past? Why have they terminated? Has he ever considered violent behaviors including suicide or homicide; if so under what circumstances? What stopped him? Did he have a plan? Knowledge of the client's life patterns are an important component in planning. Plans for someone who has held six jobs in three years, tends to "take off " when under stress, has no close friends, and uses alcohol or drugs to alleviate anxiety would be very different from someone who presents a similar picture of withdrawal and depression but whose history indicates a stable work history, close circle of friends, and a tendency to work through problems, until recently when she was laid off from a job held for ten years. Because a primary goal of assessment is to determine what is different or perceived as a problem *now*, it is necessary to know what life was *before*.

The family history is also important: specifically, information regarding the role of the client in his family, the integrity of the family unit while he was growing up and the reason for and chronology of any losses, and the existence of familial historical precedents for the client's present behavior. To this end, the client should be helped to describe, in a general way, what it was like for him when he was growing up. How did he view the people in his family? How does he think they viewed him? Is there a history of emotional illness/violence/suicide? It may also be possible to ascertain, at this time, how the client's family could be involved in treatment.

Historical precedents of behavior and their significance are essential for accurate assessment, as reactions to stress are often determined more by the emotional resources of the person undergoing stress than by the stress itself. Consequently, it is important for the nurse to understand the client's perception of the event as distinct from her perception. For example, a hemorrhoidectomy may appear to the nurse to be a relatively trivial procedure, but a client's associations and projections may transform this into a major emotional trauma. The nurse must be alert for signs of emotionally charged topics, and must be prepared to do some good detective work in pulling together seemingly unconnected pieces of historical data. Clients rarely state directly: "The reason I'm having an anxiety attack over my forthcoming surgery is that my grandfather died of cancer of the rectum when he was my age and I think that is what is really wrong with me". It is the nurse who is charged with making these significant associations by taking a comprehensive history and watching for non-verbal cues.

The objective data, the direct examination, is based upon the nurse's observations of the client's behaviors and responses—his presentation of himself. Although this data is collected through a subjective process, this does not mean that it necessarily is judgemental or value-laden. For example, in assessing the appropriateness of a client's attire, the issue is not whether it is attractive or stylish, but whether it is right for the present situation and setting; this assessment provides valuable clues for later evaluation of reality orientation. A bathing suit and sandals would not be normal for the outpatient clinic during a snow-storm if the client came in for a scheduled appointment. If, however, he was brought in by family or friends directly from the heated pool in his health club after he had begun to behave in a bizarre fashion, his attire would be evaluated differently. Thus, there are two components of the observation: 1) is it appropriate to the setting? and 2) was it appropriate to the client's place of departure?

Also, the nurse's impressions of the client's presentation of himself are described. One should observe the outward manifestations of the way that he feels. Does he look at you or away from you? If he does look at you, is he able to tolerate eye contact, or does he focus on your ear or other inappropriate location? If he looked away from you, does he stare at a particular object, or simply into distant space? Also, is this consistent throughout the interview or dependent upon the topic being discussed? Another area of concern is the degree to which he relates to you. How does he appear to view you—as a person or as an object? Does he acknowledge you at all?

In the assessment of the client's behavior, his general level of activity is evaluated through such indices as his ability to sit for an extended period of time, the degree of fidgeting, and the quality of these behaviors. Is he aware of his environment? Can he function within its constraints? Similarily, his voice and speech give valuable clues to his present status. How does his voice sound? What is the rate? Does he speak softly? meekly? Does he scream? What is the extent of tonal fluctuations? What is the rate—does he talk "a mile a minute" or is the discussion like "pulling teeth"?

A more abstract area for assessment is that of the determination of barriers to communication. A functional barrier occurs when the client is unable to discuss matters due to the intrusion of such factors as hallucinatory or delusional content, denial, hostility, or anxiety. Suppression or repression may be the operant defense mechanisms which prevent his remembering or accounting for missing information. This type of blocking may range from a simple "I don't remember" or "I can't discuss that" to a more complex withdrawal from the interview with such symptoms as word salad, neologisms, and autistic thinking. Organic barriers, too, may range from the most obvious where the client is unable to communicate due to physical deformity, to the more subtle symptomatology of organic brain syndrome and other degenerative conditions. In order to begin the process of differentiation, it is of utmost importance to note carefully the quantity and quality of memory loss, confusion, and occurrence of areas of avoidance. Oftimes clients with organic difficulties will confabulate in order to hide the memory loss. Evaluating recent and remote memory is an important basis for differentiation, and this can also be accomplished through good history taking. Also, as will be discussed later, gross testing of cognitive abilities is another basis for differentiation.

While the identification of the client's mood is relatively straightforward, the question of affect is often problematic. Affect is considered to be the visual portrayal of mood, but the evaluation should include more than a mere notation of the client's facial expression. Assessment of affect actually includes an assessment of the degree of congruity between the mood and the prevailing thought content. Are traumatic events described without expression or with an appropriate expression? Lack of facial expression is referred to as a "flat" or "bland" affect. The degree of congruity provides important clues to the quality of the client's thought content and reality orientation.

A critical area of evaluation for mental status is that of the client's thought processes. The interviewer evaluates how the client thinks, and what he thinks about. First, the quality of the client's responses to the nurse's questions are assessed in terms of spontaneity and appropriateness. The nurse notes whether there is a rapid flitting from one idea to another, whether the connections between ideas are understandable, whether there is an over-inclusion of trivial detail, and, if the words are nonsensical or irrelevant.

Next, the client's cognitive ability, his ability to deal with abstract concepts, is evaluated. Often this area of assessment is difficult to formally evaluate, as the client may feel threatened and become highly anxious if he believes that he is being tested or that the material is irrelevant. It may be helpful to acknowledge the potential anxiety by offering an introduction such as "Now I'm going to ask you some questions which may sound silly and unimportant but it is important that you answer as best you can." The client is then asked to interpret simple proverbs such as "People who live in glass houses shouldn't throw stones" or "A stitch in time saves nine". Two proverbs are usually sufficient as baseline data of conceptual ability. The interviewer should record the client's exact reponses; evaluation of the responses focuses on the degree of abstract thought evidenced in the client's interpretation. Similarly, reality testing and judgement are evaluated by asking such questions as "What do you think of the statement She kept the food warm in the refrigerator?" or "If you found a stamped, addressed letter in the street what would you do with it?"

Two readily accepted means for gross testing of intellectual functioning are "serial sevens", in which the client is asked to subtract 7 from 100 as far as he is able, and simple arithmetic problems such as making change. Reality orientation may be formally tested, if sufficient information has not been obtained through the general interview, by asking about major news events over the past week, the day's date, the president's name and so on. These questions not only regard reality orientation, but also test for recent memory and degree of self preoccupation. An excellent test of memory is to give the client three two digit numbers to remember. He is then asked to recall them after five minutes of further discussion.

In all the above examples, evaluation of performance is dependent upon the client's academic history and premorbid achievement level. A physicist who could not complete "serial sevens" would be assessed very differently than a dishwasher who had not completed the third grade. Consistent with this expectation of differing ability, one should carefully note the client's use of language throughout the interview. Is his vocabulary and ability for concept formation congruent with his education, life style, and occupation? Congruence, or lack of it, is a critical area for evaluation. One note of caution, however. This type of overt assessment, like previously noted content areas, should not be forced. In many situations it is preferable to avoid contrived test questions in favor of eliciting the data from the client's spontaneous responses. Whenever possible, of course, such formal testing should be performed, but not at the cost of the client's comfort and continued rapport in the interview.

Evaluation of thought content is extremely complex. This involves an attempt to understand the internal composition of the client's responses, concerns, and perceptions of the world. Often the nurse is more uncomfortable in questioning the specifics of this internal world than the client is in sharing his thoughts. This interview may be the first opportunity in which the client has been able to talk with someone who wants to hear his thoughts, fears, and concerns, and perhaps more importantly, does not challenge them or falsely reassure him. For this reason, although the client may show initial reluctance to share thoughts which others have found unacceptable, the nurse's non-judgemental, matter-of-fact approach will help him believe that here is someone in whom it is safe to confide.

A primary focus of the evaluation of thought content is the central theme of the interview. Not only should the nurse note any recurring areas of discussion, but also the way in which the client refers to himself. Does he repeatedly deprecate himself with such statements as "I know you have more important things to do . . ." or "I'm ashamed to tell you this but . ." or is he grandiose with such statements as "I'm certain that I'm the most interesting patient you've ever had in this place . . ." or "this must be the saddest story you've ever heard . . ."

Also included in the area of thought content is the quality of the client's insight and his level of judgement. Insight refers to the way that the client interprets his problems and his life story. Does he attempt to evaluate situations in a glib, superficial manner? Can he explain the reasons for his problems? Does he blame others or fate for his present situation? Does he display psychotic insight by ascribing his difficulties to the workings of a delusional system? An example of this is when the client claims he is a robot controlled by a computer or believes he lost his job because of a plot engineered by the FBI. Judgement, in contrast, is considered the ability to arrive at appropriate conclusions about the environment as well as one's own place in this environment. This can be evaluated both through the client's responses to questions testing cognition and abilities through his past and present history of decision-making. Does he do dangerous or risky things? Does he enjoy taking chances? What kind of chances? Does he consider the risks and possible outcomes of actions before he becomes involved? Are his life goals consistent with his past accomplishments and intellectual abilities (Bellack, 1973).

Often, a client's special preoccupations interfere with his intellectual functioning. Consequently, it is important to identify any disturbed perceptions, unusual or extreme emotional responses, obsessive thoughts or compulsive behaviors which the client experiences. For some clients it is appropriate to use psychiatric labels for such problems; they are comforted by the objectivity of such questions as "Do you have hallucinations?" For the majority of clients, however, it is more comforting and appropriate to ask about any disturbing thoughts or feelings that they may be experiencing. Questions which elicit the necessary responses include: "Do you see/hear things that other people deny? "Do you ever have trouble deciding if something really happened? Do other people often tell you that you're 'out of it'? Do you ever believe that others are saying things about you? That others can control your thoughts or read your mind? Do you hear voices when no one else is around? Do you ever feel that you have been chosen for a special mission?" and so on. The primary focus here is on how the client feels and what he believes to be true. He may not only be terrified by these feelings but may also fear that others will find them amusing or will not believe them. It is not appropriate to question or challenge the existence or validity of his beliefs, that these are beliefs which affect his behavior is sufficient unto itself. The client should not feel pressured into proving that his beliefs are true. In fact, at the time of the initial interview, not enough data is available to either confirm or deny many allegations.

For the purposes of this discussion, the final part of the assessment interview is the evaluation of the degree of suicidal or homicidal risk. It is acceptable and necessary to straightforwardly ask the client if he has ever wished that he were dead or wanted to die; likewise if he has ever wanted another person to die and if he felt that he could hurt or kill that person. What stopped him from activating this wish? Does he still feel that way? If positive responses are elicited, further information regarding past attempts, familial history, recent loss, and other provoking factors or life changes is critical to determine the degree of risk. As in past areas of assessment, when such questions are asked in a matter-of-fact tone, implying that other people also have felt this way, the questions are usually a relief rather than a challenge. If the client is not suicidal or homicidal, these questions very rarely stimulate ideas that will lead to such an act. If the client is suicidal, these questions give him permission to discuss his fears and desperation. Unless the nurse introduces this topic, a suicidal client may not bring it up as he may feel that he should not talk about this. This type of message is frequently one that he has repeatedly received from family and friends, and he has no way of knowing that the nurse feels differently unless he is told. Of course, timing of questions is important, and it may not be appropriate to ask about suicide while the client is discussing how hopeless he has been feeling.

As the initial interview ends, the nurse should recognize that the client has given a great deal of himself, and deserves something in return for this tremendous effort. Therefore, before terminating the session, a brief, objective summary of the discussion is extremely helpful. This allows the client the reassurance that he has been heard, and also permits him the opportunity to add anything which might have been missed, forgotten, or misinterpreted. In addition, the client should be told what will happen next, when and by whom he will be seen. Finally, he can be given hope if the nurse expresses concern, understanding, and appreciation of how difficult his life has become, how hard it was for him to share it, and that he has come to the right place where he will be helped to feel better.

In conclusion, mental health assessment is achieved through an interview in which the client is invited to share, perhaps for the first time, his fears, beliefs, and means of relating to the world. The nurse's goal is to gain a picture of how this person functions in the world about him in order to assist him in improving his abilities. To gain the fullest possible picture, it is essential to have knowledge of this person's present stresses and coping mechanisms as well as an understanding of earlier modes of functioning and of the various forces in his life which have contributed to his immediate situation. A firm understanding of these interlocking components is critical for the accurate interpretation and evaluation which permit optimum health planning and intervention for this person.

Addenda I

The Psychiatric Interview:
Client History and Mental/Emotional Status Assessment

I. **General Description of Client: Client Profile**
    A. Age
    B. Sex
    C. Racial and Ethnic Data
    D. Marital Status
    E. Number and Ages of Children/Siblings
    F. Spouse/Parents Ages-Still living
    G. Living Arrangements
    H. Occupation
    I. Education
    J. Description of Typical Day.
II. **Presenting Problem and History of Presenting Problem**
    (Client's perception of problems in daily living)
    A. Difficulties/Alteration in:
        1. Relationships
        2. Usual level of functioning
        3. Behavior
        4. Perceptions
        5. Cognitive abilities

B.   Increase in Feelings of:
  1. Depression
  2. Anxiety
  3. Hopelessness
  4. Being overwhelmed
  5. Suspiciousness
  6. Confusion

C.   Somatic Changes
  1. Constipation
  2. Diarrhea
  3. Insomnia
  4. Lethargy
  5. Weight loss or gain
  6. Anorexia
  7. Palpitations
  8. Pruritis
  9. Nausea
  10. Vomiting
  11. Headaches

D.   Integrative Patterns
  1. Relations to others
  2. Relations to self
  3. Relations to things and ideas
  4. Relations to present situation
  5. Relations to reality

III.   Relevant History
A.   Personal
  1. Sketch of Life History:
     A.   Previous Hospitalizations and illnesses
     B.   Educational Background.
       1. Highest grade/degree completed
       2. If leaves of absence—why
     C.   Occupational Background
       1. Presently employed
       2. Previous positions and reasons for leaving
     D.   Social Patterns
     E.   Sexual Patterns
     F.   Interests/Hobbies and Abilities
     G.   Substance Use and Abuse
       1. Food
       2. Drugs
       3. Alcohol

        H.   Unusual or Outstanding Remembered Incidents

        I.   Usual Methods of Coping with upsetting situations

        J.   Suicidal or Homicidal Attempts, Violent Behavior

  B.   Familial

      1.   Sketch of Family and Placement within Family

        a.   Significant people in home during Childhood and Adolescence

        b.   Integrity of Family Unit.

            1.   Reasons for any breakdowns

        c.   Role played/assigned within Family

        d.   Substance Use and Abuse

        e.   History of Physical and/or mental illness

        f.   Suicidal or Homicidal attempts or successes

        g.   Anything else viewed as significant

IV. Mental and Emotional Status.

  A.   Appearance

      (general impression of client)

      1.   Apparent physical condition

        a.   Physical deformities

        b.   General Health

        c.   Approximate height and weight

      2.   Dress

        a.   Appropriateness for age-sex-season-setting

      3.   Eye Contact

        a.   Where does client look

      4.   Posture

      5.   Relatedness to Interviewer

  B.   Behavior

      1.   Motor Activity

        a.   General Energy Level

            1.   Inertia

            2.   Restlessness

            3.   Impulsive

        b.   Walk and Gait

        c.   Gestures and Mannerisms

      2.   Awareness of Environment.

C. Speech
   1. Sound
      a. Shouts
      b. Whispers
      c. Mumbles
      d. Monotonic
   2. Rate
      a. Profuse
      b. Constricted
   3. Barriers to Communication
      a. Organic or Functional
D. Mood
   1. Quantitative and Qualitative Abnormalities
      a. Appropriateness to topic being discussed
      b. Overall Impression.
         1. Depressed
         2. Tearful/crying
         3. Euphoric
         4. Anxious
         5. Apprehensive
         6. Angry
         7. Hostile
         8. Sarcastic
         9. Manic
         10. Fearful
         11. Apathetic/flat
   2. Affect
      a. Appropriateness to discussion and mood
         1. Bland/flat
         2. Overdramatic
   3. Emotionality
      a. What is dominant emotion-intensity-range
E. Thought Processes
   1. Quality of Responses
      a. Appropriate/Inappropriate
      b. Tangential
      c. Concrete
      d. Flight of ideas
      e. Stereotypic
      f. Word salad

        g.   Neologisms
        h.   Confabulation
        i.   Autistic Word Usage
  2.   Cognitive Ability
        a.   Concept Formation
             1.   Proverbs
             2.   Serial Sevens
             3.   Number Repetition
        b.   Articulateness
             1.   Precision
             2.   Vocabulary
  3.   General Characteristics
        a.   Speed of Thought
        b.   Spontaneity
        c.   Flexibility/Rigidity
        d.   Distractibility
        e.   Continuity
        f.   Alertness
        g.   Blocking
        h.   Attention and Retention
F.   Thought Content
  1.   Central Themes
  2.   Self Concept
  3.   Insight into problems
  4.   Awareness of problems
  5.   Judgement
  6.   Special Preoccupations and extent to which they interfere
        a.   Hallucinations (auditory/visual/olfactory/tactile)
        b.   Delusions
        c.   Illusions
        d.   Depersonalization
        e.   Derealization
        f.   Somatic/Hypochondriacal
        g.   Obsessions
        h.   Rituals
        i.   Fears
        j.   Phobias
        k.   Grandiosity/Worthlessness
        l.   Nihilism
        m.   Morbid Thoughts
        n.   Religiosity

       7.   Suicidal Ideation
       8.   Homocidal Ideation
   G. Degree of Reality Orientation
       1.   Knowledge of time-place-month-year
       2.   Memory-remote and recent
       3.   Ability to distinguish between internal and external stimuli.
   H. Suicidal and Homicidal Risk
       1.   Wish to die/kill
       2.   History of Attempts
       3.   History of successful/unsuccessful attempts by family
       4.   Existence of plans
       5.   Intent
       6.   History of recent loss or aggravating factors
V.   Evaluation/Interpretation
   A. Need for Emergency Actions
       1.   Overt Homicidal or Violent Impulses
       2.   Potential Suicide
       3.   Inability to function
   B. Ego Strengths
       1.   Reality Testing
       2.   Judgement
       3.   Sense of Reality of World and Self
       4.   Regulation and Control of Drives and Impulses
       5.   Object Relations
       6.   Thought Processes
       7.   Functional Abilities
   C. Nursing Diagnosis
VI. Problem List
VII. Plans

Addenda II

Sample Write-Up of Mental Health Assessment.

Debra W. presents as a well-groomed thin woman aged 20 years old who both looks and dresses her age. She was dressed cleanly and neatly in a well-fitting slack outfit. She sat stiffly in her chair, holding onto the sides, while staring blankly at a point beyond the interviewer's head. She appeared very sad, her eyes brimming with tears. Debra states that she has initiated this OPD visit because she feels that she is very ill and cannot function any longer.

Debra presently lives with her mother and a 2 year old son in a 5 room apartment in a middle-income project. She does not work. Her mother, an elementary school teacher, supports Debra and her son, Donald.

Debra states that she has lost her mind and cannot remember any information about her past. She believes that she has no friends, that they have all died, and that she is totally alone. When asked for more information, she states "I'm sorry, it's too upsetting, please don't ask anymore."

Debra does note, however, that the process of losing her mind began on January 18, 1977. She denies that this date has any meaning for her other than the beginning of her present deterioration. When asked why she believes that she remembers the specific date, she replied, "Wouldn't you remember the date when you went crazy?" She then apologized for yelling at me, which she actually had not done.

Although Debra was unable to provide specific historical data, she answers direct questions cooperatively, framing each answer with tears and a query as to whether the interviewer thinks she will recover. When reassured that she can recover, she thanked me profusely, once grabbing my hands and kissing them. She attempts to engage the interviewer, yet prevents closeness, answering questions with minimal response and negligible information. She denies self-mutilative tendencies, although there are several scars on her face and lips which were allegedly received from her boyfriend; three front teeth are also absent. She denies current drug usage, but admits to snorting heroin for a year in the past.

Debra appears markedly depressed, expressing anxiety over her lack of feeling. She notes her extreme loneliness and hopelessness, feelings which are constant with no variation either in time or frequency. Her answers are very soft and slow. Her answers to questions are direct and to the point, with no voluntary expansion of answers or information; she is not, however, evasive in her answers, nor is she tangential.

She displays no ideas of reference, phobias, compulsions nor obsessions. She is preoccupied with the idea that she is dying due to her many somatic concerns. These include anorexia, severe headaches, stomach-aches, heart palpitations, and torticollis. A recent physical exam has not found any physiological basis for these complaints. She displays no suicidal ideation, but she thinks she will die from her "heart exploding". She appears overwhelmingly depressed, expressing much pessimism— "I'll never get better", helplessness and guilt—"My mother has done so much for me and I just make things worse for everyone". Also, Debra gives evidence of her own sense of inadequacy and low self esteem as she describes all that has happened is of her own doing, "I'm a totally worthless person. . . . I'm stupid. . . ."

Although she is preoccupied with her physical state and is morbidly overconcerned with the possibility of dying, she displays a marked desire and willingness to allow herself to be convinced that she will not die, that the clinic will take care of her. She denies hallucinations, but admits to intense feelings of depersonalization and derealization. She describes her mind as functioning outside her body, and everyone looking and walking as though in a dream; she feels that her body is detached from the rest of the world.

Debra was unable to perform "serial sevens", first stating that she was not good in math, then agreeing to try. She stated, "100–93– is that right so far?—86–82–76–72–68– can I please stop now?" She interpreted a "rolling stone" as "its something about ecology—I have a banner about pollution at home—is that right, did I do it right?" She then asked if we could stop talking because her head was beginning to hurt from all the thinking that she was doing.

The interview was terminated at this point as she was unable to tolerate further contact. Debra was given an appointment with a psychiatrist for the next day for further diagnostic evaluation. Also permission was obtained to contact her mother. She was instructed to call if she became overly upset before the next day.

Evaluation

Debra was not able to provide sufficient data for a complete assessment or evaluation. Little history was obtained, and there is not adequate information for an understanding of precipitating events. A meeting with her mother is essential before planning can begin. There is no need for emergency measures at this time.

Problem List

1. Incomplete data base
2. Debra's belief that she has "lost her mind" on January 18, 1977
3. Somatic Complaints
   a. Palpitations
   b. Anorexia
   c. Headaches
   d. Torticollis
   e. Stomach-aches.
4. Anxiety
5. Depression
6. Hopelessness
7. Social Isolation
8. History of Heroin Use
9. Past destructive relationships

10. Confusion
11. Morbid Preoccupation
12. Poor cognitive performance
13. Inability to tolerate interview
14. Depersonalization
15. Derealization

Bibliography

Bellack, Leopold., et al *Ego Functioning In Schizophrenics, Neurotics, and Normals.* New York: Wiley and Sons, 1973.

Cadoret, Remi, and King, Lucy. *Psychiatry in Primary Care.* St. Louis: C. V. Mosby Co., 1974.

Matthews, and Stevenson. "The Art of Interviewing:, cited in *A Manual for Psychiatric Case Study* by Karl Menninger, New York: Grune and Stratton, 1952.

MacKinnon, Roger, and Michels, Robert. *The Psychiatric Interview in Clinical Practice.* Philadelphia: W. B. Saunders Co., 1971.

Menninger, Karl. *A Manual for Psychiatric Case Study.* New York: Grune and Stratton, 1952.

Sullivan, Henry S. *The Psychiatric Interview.* New York: W. W. Norton and Co., 1954.

THE FAMILY AS A SYSTEM: A NETWORK OF RELATIONSHIPS

Rae Sedgewick, Ph.D., R.N.

IN ORDER TO BETTER UNDERSTAND THE FAMILY AS a unit, let us begin by looking at the family as a system of relationships. Families are made up of relationships between people whose interactions and patterns of living influence each other. A family then, is an integrated system of interdependent structures and functions, is constituted of relationships, and consists of people who must learn to live together.

Each person, in a healthy family, must be capable of transmitting messages and responding sufficiently so that others are aware that a transmission has occurred. Each person responds predictably, with some pattern to the behavior. These patterns of behavior compose a network of relationships which may be referred to as a system. Patterns of behavior may be referred to as components or units which in combination with other components interrelate to produce the overall system known as the family. These units or patterns of behavior reveal via symbols, verbal and nonverbal, what is going on within respective belief systems. These patterns of behavior are transmitted via symbols, from generation to generation. Each member of each generation is, in some way or another, an origin of values, beliefs or attitudes. Each originator or origin acquires tools, skills and expertise which will facilitate or hinder the transmission or articulation of these values, beliefs and/or attitudes.

Since this view of the family differs from traditional approaches and has concomitant implications for social, psychological and health oriented interventions, it is helpful to describe more fully the family as a network or

Reprinted, with permission, from *Journal of Psychiatric Nursing and Mental Health Services*, March–April 1974.

system of relationships. Viewing the family as a system of relationships can be contrasted with viewing the family as made up of individual people with stereotypic role functions. The latter approach, as is well known, describes the family as a biological unit and calls into play those principles which have been traditionally utilized to understand biological units, *i.e.*, one in which the members are bound by fixed rules and role expectations based on biological functions and explained by historical precedents. The former view entails describing the family as a social unit, and of employing principles and dynamics of group development or social units to understand the overall process.

If we regard the family as a system of relationships, we seek to understand development of relationships, of group norms and expectations, of communication skills, of group decision-making and of group methods of dealing with individual needs and group expectations. If, on the other hand, we regard the family as a biological unit, we seek only to know the traditional expectations of each role or function and any dysfunction is attributed to the individual's inability to properly execute or fulfill those traditional expectations.

A further elaboration is helpful. The family has been traditionally viewed as a biological unit meaning there is a male-father, female-mother and as a result female and/or male offspring. The family is not "complete" without such members. While this is a sound biological description of a "family," parenting is predominately social. Parenting is a process which not only begins with conception but extends throughout the life span. Parenting need not be biological but rather can be quite logically based on social and emotional responsibility. Fathering is traditionally associated with those qualities or characteristics assumed to be typically masculine, *i.e.*, decisive, dominant, aggressive, strong, intellectual, and work-oriented. Mothering, on the other hand, is traditionally associated with those qualities or characteristics assumed to be feminine or womanly, *i.e.*, tender, caring, gentle, submissive, cooperative, tactful, and home-oriented.

The roles emerging from the traditional biological approach are analogous to the hierarchal structure in industry: manager-policy making and labor-policy implementing. This structure is best understood by knowing tradition and making comparative analyses between what are traditionally or historically acceptable roles and the present role enactments. The understanding gleaned from this approach has very little to do with what actually goes on in any given *group* or family. This approach, while accepted by many lay people, health professionals, and behavioral scientists, has added little to our conceptual or practical knowledge of families. It is an approach based on generalities and stereotypes. A family cannot be understood by looking at traditional roles and expectations and inference applying this analysis to all other families.

On the other hand, if we approach the family as a system, organizational theory and principles of psychosocial learning become our conceptual framework. The family can be viewed as a social unit made up of interdependent relationships and as a social unit in which decisions must be made, policies determined, feelings honored, skills respected, and comfort given. Each person needs space for individual growth and development; but each has group or family obligations as well. Parenting is no less important in this framework. As in every group, leadership is imperative. Those who are best prepared should assume that role. As in other organizational models, there are managerial decisions, labor implementations and consumer/user needs. While traditionally these roles cited above have been filled by father, mother and child, respectively and exclusively, in the systems model these roles need not be so rigidly defined and assigned. Clarity of role is both necessary and useful, however clarity of role in the traditional approach frequently implies rigidity as well; *i.e.*, one person exclusively fills one role. The social approach allows more flexibility, *i.e.*, one role can be filled by different persons under different situations. The role fulfillment then becomes dependent on an individual's strengths and weaknesses in particular situations. Stress can severely limit one's ability to be protective in one particular instance while that same individual may be very protective and supportive at other times. While roles are necessary for effectiveness, role assignment need not be traditional.

Task and expressive roles are the most commonly agreed upon roles necessary for group effectiveness.[1] Expressive roles are those primarily centered on interpersonal tasks, which are concerned with maintaining and strengthening interpersonal relationships. This is what is meant by being "people centered," so frequently associated with mothering. By contrast, task leaders are primarily involved with task or job accomplishments, with things rather than people and with solutions to problems rather than with interpersonal relationships. Traditionally, it has been assumed that the father will assume a greater degree of leadership in the task area, while mothers tend more often to take the role of mediator, conciliator and comforter. However, regardless of who is assuming a leadership function, effectiveness in group functioning is dependent on a high level of cooperation and support from the partner not assuming that role.[2] This can be contrasted with disturbed families where patterns emerge which are fixed, static, and often extreme, *e.g.*, authoritarian, patriarchy. In the healthy family, roles are not fixed and static, but are assumed by the person with the greatest time and inclination for fulfilling that particular role at that particular point in time. Role fulfillment is flexible, *e.g.*, little Diane falls and scrapes her knee, daddy being available picks her up, comforts and soothes, and she's off again. Mother, having taken a course on *Care of Your Car* is making a decision on when and where to have the car serviced.

Dysfunction of the family, using the systems approach, assumes the dysfunction to be either within the particular family system *e.g.*, lack of role clarity, vagueness of expectation, unresolved conflict or some disturbance between the family systems and other systems such as church, police, school. Dysfunction is not taken to be within one individual, *e.g.*, the identified patient, but the result of some system deficit. Additionally, a dysfunction in any one part of the family system or any impinging systems, *e.g.*, school, has an affect on all systems involved. The child who demonstrates behavioral problems in the classroom or at home is frequently an indication that something is amiss in one of the systems, *e.g.*, parental disharmony, teacher-principal conflict, vagueness of policy or inadequate role definition.

Several indices can be employed to examine relationships within a group, social unit or family.[3] Five common yardsticks are: productivity, decision-making, utilization of information or data, implementation of decision-making, and resolution of conflict or disagreement.

Productivity relates to a family or group's ability to complete a task. For example, if a family has defined priorities for itself, how able are the members as a group to carry them out? Observation should be made of how the family decides what a task will be, who decides how a task will be carried out, and who participates in the task solution.

Decision-making is inextricably linked with how the family utilizes information in their environment, how they refer to each other and how they identify, mobilize and utilize their own resources within the family. It is undoubtedly obvious that the healthy family is better at making decisions than unhealthy families. How these decisions are reached is also more apparent in the healthy family. In the effective group and healthy family, there emerges a pattern of decision-making which is observable. It is one in which a leader assumes final reponsibility. I would interject that while i⁻leally each member has input, parents act as ultimate leaders or responsible people in the process. There must be a point, it seems to me, at which the parent or leader assumes a firm-footed stance, based on experience, expertise and justice. While each member in the family should be heard and allowed decision-making responsibilities for which they are prepared, there are certain times and particular areas for which parents or leaders should assume final responsibility and assume leadership in the implementation. I would suggest that in unhealthy families roles of adultness are not assumed by the parents and frequently fall to the children, who are ill-prepared for the roles and responsibilities. In terms of decision-making, one would want to observe who takes responsibility for making decisions, who initiates, who follows, who suggests, who addresses whom, and who listens.

Utilization of information means seeking, sharing, listening, and utilizing each other, outside agencies and other people, to achieve the best decision, *i.e.*, how open is the family to outside influence? Here one would want to observe what kinds of information are useful to the family; with regard to that information, who seeks, sends, clarifies, inquires, and deciphers the data. It is important to observe whether the family seeks information which supports what they already know or which raises questions which allow for growth or change.

Implementation of decision-making is barely separable from gathering data and making decisions. However, we all know families or groups who make decisions, but who never seem to carry them out. This may be related to: (1) the decision-making process, (2) who feels and who assumes responsibility in the group, (3) lack of specification about who is supposed to be doing what, or (4) uneven allocation of responsibilities within the family.

Resolution of conflict is an extremely important index because unhealthy or ineffective groups tend to ignore, deny, and push under the surface any conflict, thereby failing to identify problem areas and hence solutions. This type of behavior is somehow based on the mythical notion that harmony is characteristic of healthy families and that conflict is an adaptive failure. Harmony is *not* equivalent to stability nor is conflict necessarily a sign of dysfunction.[4] A family, as a group, which does not deal only with conflict, problems or disagreements, may resort to backbiting, deception, undermining and disillusionment. Careful observations to make here are how able the family members are to challenge one another's ideas, how open and honest they are, how often deception must be resorted to in order to maintain pseudo-harmony and how able they are to seek differing opinions and utilize information available to them. Don't be surprised if you find that the mode most frequently employed is denial that any conflict exists. To many people, conflict means denial of love or potential rejection and while it need not be so, it is a very real fear of many people.

We have thus far explored the family as a psycho-social unit of relationships, affected by and having influence on other systems. Maladjustment is taken to be a manifestation of dysfunction within the system itself or in some system influencing the family, thereby removing the blame or responsibility for the "problem" from the "identified patient." One implication of the psycho-social approach is that the counselor, public health nurse, community mental health nurse or other health related personnel operates from a knowledge base of organizational and group dynamics, and learning theories of behavior. The role of such an intervener becomes one of consultant and of social change agent in an ever evolving, ever changing family unit or system. Applying the social system approach to the family implies some changes in traditional role assignments, some re-thinking of traditional givens for men and women, an expanded role for the mental health nurse, and can result in greater effectiveness in identi-fying solutions for social and family problems. Some indices of effective family behavior have been identified, with some specific references to im-portant observations and assessments for the health professional to make. Attention must now be turned to explicating effective health interven-tions.

References

1. Johnson M, Martin H: A sociological analysis of the nurse role. Amer J Nurs, March 1958, pp. 373–7.
2. Murrel SA, Stachowiak JG: Consistency, rigidity, and power in the interaction patterns of clinic and nonclinic families. J. Abnorm Psychol 72:265–272, 1967.
3. Cartwright D, Zander A (eds): Group Dynamics: Research and Theory. New York, Harper and Row, 1968.
4. Kelly J: Make conflict work for you. Harvard Bus Rev, July–August 1970, pp. 103–113.

Bibliography

Bell JE: *A theoretical position for family therapy.* Family Process 2:1–14, 1963.

Laing RD: *The Politics of the Family.* New York, Vintage Books, 1972.

Satir V: *Conjoint Family Therapy.* Palo Alto, California, Science and Be-havior Books Inc, 1967.

3 GUIDE TO ASSESSMENT OF FAMILY FUNCTIONING

Nathan W. Ackerman, M.D.

Note: For each category of information provide the relevant historical background.

  I. A. Presenting problem
       B. Level of entry
          1. Disturbance of family member
          2. Disturbance of family relationships
          3. Impaired family functions
          4. A special stress situation which precipitates the referral, inside or outside the family
       C. Attitudes toward the family problem and toward professional intervention
 II. Identifying data
       A. Composition of family: age, sex of family members and other persons in the home
       B. Physical setting: home, neighborhood, geographical mobility
       C. Social and cultural pattern: occupation, income, education, ethnic and religious status, social mobility
       D. Special features: e.g. previous marriages, separations, pregnancies, health problems (mental or physical), significant deaths.

FROM THE PSYCHODYNAMICS OF FAMILY LIFE: DIAGNOSIS AND TREATMENT OF FAMILY RELATIONSHIPS, by Nathan W. Ackerman, M.D., from Chap. 9 "Guide For Data Leading to Family Diagnosis", © 1958 by Nathan Ackerman, Basic Books Inc., Publishers, New York.

III. Family as a group
   A. Internal organization
      1. Describe emotional climate, communication, shared goals, activities, pleasures, lines of authority, division of labor, child-rearing attitudes, problems, etc.
      2. Evaluate:
         a. Identity of the family group: strivings, expectations, and values
         b. Stability of the family (identity and stability as imaged from within)
            1) Continuity of family identity in time
            2) Conflict in family relations, mechanisms of control and interplay of defenses
            3) Capacity for change, learning, development, complementarity in family role relations
   B. External adaptation of the family to community
      1. Describe associations and transactions of the family with the community as a group, as marital and parental pairs, and as individuals
      2. Evaluate identity and stability as above (as perceived from without)
      3. Conflict and complementarity in the requirements of intra- and extra-familial roles
IV. Current family functioning:
   A. Current marital relationship
      Describe interaction as marital partners, perception of own and partner's role adaptation, describe components of marital role relations at sexual, social and emotional levels, quality of love and related satisfactions, image of future relationship, including children
      2. Evaluate identity and stability of marital relationship as above
   B. Current parental relationship
      1. Describe interaction as parents and with children; describe perception of own and partner's role adaptation
      2. Evaluate identity and stability of parental relationship as above
   C. Current parent-child relationship
      1. Describe relations of parental pair and each parent with child, influence of parental pair and of each parent on the child, and vice versa

      2.   Evaluate identity and stability of parent-child relationship as above

    D. Sibling pair relationship, as in IV C.

V. Personality make-up of each individual member

    A. Appearance, attitudes, behavior

    B. Personality structure; evaluate identity and stability as above

    C. Evaluate pathogenic conflict, anxiety, symptoms and patterns of control in the frame of total functioning and integration into the family group

VI. Relations with primary parental families

VII. Developmental history of the primary patient; problems in relation to mother, father and family group

VIII. Summary interpretation of the mental health of the family group and interrelations between individual and family mental health

4 ASSESSMENT OF A FAMILY'S POTENTIAL FOR CHILD ABUSE

Mary Louise Kidd Kohrt,

M.S, R.N.

CHILD ABUSE HAS REACHED EPIDEMIC PROPORTIONS
IN THE United States. Ray Helfer, a pioneer in the field of child abuse
estimates that between 1973 and 1982 there will be one million potential
child abusers, 300,000 permanent injuries to children, 50,000 deaths, and
over 1.5 million reports of child abuse. Nurses must become aware of the
extent of this problem and learn to identify families with the potential for
child abuse, as they will encounter abuse in all health care settings from
public health facilities, psychiatric settings, and schools, to inpatient and
outpatient services and hospital emergency rooms.

This paper will present a framework for the assessment of child abuse
potential. The term "child abuse" will be used to cover a multitude of
problems which include the passive abuse of child neglect, the more active abuse of battering, maternal deprivation and failure to thrive. It is
important to consider that this syndrome encompasses a total continuum
beginning with the potential for abuse, and ending with the child's death.
Intervention is possible at any or all points of this continuum, but the optimum point is to assess potential and intervene before this child is
harmed in any way. The concepts and principles of child abuse and the
assessment of its potential will be presented in a general manner so that
the nurse can tailor the interview to her particular professional setting. It
is expected that the nurse has a working knowledge of basic interviewing
techniques and is familiar with the mental health status assessment.

Thus, although the above listed terms have different medical and legal
definitions, they will be discussed under the rubric of "child abuse" since

---

this syndrome has implications for all. Prior to a specific discussion of the assessment of the family for child abuse potential, the nurse needs an understanding of the child abuse syndrome. Through the research that has been done in the field of child abuse there seem to be commonalities among the families. Child abuse does not seem to have cultural or socioeconomic preferences. These parents do not fit neatly into a psychiatric diagnostic category, nor do the majority respond to traditional psychiatric intervention. Only 10–15% of abused children have parents with serious mental illness, psychosis, or aggressive psychopathology.[1]

The major areas of concern in the child abuse syndrome are 1) parent's childhood, 2) level of ego function, 3) interpersonal support system, 4) the special child, and 5) the crisis. The primary component of the child abuse syndrome is negative childhood experiences. However, all abusing parents were not necessarily beaten as children. These include parents who cannot recall a warm trusting relationship with their parents. In some aspect, their own parenting was inadequate. These individuals' physical needs may have been met, but not their emotional needs. The maternal experience for these parents was not sufficient for them to have developed even basic trust. The vulnerable child grows into a vulnerable adult–withdrawn, indecisive, anxious, depressed, phobic and obsessional. The parents, as children, may have had the additional stress of foster care, broken homes, numerous siblings, death of a parent or any event that may have effected their childrearing. Their parents may have placed excessive demands on them. They were expected to meet the needs of their parents, that is, to provide nurturance for the parent. The expectations for these abusing parents as children were unrealistic. Their parents had a poor understanding of age appropriate behaviors and the normal growth and development of a child. Consequently, as children, the abusing parents constantly failed, were criticized and became "bad" children. It is of interest that some of these parents can describe similar relationships between their own parents and the grandparents.

Thus, abusing parents do not seem to have had positive childhood experiences. They reached adulthood without having experienced a true childhood. They have not learned to trust others, nor have they developed a sense of self-competency. They have poor self esteem. They see themselves as unlovable and unworthy. Their ego developed defensively rather than developing normal autonomous ego function. They may have become constricted, obsessive compulsive adults. Similarly, abusing parents tend to lead isolated, alienated lives. They have not learned to identify their needs, to express them, to share them, or to seek help and

---

[1]Kempe, *Helping the Battered Child & His Family*, p. 96.

accept help. There has been no one to turn to with the normal every-day crises. As adults, abusing parents need constant reassurance and support. Somehow, there is never quite enough of this for many abusing parents because their basic needs are so extensive.

It seems to follow then, that as adults these individuals are attracted to mates who accentuate their problems. The symbiotic relationship between the parent and child was neither fulfilling nor resolved. Consequently, these parents seek that symbiosis from each other. Each expects the other to nurture him. There is competition for attention and comfort. Each looks to the other to be dependable and responsible. Because of these dynamics, frequently there are no relatives or friends to turn to for support.

At last there is a child: one last salvation. They hope the child will meet their extensive needs for love and comfort. The birth of a child makes a family of three children, each with basic needs and demands. It follows that child rearing, disciplining and decision making are difficult, emotionally charged areas for these families. Unlike most parents, abusing parents do not have positive childhood experiences to draw upon. In essence, the parent expects and demands of his child what was expected and demanded of him as a child. The individual characteristics of the child will determine his ability to "survive". Premature infants, infants with congenital anomalies, colic, etc., are more likely to place additional demands on the parents and less likely to begin to meet the parents' needs. The infant or child's resemblance to his parents will also affect his vulnerability. The child who is perceived by the parent as different or "bad" is more likely to become the abused "special child".

The last major component of the child abuse syndrome is the crisis event. Drs. Justice discuss "Life Crisis as a Precursor to Child Abuse".[2] They believe excessive changes necessitating constant readjustments constitute a "prolonged life crisis". These include the maturational crises of childhood, adolescence, marriage, pregnancy, divorce, death, and the situational events of every day life such as job concerns and child rearing problems. These prolonged series of crises have the individual exhausted, unable to adjust, and constantly on the brink of losing control. With the addition of a seemingly minor event such as a child wetting a diaper, a disapproving glance from a spouse, or an infant crying, the parent loses control and abuses the child.

As was stated above, child abuse seems to have a generational quality. Abused children can grow up to become abusing parents. Thus, the cycle is perpetuated. There is a need for early and complete assessment of

---

[2]Justice, *The Abusing Family*, p. 25–34.

these families with abuse potential so that intervention can be planned, abuse and neglect prevented and the cycle broken. It must be re-emphasized that the elements common to the abusing families can be present in any family; however, it is the extent of their expression that leads to the abuse situation.

Interviewing the Family

The goal in interviewing the family is two-fold: 1) to determine the abuse or neglect potential and 2) to demonstrate to the family the desire to help, the ability to be honest and trusting. Assessment is the first step of intervention. Good basic interviewing techniques must be utilized. A relaxed, nondirective, nonjudgemental approach is bes.. It must be remembered that these families have not learned to trust others or to turn to others for help. They may be either cautious and resentful or too compliant. The ideal place for the assessment of the family is, of course, the family's home. There the family is on its own turf. In addition, the nurse can learn much about the family by observing its living conditions, health and safety standards, and the living arrangements of the children and parents.

The nurse must not expect to make a complete assessment of the family with one interview. With a good understanding of the significant areas outlined here and some experience interviewing families, the nurse should be able to make a judgement concerning the safety of the child in the home. Under optimal circumstances several short interviews averaging a half hour in length are desirable. Many abusing parents cannot tolerate the demands of lengthy one hour or more interviews without losing the therapeutic benefits of the assessment. It is helpful initially to follow a structural format in assessing the family. The significant areas of assessment are:

1) Parent's Childhood
2) Level of ego function
3) Interpersonal support system
4) Special child
5) Crisis event

Care must be taken throughout the interview to support and reassure the parents wherever possible and to avoid judgments and criticism. Above all the nurse must be honest and straightforward about her role and the sharing of information learned from the family.

Parent's Childhood

Because abusing parents may have been abused children, the parents' recollections of their childhood is extremely important. One or two leading questions and empathetic direction should encourage the discussion of this significant period for the parents.

What was it like for you as a child?
How would you describe your relationship with your mother and father?
Did you feel loved?
What did you do on your birthdays, holidays?   .
How were you punished as a child?
Did you deserve it?
Were you a "bad" or "good" girl/boy?
Do you feel your parents enjoyed you?
What did you do to please your parents?
How did your parents feel about you in relation to your brothers and sisters?
What kind of relationship do you have with your parents now?
Are your parents happily married?
Do you remember anything about your parents' relationships with their parents?

Certainly nothing is benefited by forcing parents to discuss areas of anxiety initially. The nurse should not be looked upon as a curious interrogator, but rather as one genuinely concerned about the parents and the difficulties they may have had as children. An approach to this emotionally charged area is to offer an interpretation of the parents' behavior. For example, if a nurse observes a parent expecting too much of a child she might respond, "It must have been difficult for you as a child to have been expected to do so much around the house."

From this type of discussion the nurse should have some impression of the quality of the attachment between these parents as children and their parents. Do they have a trusting, nurturing, loving childhood they can fall back on or do they feel rejected, unloved, worthless, incompetent? The histories of abusing parents may include foster home placement, prolonged hospitalization, criminal records, runaway, divorce in the family, single parent families, addiction, or teenage pregnancy. Each of these within themselves would test the emotional strength of an individual; however, for an individual with poor or inadequate parenting, it is further proof of failure and the undependability of others.

Level of Ego Function

Because of inadequate parenting as children, abusing parents have a variety of personality charcteristics in common. Their ego structure is weak. Defensive functioning of the ego may lead to isolated, withdrawn lives. They may be wary of others, unable to seek help for solutions to everyday problems. Other parents may be outwardly belligerent and hostile. The nurse must remember that under this angry aggressive facade is a child with an intensive need for nurturance. They may have a poor self image. Observe the dress and physical appearance of the parents. Do they take pride in their appearance? Is their dress appropriate for their culture, season, and time of day? Is makeup worn appropriately? Is their hair combed? Are their teeth cared for? Do they have many physical complaints?

Abusing parents may have a limited self-observing function of the ego. Can they identify their needs and their problems? Can they express goals for their lives? Can they identify what feelings and events may trigger loss of impulse control? Many parents can identify the minor event that triggers abuse or excessive inappropriate punishment such as a toddler soiling a newly scrubbed floor; however, they may not be able to identify the component feelings of loss, desperation, and anger. Because the parent may not be able to identify any feeling beyond the anger, the nurse can offer a therapeutic interpretation, such as: "You must feel hurt, unloved. Is that how you felt when you were a child and did something that did not please your parents?"

Interpersonal Support System

To reiterate, abusing parents have not learned basic trust. Children with such inadequate parenting tend to select inadequate partners. Thus, we have two needy, dependent inadequate adults with an unhealthy symbiotic relationship. Each looks to the other for nurturance. Each expects the other to make the decisions and carry out mutual responsibilities. One of the parents may assume this over-adequate role while the other inadequate personality acts out the abuse. Both spouses are either overtly or covertly involved in the abuse. If an adult with poor parenting experiences happens to marry a "healthy" spouse, then of course abuse is less likely to occur. Discussion of the following areas should give the nurse an impression of the quality of the relationship between the parents:

> What initially attracted you to each other?
> Is your marriage (relationship) what you expected?
> Are you happy with each other?
> How do you spend your time alone together?
> Can you rely on each other for support?
> Can you tell when your spouse is upset and help him/her?
> Can you identify each others needs?
> What happens when you disagree with each other?
> Does your spouse help you care for the child?
> Do you have a babysitter?
> Do you go out without the children?
> How do you enjoy spending your leisure time?

In many cases abuse occurs in broken homes or in one-parent homes. It is especially helpful with these families as well as with two-parent families to have an awareness of the parents' relationship with their relatives and other individuals. As has been emphasized, abusing families usually lead isolated withdrawn lives. If relatives are available they cannot meet their needs. Questions about the availability of relatives and friends in the times of stress are significant. Remember, abusing parents have difficulty not only asking for help, but also accepting help.

The Special Child

The interview should focus primarily on the parents, secondarily on the child. If, of course, the child is in immediate danger then a thorough examination of the child must come first. However, when it is not an emergency and the nurse's goal is to identify abuse potential and provide therapeutic aspects from the assessment, then the focus must be on the parents. Focus on the child may lead the parent to compete with the child for the attention of the nurse to the extent of abusing the child. It must be remembered that abusing parents are as needy as their children.

In obtaining the history it is important to get an idea of the meaning of the child to the parents beginning with the pregnancy. Try to get a detailed obstetrical history.

> Did you want children? Why?

Have you had any miscarriages, abortions, stillbirths?
How would you describe your pregnancy?
How did you feel physically and emotionally?
Were there any complications?
Were the pregnancy and delivery what you had expected?

Many "special" children seem to have been labeled as "bad" from conception, causing morning sickness, fatigue, head aches, a long labor, etc.

How did you feel when you first saw your baby?
Was the baby the sex you wanted?
Did he/she have any problems at birth?

The nurse must try to help the mother identify her feelings and the parents' expectations throughout this significant experience. Remember, for an abusing parent this baby may be their last salvation for love and comfort. The nurse can also determine how realistic the parents expectations are. This helps the nurse not only to identify abuse potential, but also to plan health teaching intervention that may prevent abuse. The initial interview is not usually the time for extensive instruction in child care unless a specific area is of immediate concern to the parents.

Can you describe your initial contact with your baby?
Did your baby have his eyes open? Did he look at you?
Were you separated from your baby for any amount of time?
Did your baby have any breathing or feeding problems?
Was he easy to care for?
Was he fussy? Did he cry a lot? Did he have colic?

This initial contact and the entire neonatal period is extremely significant in terms of mother-infant bonding. If the experience and the baby lived up to the mother's expectation and the child was easy to care for, then an abuse situation is less likely. Premature infants, infants with congenital anomalies, feeding problems, colic, or anything that makes them different or more difficult to care for have a higher probability for becoming a special child in the eyes of the parents. That special child has a higher risk for becoming abused.

Does your baby cry a lot?
How does that make you feel?
What do you do?

The significance of the baby's cry to the parents cannot be over-emphasized. A crying infant is asking for help and it certainly is not comforting a parent. Most parents will try a series of actions to alleviate the crying: check to see if the baby is hungry, check to see if the baby is wet, and perhaps rock the baby. Most babies will stop crying with one of these measures. For the abusing parent, a crying infant sets them into a panic. It recalls their own painful childhood. If the child does not become quiet, then it further demonstrates to the parent his inadequacies. Some abusing parents truly believe that an infant is crying deliberately to hurt them.

This area must be discussed not only because of its significance in determining abuse potential but also because of its richness for skilled nursing intervention. The nurse is striving to support and reassure these parents and to help them to become more competent in caring for their child.

If there are several small children in a family, a separate history of each is important. Usually one child is singled out as the special child and abused. However, this is not always the case. Similarly, should the special child be removed from the family, a second child will take his or her place.

Is your child "bad"?
What does he do that is "bad"?
Do you worry about his becoming "spoiled"?
What makes him that way?
Is your child doing what you think he should for his age?
When and how did you toilet train him?
How do you punish him? Is it effective?

In this discussion the nurse hopes to gain information about the parents' expectations for the child, their reality base, and the discipline techniques they employ. Toilet training is usually a highly charged area of child rearing. Most important, does the child provide the comfort, the love, and the attention that the parents expect, want and need?

Infants and children need to be assessed for failure to thrive. A length and weight must be taken and plotted on a growth chart. Failure to thrive and malnutrition can be associated with problems in parenting. Failure to thrive without an organic cause is usually linked with child neglect. Recent studies associate some cases of failure to thrive with inadequate calorie intake.[3] This is a valuable area for nursing intervention.

---

[3]Charles Whitter et al, "Evidence that Growth Failure from Maternal Deprivation is Secondary to Undereating", *J.A.MA.* Sept. 1969, p. 1675–1682.

The nurse must constantly note the parent-child interactions. In assessing infant-mother interaction, does the mother hold the baby comfortably? Does she talk to him? Do they make eye contact? Does she stroke him? Does she feed him a bottle at his own pace or force it on him? There has been considerable research in the area of infant-mother communication and the significance of eye contact and stroking. Eye contact usually becomes more prolonged with the initiation of talking or cooing to the infant. Stroking usually begins peripherally with the toes and fingers and leads to comfortable holding and rocking of the entire body of the baby. An infant will pause as he eats, to rest, to look at his mother—the very beginnings of communication. Does the mother respond appropriately to her infant's cry? How does the father interact with the child?

In assessing the child 18 months of age and older, the nurse should be alert to the role that child plays in the family. Is the child expected to wait on the parents and to meet their physical as well as emotional needs?

Some children actually learn to become "compliant". That is, they learn to meet their parents' needs and thereby avert abuse. An example was a parent who became anxious and began to cry. The two year old child ran up to her mother, hugged her and began rocking and patting her gently on the back. This child responded the same way when held by an adult. The child had learned at a very early age to mother her own mother.

Children pass through many different developmental stages, each with its own rewards and stresses. The majority of abused children are under three years of age, half of these are less than a year.[4] In interviewing parents it is helpful to determine which developmental stages they enjoy, which are most rewarding and which are most difficult. Most abusing parents find the early stage of dependency needs of the baby most difficult. A second trying time is ambulation and toddlerhood; and the toilet training is most difficult. (Usually because it is expected at too early an age.) For other abusing parents the toddler who has "learned his role" is not as difficult as the crying infant. Conversely, some find the cuddly baby more rewarding than the independent toddler.

Crisis Event

Frequently there is a single event which causes the parent with inadequate parenting, poor ego development, and lack of interpersonal supports, to lose control and abuse the special child. As has been stated, it is not necessarily the major crisis of loss of a job or prolonged illness, but can be a seemingly minor event such as a child crying, child wetting a newly

---

[4]Justice, The Abusing Family, p. 25–34.

changed diaper, toddler turning on the TV, washer breaking, or a spouse arriving late for dinner that causes the abusing parent to lose control and strike out at the child. Pollack and Steele[5] describe two elements in a family crisis. One is readily identifiable relating directly to an incident such as diaper wetting, however, this is usually precipitated by a more subtle yet more significant crisis such as a loss. The abusing parent's ego is so fragile that any possibility of loss of affection can recall all the desperation felt in childhood. The process of helping the parents to identify these events and their concommitant feelings is therapeutic. The next step is to help them find alternatives to abusing the child when these feelings and events occur.

Child abuse and neglect is a devastating health problem. Nursing has many roles in addressing this problem. The premise has been presented that abusing parents had poor, inadequate parenting as children, they consequently did not develop ideal ego functioning, they married similarly deprived adults, they lead isolated lives without interpersonal supports and they have a special child who is viewed as their salvation for nurturance. A specific crisis to this family unit causes the child to be abused. It is hoped that the nurse assessing these significant areas in a family will be able to determine their potential for abuse and provide intervention. It must be stressed that these factors are not unusual in themselves, but the degree to which they are expressed is distinctly excessive in the abusing family. The family interview is an integral part of the assessment process and the beginnings of a therapeutic approach to helping these families.

Bibliography

Anthony, E. James. "The Syndrome of the Psychologically Vulnerable Child", from *The Child in His Family: Children at Psychiatric Risk*, Anthony, E. J. and Koupernik, Cyrille Eds. John Wiley and Sons, New York. 1974.

Escalona, Sybil. "Emotional Development in the First Year of Life", from *Problems of Infancy and Childhood*, Senn, M. Ed. Josiah Macy Foundation Publications, New York. 1953.

Fontana, Vincent. *Somewhere a Child is Crying; Maltreatment-Causes and Prevention.* Macmillan Publishing Co., Inc. New York. 1973.

[5]Kempe, *Helping The Battered Child and his Family*, pp. 6–7.

Freud, Anna. *Ego and Mechanisms of Defense.* International University Press, New York. 1936.

Goldstein, Joseph, et al., *Beyond the Best Interests of the Child.* Free Press, New York. 1973.

Glaser, Helen, et al., "Physical and Psychological Development of Children With Early Failure to Thrive", from *Journal of Pediatrics,* Nov. 1968. Vol. 73, No. 5, p. 690–698.

Helfer, Ray. *The Diagnostic Process and Treatment Programs.* Washington, D.C.: U. S. Department of Health, Education and Welfare, 1970.

Justice, Blair & Rita, *The Abusing Family.* Human Sciences Press, New York, 1976.

Kempe, C. Henry, and Helfer, Ray E., Eds. *Helping the Battered Child and His Family.* Chicago: The University of Chicago Press.

Rexford, Eveoleen, et al. Eds. *Infant Psychiatry: A New Synthesis.* Yale University Press, New Haven. 1976.

Visiting Nurse Association of Chicago. "Descriptive Statistical Study: Child Abuse Intervention Program (July 1, 1973–June 30, 1975)", Prepared by Melva Rowe and Carole Anderson. Child Abuse Coordinator, 1976.

5 QUESTIONS FREQUENTLY ASKED ABOUT THE PROBLEM-ORIENTED RECORD IN PSYCHIATRY

Linda C. Smith, B.S., R.N.

Christine J. Hawley, B.S., R.N.

Richard L. Grant, M.D.

THE WEED SYSTEM OF PROBLEM-ORIENTED MEDICAL RECORDS was adopted in September 1971 by the department of psychiatry of the University of Vermont College of Medicine. One of the authors (RLG) had previous experience with the problem-oriented record,[2] and was a consultant to the staff during the transition period. Later the other two authors became teaching associates on the use of the problem-oriented record.

The change from the traditional source-oriented records to problem-oriented ones brought many questions from the residents and inpatient nursing staff. Answers to some of the most frequently asked questions were worked out by the ward staff and the authors and are presented

Reprinted, with permission, from *Hospital and Community Psychiatry*, Vol. 25, No. 1; January, 1974.

[1]L. L. Weed, *Medical Records, Medical Education, and Patient Care*, Press of Case Western Reserve University, Cleveland, 1969.

[2]R. L. Grant and B. M. Maletzky, "Application of the Weed System to Psychiatric Records," *Psychiatry in Medicine*, Vol. 3, April 1972, pp. 119–129.

here. The questions are organized according to the four components of the problem-oriented record—the data base, the problem list, the initial plan, and the progress notes.

The Data Base

What is a minimum data base? A minimum data base is a predefined body of information elicited from those who seek health services in a particular setting. It serves a screening function by identifying categories of health concerns that the setting decides it cannot afford to miss; after they are identified, then more specific questions are indicated. It also is a record of the development of present illness. Both kinds of information generally are gathered in an initial interview or work-up and are recorded together in the data-base section of the record.

When a health-care setting defines psychosocial or mental health care as part or all of its task, then gathering the minimum data base includes using either specific screening questions related to such care or an outline of the areas in which questions are to be asked. At Vermont, the specific content for each category outlined as minimum baseline data has been defined in a standard data base so the user knows what information he is expected to collect.[3] Such defined content makes it possible to audit the data base for completeness.[4]

Who collects and records the data base? That is determined in part by the form of the data base itself and organizational decisions about who should be responsible for collecting data. The information may be elicited from the patient verbally by an interviewer, as is usually done in our department, or the patient may be asked to complete questionnaires or checklists. Anther possibility is an automated screening questionnaire.

Regardless of the form in which the data base is recorded, one individual is usually considered responsible for the over-all management of a patient's care and the keeping of his record. In psychiatry, it has traditionally been the physician. However, social workers, nurses, and other

[3]Copies of the minimum-data-base outline and a preliminary screening questionnaire are available on request from the Department of Psychiatry, University of Vermont College of Medicine, Burlington, Vermont 05401.

[4]C. J. Hawley, L. S. Smith, and R. L. Grant, "Initiation of an Audit System for Problem-Oriented Psychosocial Care," in *Applying the Problem-Oriented System*, H. K. Walker, J. W. Hurst, and M. S. Woody, editors, Medcom, New York City, 1973.

professionals are assuming increasing responsibility within the treatment team, and the task may be delegated to any one of them. This primary therapist or patient-care manager is then responsible for the completeness of the record. In our department, he may choose to collect all the data himself, delegate other team members to obtain specific kinds of data, or ask the patient to provide them through questionnaires.

Is it necessary for the section of the data base dealing with present illness to be problem-oriented? No, but it helps. In psychiatry, emphasis has been on the chronological narrative of present illness, which some maintain gives a more complete picture of the patient. As originally conceived, the problem-oriented record required that problem areas be organized as subjective information, objective information, plans for treatment, and significant problems. In our system, it is permissible to make a narrative record of present illness, but therapists are encouraged to attempt to develop specific topic headings, not necessarily problem titles, that help organize the account of present illness. A narrative form should not be used when a defined problem list is available from the patient's previous admission.

What use is made of a psychiatric data base already collected? When a patient is readmitted or re-enters therapy after some length of time, the existing data and record are reviewed against the required minimum data base. Previously omitted information is collected. Interim information is obtained in those areas where changes may have occurred since the original data were collected. They might include such items as results of a routine physical examination and changes in social history. An inclusive problem-oriented progress note should be written on each active problem, summarizing its course between termination and resumption of therapy. In essence, the existing record is simply updated.

If the patient is transferred from a nonpsychiatric facility, the information is handled the same way as for readmissions; the data base is reviewed and added to as necessary. We usually find that many additions need to be made in the psychosocial area, because general health-care facilities do not gather such data in as much detail as our minimum data base requires.

What do you do if you can't complete the minimum data base? We found that an arbitrary time limit needed to be established for completing the data base. On the inpatient service, the staff suggested a period of 24 to 48 hours after admission. On the outpatient service, data collection is usually completed in the first two interviews. If completion is not possible within those time limits, then a problem of "incomplete data base" is recorded. In the corresponding progress note for this problem, the missing data are specified, the reason for incompleteness is stated, and a plan for completing the data base is outlined. When the missing data are collected, they should be entered in the data-base portion of the record, with the date of entry noted. Another progress note is then entered, indicating that a further data-base entry has been made.

Doesn't all this emphasis on completing the data base result in less attention to effective interviewing skills and the formation of a therapeutic relationship? Medical students and other beginning therapists have told us that they did, at first, feel pressured to have a complete record, and sometimes ignored other relevant concerns in the interview. They said they felt much less pressured when we pointed out that a judgment may be made to institute some type of therapy or intervention immediately, based on whatever data is collected. Teaching problem-oriented data collection should closely parallel the teaching of the skills of interviewing and establishing a therapeutic relationship. When the therapist considers it inappropriate to continue to use the interview to collect data, all that is necessary in the problem-oriented system is that the missing base-line be noted with a plan to collect them.

Should information about a special meeting, such as a staff session with the patient and his family, be included as part of the minimum data base? Yes, if the meeting's purpose is to gather baseline information. If it is held after treatment goals have been established and is related to one of the patient's specific problems, then a description of the meeting is more appropriately recorded in the progress notes under the title of that problem.

The Problem List

How do you date the problem list? Once the data base has been collected, the next step is to list and number all the patient's problems. The forms used by our hospital call for the date of onset of the problem, and the date it was defined or formulated. The latter date is useful since it indicates when the first progress note for that problem was written. As new problems are added to the list, the date defined allows the reader to quickly locate the first progress note pertinent to the new problem. Figure 1 shows a sample master problem list, with the dates indicated by the letters A and B.

Who formulates the initial problem list and who enters new problems? On our service originally, only the resident responsible for the patient's care entered problems on the list. Other staff members suggested additions or entered temporary problems in the progress notes as suggested by Weed. However, as the team approach to patient care became increasingly emphasized, various team members assumed the role of primary

FIGURE 1   Sample problem list

MASTER PROBLEM LIST
Medical Center Hospital of Vermont

Date: Onset Noted		Active Problems	Date Resolved	Inactive/Resolved Problems
8/71 A 9/8/71B	1.	LOWER (R) ABDOMINAL PAIN——10/10/71——▶ (R) OVARIAN CYST———————	 1/25/72 ——▶	S/P OVARIAN CYSTECTOMY
6/6/72	2.	CIGARETTE SMOKER		
6/6/72	3.	HEADACHES——11/8/72–D–▶MULTIPLE—— SOMATIC SYMPTOMS——◀–G–	1/10/73 ——▶ 2/10/73 3/14/73 ——▶	
6/6/72	4.	NAUSEA-VOMITING ————— E —————	11/8/72 ——▶	REDEFINED TO #3
6/6/72	5.	SHORTNESS OF BREATH ——— E ———	11/8/72 ——▶	REDEFINED TO #3
6/6/72	6.	PALPITATIONS ————— E —————	11/8/72 ——▶	REDEFINED TO #3
9/20/72	7.	DEPRESSION——10/4/72–▶DEPRESSIVE H SYMPTOMS ——	1/10/73 ——▶	
10/4/72	8.	SUICIDAL IDEATION———————	11/8/72 ——▶	
10/4/72	9.	INCOMPLETE DATA BASLTIES ———	11/8/72 ——▶	
10/4/72	10.	DIFFICULTY WITH SPOUSE——11/8/72 ——▶ DIFFICULTY WITH COMMUNICATION C WITH HUSBAND——	 5/16/73 ——▶	
10/4/72	11.			HISTORY OF MARIJUANA USE
10/4/72	12.	SURASSERTIVENESS		
10/4/72	13.	DIFFICULTY EXPRESSING FEELINGS DIRECTLY		
10/4/72	14.	NOT WORKING OR ATTENDING SCHOOL—— F	1/10/73 ——▶	
10/4/72	15.	SEXUAL DIFFICULTIES ———	5/16/73 ——▶	
3/14/73	16.	UNWANTED PREGNANCY———————	4/18/73 ——▶	S/P ABORTION

Temporary Problems (w/dates)					D.			
A.					E.			
B.					F.			
C.					G.			

Note: All problems necessitating or prolonging this admission must be so in-   Copy Date:
dicated by a circle around the problem number.

therapist. As a result, the staff decided that the primary therapist would be responsible for entering the initial problem list, and that any team member could add new problems to the list as they arose. Entering a new problem required that a progress note be written defining the problem and suggesting a plan. The primary therapist, in conjunction with the team, was then responsible for the decision about managing the new problem.

Initially the staff were hesitant to make the problem list open to all team members. Primary therapists were concerned that it would become too long and unwieldy. Staff members who had never entered problems felt they couldn't adequately define them. As a result, we suggested using a practice problem list in addition to the permanent list.

The practice list was placed in the record immediately behind the permanent problem list, and served as a work sheet. Team members entered problems on this list the same way as on the permanent list and wrote a progress note. Suggested problems included the letter "P" before the problem numbers to make them readily identifiable as suggested problems. The primary therapist was then responsible for reviewing the practice problem list and deciding whether or not the problems should be added to the permanent list, either separately or as subcategories of other problems.

The practice list was used for a few months on a trial basis. It proved to be a helpful way for inexperienced staff to learn to define problems. The major drawback was the confusion that sometimes resulted from having two lists. We recommend using a practice problem list as a training device for staff new to the problem-oriented system, but not as a permanent part of the system.

How should problems be defined? Weed outlines four levels at which a problem may be defined; they are a diagnosis, a pathophysiological finding, an abnormal laboratory value, and a symptom or physical finding. He stresses that a problem should be defined at its current level of understanding; no entry should be made for a possible problem, for one that is questionable, or for one that can be ruled out. Instead the specific symptom, behavior, or abnormal finding should be entered on the list.

In the psychosocial area, the problem titles are most useful in planning treatment and evaluating progress when they are defined at a pragmatic, functional level clearly indicating what the patient's problems are. A problem title of schizophrenia is a broad generalization that says little about the individual patient's behavior. Titles such as withdrawal, angry outbursts, neglect of personal hygiene, auditory hallucinations, and self-mutilation specifically describe the patient's problems and indicate where treatment needs to be focused.

How do you redefine a problem title once you have entered it on the list? Since problems are defined at the current level of understanding, the need frequently arises to redefine them as more data are gathered. That is done by listing the new title after the initial entry of the old one, drawing an arrow between them, and writing the date of redefinition above the arrow. (See Figure 1, C.) That change is made throughout the record, in every place where the old title appears.

What if you have several problem titles that you later decide are all related to one major problem? A procedure similar to the one above is used. For example, suppose four problems are defined initially; they are headache, nausea and vomiting, shortness of breath, and palpitations. Later they are all judged to be manifestations of one problem, such as multiple somatic symptoms. An arrow is drawn from the first problem, headaches, to the new definition of the problem, and the date of redefinition is recorded over the arrow. (Figure 1, D.) Arrows are drawn from other related problems and a notation is made that they have been redefined to problem number three; again the date is written over the arrow. (Figure 1, E.)

When should problems be combined, and when should they be listed separately? If the relationships between problems are unclear, they should be listed separately. Thus constipation should not be incorporated within a problem of depression unless other conditions associated with constipation have been ruled out.

Another guideline we have used in defining problems relates to treatment. If two problems are related but require separate treatment and management, then Weed suggests that they be listed separately.

What do you do with a problem that is resolved or is no longer active? That is indicated on the problem list by drawing an arrow from the active column of the problem list to the inactive or resolved column. A final progress note is written explaining the change in status. Again the date should be included above the arrow, indicating when the problem became inactive and when the progress note describing the change in status was written. (Figure 1, F.)

What if a problem that has been declared inactive becomes active again? That is indicated by drawing an arrow from the resolved column to the active column, again writing above it the date the problem became reactivated. (Figure 1, G.) A progress note is also written. If a problem occurs repeatedly over time, then the title is redefined to indicate its episodic nature, such as episodic suicidal ideation or repeated suicide attempts. The problem then remains on the active list, and its current status is described in the progress notes. When an episode occurs, progress notes about symptoms and management are written until the episode is resolved. No additional notes are necessary until the next occurrence. Defining the problem in this way eliminates the need to continually reactivate the problem title as episodes arise.

Do you make up a new problem list for each admission of the same patient? No. The previous problem list should be used to maintain continuity. The list can be updated as necessary by redefining, reactivating, or adding problems. The Medical Center Hospital of Vermont has established a master problem list for each patient; it is kept on file in the record room, separate from the patient's chart, which also contains a copy of the list. That makes the established problem list immediately available to the services whether the chart is or is not. Using the same list helps avoid the confusion that results when the same problems are defined on different lists and assigned different numbers.

How do you use a problem list defined by another service or facility? It should be handled the same way as a list from a previous admission. Again the list may require redefinitions, changes in active or inactive status, or additions. Problem titles should not be erased or deleted from the problem list. If psychosocial problems are not clearly or accurately defined, they should be redefined and accompanied by progress notes that explain the change in thinking. (Figure 1, H.) Thus the evolution of problem definition can be seen over time.

Plans and Progress Notes

What is included in the plans? Weed has divided the plans into three areas of emphasis: gathering of more data, approaches to treatment or management, and patient education. The first can include additional information about the development of the present illness, the results of lab tests or special studies, or the need to obtain old records. The treatment category includes medication, procedures, or specific plans of action. In psychiatry, a description of a behavior modification program or the type of psychotherapy to be used is included here, as are suggestions for staff interactions with the patient. Goal expectations may be outlined and used later to measure treatment outcome.

The third area of emphasis, patient education, is often overlooked in the plans. It is useful to record what the patient will be told about the problem, diagnosis, or treatment, for his or her own information, so that it can be communicated to all staff through the record.

How can initial plans for patient management be written so that they include an assessment of the problems? In the Weed system, there is a section in the data base for initial plans, but no assessment is included. In psychiatry, we have modified this to allow for the psychiatric assessment or formulation along with the initial plan. We have called this modification the initial progress notes. Such notes are written for each problem defined, and are the first entry in the progress-notes section. They include a summary of subjective and objective information obtained if the present illness is described in narrative form. If the illness has been broken into problem areas and is already described in subjective and objective terms, only a note to "see present illness" is made. Next the assessment of the problem is written. It leads naturally into plan definition, which is the final part of the initial progress notes, as illustrated in Example A.

What is included in the assessment? This is the area for analysis or formulation of the problem area. It should be backed up by subjective and objective data and should summarize the therapist's current understanding of the problem. If the problem is not clearly understood, a statement to that effect should be made. The initial assessment should attempt to answer questions such as:
- Why is this a problem for the patient at this time?
- How does the problem disrupt the patient's functioning?
- What needs to change and how can the change be effected?
- How is this problem related to the patient's other problems?
- How did the patient come to have this problem?

In auditing initial assessments, we look for answers to those questions supported by information from the data base. Once a thorough analysis of the problem has been documented in the initial assessment, then continued follow-up assessments focus on patient progress and the effectiveness of the initial plan. Follow up assessments do not attempt to answer all the above questions unless continued data collection leads to changes in formulation of the problem.

What information is considered subjective? The patient's own statements about his feelings or moods, activities, plans, and concerns, as well as his evaluation of the treatment and his progress in resolving the problem, are subjective information. Such information may also come from family members, friends, and others not professionally involved with the patient.

What information is considered objective? Staff observations about the patient's appearance, activity, and behavior, as well as findings from the mental status examinations and laboratory reports, are included. Previously formulated plans that have been carried out, such as special nursing care, are also recorded in this section.

Can you combine subjective and objective information in writing a progress note? A difficulty in the application of the problem-oriented record to psychiatry has been recording interactions. It is often difficult to record what the patient says together with what the interviewer says and observes about his behavior without losing continuity. Sometimes recording specific behavioral observations, such as crying in response to a statement, leads to repeating some of the information. To avoid that, we have suggested recording the interaction under the subjective note, with specific behavioral observations in parentheses after the corresponding verbal statement. (See Example B.) Thus specific behaviors can be linked with their verbal counterpart, leaving the objective category for general observations.

How is a progress note written on a new problem? Whenever a problem is defined on the problem list, the date defined serves as an index to the first progress note on that problem. In the progress notes, the date is noted with the new problem title, followed by the notation "new problem." That is the only time such a designation is made. A complete description of the problem (subjective, objective, assessment, plan) would be recorded the same way as an initial progress note.

How can you quickly ascertain the status of a specific problem without having to read all the progress notes on that problem? One solution has been for each service to set an arbitrary time interval for recording a summary progress note on each active problem. On the inpatient service recording is done weekly; on the outpatient service, every three months. The primary therapist is responsible for seeing that the summary notes are done. If they are, it is easy to review the progress of treatment for all problems or one, returning to the previous progress notes only if further detail is needed.

How do you record routine observations made at hourly or more frequent intervals? They may be recorded on graphs or flow sheets. For example, one of our patients was noted to have frequent episodes of severe agitation. There was some speculation that they might be a paradoxical reaction to phenothiazine because some were reported to occur after administration of the medication. We decided to observe the patient's activity level at 15-minute intervals and rate the activity on a scale ranging from 1 for sleep to 5 for severe agitation. The specific behaviors for each rating were outlined in detail. Recording the ratings merely required making a dot on the proper place on a graph for every 15-minute interval.

We were able to determine that episodes of severe agitation in fact preceded the administration of medication, while periods of sleep or quiet activity followed soon after the patient received medication. She improved after the dosage was increased. Through the use of such a flow sheet, many observations can be quickly recorded without writing out an entire progress note. The flow sheet then serves as a progress note in itself. A summary of the observations from flow sheets is recorded in the progress notes by the primary therapist.

Where does the nursing staff record observations about activities of daily living? All progress notes should be problem-oriented, and therefore observations should relate to specific problems. However, some agencies require the recording of certain routine observations such as temperatures or participation in activities, whether they are related to problems or not. Such observations can be recorded on flow sheets in the manner described above.

What is an interim progress note? It is a summary note written on all active problems when a patient resumes therapy after a period of no treatment.

Is the discharge summary supposed to be problem-oriented? Yes. It is a final progress note briefly summarizing the course of the problems. Not all problems need to be summarized; those that do include active or inactive problems for which action was taken during treatment, problems that require continued treatment after hospitalization, and those that require special plans to prevent difficulty. All other problems are simply listed by title either in the order of occurrence on the problem list or in a group at the end of the summary notes. If a problem has been redefined or updated, only the most current title is listed.

EXAMPLE A   Initial progress notes

6/1/72   #1 Compulsive eating
SUBJECTIVE: See present illness. In summary, reports history of episodic compulsive eating resulting in weight gain of as much as 50 pounds. Currently reports eating is "out of control."
OBJECTIVE: See present illness. Height 5′4″. Weight 195 pounds. An increase in 30 pounds in past month.

ASSESSMENT: Patient is overweight and gaining steadily as a result of current eating patterns. This behavior leads to increasing social isolation, since patient spends more time eating and eats only when alone. It also leads to increasing self-derogatory comments as sees self as "fat and ugly." Episodes of overeating seem related to difficulties in relationship with parents because these episodes occur at times when patient perceives parents as not caring and "wanting to be rid of me." Needs some external controls to reduce amount of food consumed, therefore will hospitalize. Will aim only for weight maintenance for now.

PLAN: 1.   Gather more data: obtain records from former therapist in Kansas.
    2.   Treatment
       a.   admit to hospital
       b.   place on weight maintenance diet for frame and height
       c.   restrict from ward kitchen and dining room to provide external controls on overeating
       d.   send meals on tray to room with staff member present
    3.   Patient education: above plans to be discussed with patient by J. Brown, R.N.

EXAMPLE B   Progress note combining objective-subjective information

---

#2 Marital conflict

SUBJECTIVE: Talked at length about fear that husband would leave her because of her illness. Stated he often would shout at her because she didn't feel well enough to do housework. (Cried for several minutes.) Said children often become frightened and cry during arguments. Said at times feels the children are her only friends. (Smiles.) Said she feels meeting with husband would be helpful.

OBJECTIVE: Sitting in chair, wringing hands constantly, no eye contact.

ASSESSMENT: Think marital counseling sessions should be started as soon as possible to deal with the reality of marriage situation, identify further problem areas, and evaluate husband's interest in help of this type.

PLAN: Discuss with team; if acceptable, set first session time, notify patient and husband.

MANAGEMENT

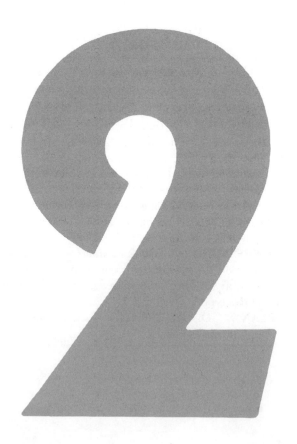

Introduction

Several questions frequently asked by beginning practitioners in psychiatric nursing are: What is my role as a nurse? What will I do all day, just talk? Will I say something which will hurt a client? How should I respond to unusual behavior? It is tempting to look for an instant "cookbook recipe" answer to these questions. Indeed, at times immediate intervention must occur. However, in many situations in psychiatric/mental health nursing practitioners need to evaluate what has happened in each nurse-client interaction. An assessment of one's own responses and feelings, as well as the client's, is important. Supervision from an objective third person is needed. Review of the literature regarding what other nurses and colleagues have written about a particular problem area can be helpful. A consistent evaluation of the on-going interpersonal process between nurse and client is necessary.

It is in the actual process of learning psychiatric nursing through theoretical content, clinical practice, and supervision that practitioners begin to answer for themselves some of the above questions and, indeed, to find that even more questions are raised. For example, if an intervention which was effective in helping one client describe his feelings was not effective with another client—what was different in the two situations—how did the clients differ and how did the nursing approach differ? Why is it that a particular nurse seems to work well with withdrawn clients and not so well with clients expressing hostility? How does a practitioner begin to try to understand a client's symbolic language? In the following chapter we have attempted to select articles which provide nurse practitioners with clinical approaches to nursing care based on theoretical content. The nurse-client relationship is seen as the nucleus from which care and intervention evolve.

Fagin (1967) describes the unique role of the nurse in psychiatry and how this role differs from that of other therapists in different disciplines. The professional nurse needs to be aware of herself and her feelings and expectations of others. An essentially interpersonal philosophy of psychotherapeutic nursing emphasizes the nursing role as being one in which the nurse helps the client establish more comfortable interpersonal relationships. The methodology of implementing this role is discussed.

The significance of the collaborative relationships between nurse and client is discussed by Bayer and Brandner (1977). In their description of the peer practice of nursing, the authors point out how the nurse and the client work together in the problem-solving process, discovering the client's healthy strengths as well as looking at what behavior responses the client has "chosen" to preserve his human system. The nurse and client then look at what choices and solutions the client has to his problems and the client can decide which choice appears most appropriate. A primary focus in the peer practice of nursing is that the health and strengths of the client are supported. The reader is referred to "Safecracker," a poem by Diane Drapeau (*American Journal of Nursing*, Vol. 77, No. I) for an excellent first person account of a client's response to Bayer and Brandner's therapeutic intervention.

Moscato (1975) believes it is important for nurse therapists to move beyond the "good mothering", primarily supportive role in care for chronic patients and away from the medical-disease model of treatment and the stereotyped caretaking functions of women. Moscato worked as the nursing member of an interdisciplinary team in an adolescent outpatient service, and she outlines her functions in that setting. The article concludes with specific recommendations for implementing the outpatient therapist role, including provisions for supervision, support and self-exploration, with the author again using her own practice as an example of how these things can be accomplished.

Practitioners, in an attempt to show their acceptance and non-judgemental attitude toward clients, often experience some difficulty in setting limits. What is an appropriate intervention if a client takes off his clothes, or gives you a gift, or kisses you? Lyon (1970) explains why there is a need for limit-setting and how this can be used as a therapeutic tool. Limit setting is one part of the nurse-client relationship which can help the client reduce his anxiety and reestablish himself to function in a more comfortable and acceptable way with others.

Underwood (1971) discusses how role-playing may facilitate communication between a nurse and a client. She defines role-playing as a learning experience in which nurse and client act out a situation either in the past or present as if it were actually happening. Pertinent dialogue from several role-playing sessions illustrates how this technique may be utilized. This article also points out how the process of the nurse-client relationship helped the client to develop appropriate assertiveness.

In the article by Davitz (1971) it is possible to see many problematic areas that may be encountered in a nurse-client relationship. The article is in the format of a dialogue between a psychiatric nurse and a client in an outpatient setting. At the onset of the relationship, differences in the therapy expectations of nurse and client block communication. This block is further intensified by difficulty in looking at the social and cultural differences between the two participants. The client utilizes many resistance maneuvers which are not dealt with by the nurse. The nurse's problems of counter-transference are evident as the dialogue develops. It is clear from reading the interactions that supervision is needed at all levels of psychiatric nursing practice in order to realistically evaluate what is happening in the nurse-client relationship and to plan continued appropriate intervention.

Fowler, Fordyce and Berni (1969) describe how operant conditioning can be utilized to help clients change their behavior. If sick behavior is rewarded, clients will most often display sick behavior. However, if well behaviors are rewarded, it may be expected that clients can be helped to drop sick behaviors. The authors give examples of operant conditioning utilized in helping three different clients change their behaviors. While the examples given are those of clients with chronic illness, the principles of operant conditioning may also be utilized with clients having psychiatric problems.

Kroah (1974) attempts to classify and move toward clarification of the language and thoughts of clients with schizophrenia. She includes some theories about the language and thought processes in schizophrenia, including the theories of Sullivan, Haley, Kosanin and Whorf. The strategies she presents for intervention, based on the above theorists' ideas, are those which have been applied to psychotherapeutic nursing by Peplau. Varients of language and thought disorders, such as scattering, circumstantiality, and idiosyncratic language are presented in terms of actual dialogue with clients and nursing interventions in these behaviors are presented.

Schwartzman (1975) analyzes the hallucinatory process by attempting to answer such questions as why does the person show this behavior? What needs are being met for this person by using hallucinatory behavior? What does this experience mean for this person? What is the nurse's role in response to it? Sullivanian theory is presented as a theoretical framework. A detailed account of the author's relationship with a client who had hallucinatory behavior is discussed, both in terms of the client's past history and the relationship of hallucinations to this, and in terms of the present nurse-client relationship and nursing interventions. Other treatment modalities which may be considered in conjunction with the nurse-client relationship are medications, a group experience, and family involvement in the treatment plan.

Communicating with depressed clients can evoke feelings of helplessness and hopelessness within the therapist. Swanson (1975) discusses the communication patterns, both verbal and non-verbal, which develop between the depressed client and the nurse. She also reviews the psychoanalytic and interpersonal views that explain the dynamics of the frustration and anger underlying the behavior of depressed persons. In interacting with a depressed client, the nurse should remember that the client greatly needs human company and communication even though he may seem to have a total lack of interest in both.

Caring for a hospitalized client who has a potential problem of aggresive behavior, or who is currently experiencing loss of control requires all members of the health team to work together in formulating a treatment plan. Nissley and Townes (1977) discuss the significance of getting to know the client and intervening at the first signs and symptoms of escalation in his anxiety. If the client is physically out-of-control, staff needs to be aware of his feelings of fear as well as their own feelings of anxiety and fright. Guidelines are presented as to how to work with such a client, and the use of the seclusion room as a therapeutic modality is discussed. It is imperative that staff agree among themselves as to how seclusion will be utilized with each client for whom it may be indicated, since clients readily pick up on staff ambivalence and may become more excited and aggressive because of this.

The termination of a student nurse-client relationship often involves the ending of a process that has been a learning experience in meaningful human interaction for both people involved. Sene (1969) presents information which is helpful to both the instructor and the student in the termination phase of the student's one-to-one relationship with a client.

Concepts of separation anxiety and object loss need to be considered in this phase, as does the fact that both student and client need to mourn a loss. Client behaviors in response to this termination are often seen in terms of increased anxiety, regression, and withdrawal. Student reactions to termination may be seen in discussions of feelings of guilt, frustrated goals, and anger at having to leave the client. Sene presents some therapeutic guidelines from which each therapist may select those approaches best suited to each individual relationship in regard to termination. Two significant concepts in these guidelines are that the nurse needs to establish with the client the realistic fact of the impending separation and the actual termination date and the importance of the nurse in utilizing supervision at this time.

This chapter has looked at various components of the nurse-client relationship and at nursing interventions planned in response to clients' needs. It is evident that theories of nursing care are developing in psychiatric/mental health nursing and that practitioners can refer to their colleagues in nursing and nursing literature, as well as in other disciplines, to seek answers.

6 PSYCHOTHERAPEUTIC NURSING

Claire M. Fagin, Ph.D., R.N.

PSYCHOTHERAPEUTIC NURSING CONSISTS OF THOSE ACTS, THOSE INTERVENTIONS through which nurses help patients use new or healthy patterns in consistent and continuous ways. To do this the nurse moves on three avenues of approach: through the milieu, that is, through manipulating the organization of the social system in the patient setting; through her one-to-one relationship with the patient; and through her interactions with groups of patients.

The nurse may work in all these ways simultaneously or in one way exclusively. For example, she may have a one-to-one interview with a patient in a structured setting where she is aware of the social system which affects the patient but is not a part of it. Or the one-to-one relationship may occur within the context of a milieu—home, hospital, or institution of any kind—which the nurse may attempt to change.

The place of treatment need not be the hospital. It could be the home, the community center, the storefront. And within this frame of reference, it is not only the patient who is deemed sick; his family also, as a social system, is seen as functioning in a pathologic way. There is, in other words, an integration constructed within this family unit which serves to elicit and continue disturbing behavior on the part of the patient.

The nurse's intervention with groups of patients also has a specific configuration. Even though she may work with groups of patients in the same structured way as other therapists, she also works with groups of patients and plans intervention with groups on the ward or in the home where the setting is far less structured. It is in these less structured areas that our theoretic frame of reference regarding nursing therapy is not well developed. In the more structured aspects of individual and group interviews, nurses can borrow and adapt from the approaches of other professional workers. However, in our manipulations of the more typical nursing roles, we are less scientific even though we have much pragmatic evidence. But, this has neither been shared nor researched.

For example, seven dimensions of nursing practice may be identified:

TIME SPENT WITH PATIENTS   Nursing personnel live with their patients within the hospital for an entire tour of duty. If we think of the concept of anxiety, it is obvious that one cannot live with anxiety for extended periods—neither patients for their twenty-four-hour day nor nurses for their eight. Nursing personnel must, therefore, be able to intervene in anxiety-producing situations wherever these occur—in the hospital, in the home, or in the clinic.

THE SPATIAL AREA   Nursing personnel have to be able to participate effectively in areas as varied as bedroom, bath, dining room, living room, or recreation area. This is in sharp contrast to the psychiatrist or social worker, whose spatial area generally is structured.

VARIETY OF PATIENTS   The nurse must relate simultaneously with many individuals who have varying degrees of health and illness with multiple and possibly conflicting needs.

CARE FOR THE WHOLE PATIENT   The nurse's ability in relation to patients' physical as well as emotional care needs can be extremely useful in her psychotherapeutic efforts. It can also pose a problem, however, of too great intimacy for the patient and a lack of clarity of role for the nurse. Again, this is in sharp contrast to the psychiatrist or the social worker whose roles tend to remain more or less constant.

RAPID ADJUSTMENTS   Throughout her working day, the nurse moves frequently from relating to individual patients to relating to groups of patients. Her effectiveness is determined by her ability to make rapid adjustments to these changes in situations and to creatively utilize and influence the interactions. In other words, the movement from individual therapy to group therapy and vice versa should not be seen as an interference with the relationships but as a learning experience in the daily life of the patients.

CARE FOR PATIENTS AS A GROUP   Frequently nurses are involved with groups of patients. Group interactions are inherently complex, especially in terms of the meaning of relationships and communications between nurse and patients, patient and patients, and nurse and family.

ON-THE-SPOT DECISION MAKING   The nurse has to make moment-to-moment decisions, compromises, improvisations, and take risks for prolonged periods of time.

Although each nurse may add to this list on the basis of her own experience, considering these seven dimensions has been useful in thinking through nursing roles and relationships.[1]

To achieve therapeutic effectiveness, the first step the nurse must take is to look at the preconceptions she brings to the situation. What is of particular concern is her concept of illness which, overtly and covertly, influences her philosophy of nursing and her approach to therapy. The nurse must understand the meaning of illness in our society and, more particularly, the meaning of mental illness.

ACTION FOR MENTAL HEALTH   The report of the Joint Commission on Mental Illness and Health, noted sharply that attitudes about mental illness were obstacles to therapeutic efforts. They found an underlying attitude of rejection and disapproval of mental illness and the mentally ill which frequently engendered more rather than less estrangement of the sick person (1). The patient, too, holds these attitudes and, therefore, he tends to reject himself for some of the same reasons that others do: fear of his acts, his destructive impulses, his anger, and his helplessness. Lack of awareness of our own feelings about mental illness and the mentally ill covertly influences our behavior. This is true, of course, of preconceptions in general.

By way of illustration, let's take the preconception some people have of nurses. Occasionally, it is said that nurses are authoritarian and cold-hearted. The nurse who is not authoritarian may provoke anxiety in patients who think this. Such a patient comes to the nurse expecting that she will give him answers and tell him what to do. If, instead, the nurse is warm and spontaneous and tries to make decisions *with* the patient instead of *for* the patient, his preconceptions may clash with reality. But if this nurse also notes the cues to the patient's anxiety and tries to understand and clarify with the patient what is going on, there is possibility for growth.

The nurse's concepts and attitudes also are relevant. For example, the nurse working with a specific cultural group needs to examine her precon-

---

[1]This list is based on but is not identical with that developed through collaborative efforts with Gwen Tudor Will and Agnes Middleton.

ceptions about this group, test them with reality, and then attempt changes if her findings so dictate.

The recognition and subsequent alteration of one's preconceptions are essential modes of behavior in any area in which the nurse finds herself. And unless she is clear on the degree to which her preconceptions are accurate and on how they influence her thinking, she cannot begin to be therapeutically effective in any relationship: one-to-one, group, or milieu. Morris Schwartz points out:

There has been increasing acceptance of the idea that non-organic mental illness is not a disease entity lodged within the patient. Rather, it is seen as a pattern of difficulty that the person manifests in relating to himself and others. This pattern of difficulty is seen not only as a product of what a patient "is" but of what he does and what others think about him and do to, and with, him. This line of thinking further maintains that, if the patient's difficulties are to be alleviated—his thinking and behavior changed—not only must the patient do something about himself but personnel who are part of his daily social environment must develop attitudes and behavior toward him that best fit his needs and are most appropriate for his current and changing condition. (2)

This concept leads to the view that is within the behavior, within the interpersonal relations which develop between staff and patient, that the patient can learn and grow and, therefore, get well. Such a concept can determine a philosophy of psychotherapeutic nursing that is essentially interpersonal. It is, for example, no longer believed that a therapeutic hour each day, alone, helps the patient get well but, rather, that one or many persons in many situations with the patient can bring about therapeutic results. Patients, and their families as well, are seen as active participants in treatment.

Quite simply, one might say that a patient comes into contact with psychiatric personnel because he is having difficulty in living; specifically, difficulty in living with other people. One of the purposes of nursing intervention, then, is to provide experiences in living which will enable the patient to establish relationships that are less anxiety provoking and more comfortable, making possible other less threatening, less forbidding relationships.

Methodology

The obvious question then is, "How does the nurse do this?" First of all she *observes* and *collects data.* Part of this data is theory: information about personality development, interpersonal interaction, the concept of anxiety, and how social systems operate (3). She acquires this knowledge from the literature and from her own observations and research.

In addition to theory, the data include specific observations about the patient: his verbal and nonverbal communications; that is, his words, actions, expressions, and gestures. The extent to which the patient uses gestures rather than verbal communication, for example, will indicate something about the level of personality development at which he is operating.

In addition to these observations, the nurse needs to look at her own words, actions, and gestures and, even more important, at her thoughts and feelings for the clues they give. Thoughts and feelings of patients are not always obvious yet they often are the first clues that something is amiss with patients, the group, or the social setting. They may, on the other hand, tell us that things are going well and that the situation is comfortable.

Harry Stack Sullivan said that two overall goals in interpersonal relations were satisfaction and security (4). These two broad categories are helpful in grouping patients' needs. Satisfaction, for example, is produced when needs that are primarily biologic are met; security when needs that are primarily interpersonal are fulfilled. Both of these categories are of concern in nursing since a patient's problems often are entwined with frustrations in both biologic and interpersonal areas. A patient on a special diet who is always hungry may feel a lack of physiologic satisfaction but, since food plays a significant role in our interpersonal context from birth to death, he also may have his need for security breached. Or a man seriously mutilated in an accident may be more troubled by the change in his self-image than with his severe pain.

Needs which have to do with maintenance of the self, that is, who we are and what we are, are included in the category of security needs. For example, such needs as the feeling of respect for oneself, for approval, prestige, love, friendship, recognition, power, and so forth, obviously deal with personal security. When these needs are unmet or, in other words, when there is a threat to the self-esteem, a feeling of anxiety may be experienced. All of us are familiar, in one degree or another, with the discomfort of anxiety, as well as with the desire to avoid such discomfort. The wish to avoid anxiety gives rise to patterns of behavior that will meet needs or, at least, preserve the self with a minimum of discomfort.

Anxiety is essentially an emergency emotion that warns the individual that something is likely to interfere with the self-concept. This emotion can be generated interpersonally by co-workers, patients, family, or others in the situation, or it may be generated by something in the present situation which unconsciously reminds the individual of a painful experience in the past.

People have different ways of seeking relief from the feeling of help-lessness that arises with anxiety. Some persons may become more de-pendent and submissive, clearly demonstrating the helplessness that they feel. Others may respond with defiance or stubbornness, or they may be-come demanding. Each response that a person makes is apt to bring a response from others which may reinforce the way the person feels or alter it.

Most people have experienced anxiety from being with a very anxious person. But this reaction often is not realized until a later time. This process—one person's anxiety being communicated to another person—may become circular if there is no awareness of the anxiety and no under-standing of it. Self-observation, therefore, is crucial in being therapeutic.

The second function is to *make inferences* from the data gathered. Here the nurse looks at the data and tries to relate her own observations of the situation to the theory and also to past situations she and others have observed. She makes an attempt to decode and infer meaning from the communications, and to look at the whole: herself and the patient, the nonverbal and the verbal communications, and at the theory.

Third, the nurse *structures her interventions according to her in-ferences*. These three—collecting data, making inferences, and structur-ing nursing interventions—may occur on a rapid moment-to-moment basis or over a long period of time. The nurse working with a patient thinks about what is happening and plans her interventions accordingly. But she also thinks about the relationship of today's activities with those of the week before and the weeks to follow; she thinks of the continuous process, the themes that emerge, the unique patterns, the recurring pat-terns.

Fourth, she also *evaluates*. The correctness or incorrectness of particular interventions or of inferences she draws about the patient's responses, the feeling tone of the group, progress, regression, obvious or subtle changes, or even no change are looked at in this process. Evalua-tion is a separate function, yet it also is a part of the nurse's other thera-peutic functions.

The nurse cannot practice psychotherapeutic nursing unless she is able to take these four steps independently as well as interdependently. Un-less she can use her own intellectual abilities, she will function only in rote fashion and not consistently and continuously in terms of the specific situation in which she is interacting with the patient.

For example, if the principle is accepted that behavior is reciprocal—that is, what we do with patients influences their responses—the nurse can alter her behavior on the basis of what she knows about the situation. But this may elicit any of a variety of responses from the patient since no set response to a particular behavior can be predicted. In determining a correct and useful response to make to the patient, the nurse uses the skills with which understanding is built—observing, listening, studying, decoding, inferring, acting, and evaluating. Patient's needs, however, are often expressed in obscure and confusing ways, and any conflict between the nurses' and the patients' interpretation of what is being communicated must be resolved if there is to be understanding of the problems the patients are facing.

So far this paper has focused on the ideas which are relevant to the three avenues of approach in psychotherapeutic nursing intervention—the one-to-one relationship, group relationships, and the milieu. The remainder of the paper will identify some specific techniques that can be used in each of these three areas.

Individual Therapy

A useful beginning in individual, or one-to-one therapy is to look at how the patient might see the nurse. Every patient will have ideas about the nurse and her job because of the cultural stereotype. But each nurse needs to examine this stereotype for herself. If the patient has had pleasant experiences with nurses, he might see the nurse as someone who cares for or helps people, who goes out of her way to do something for someone. This concept of doing something for someone may be of positive value with patients who are dependent, yet unable to express their dependency in a way that will get them constructive help. Such a patient may find it difficult to seek help or to express his needs for help. The nurse, on the other hand, can go to the patient. Some writers describe this approach to patients as positive aggression (5). That is, the nurse goes after the patient and meets the patient on his own terms. The one-to-one relationship, thus, may be started in an unstructured way and continued on an appointment basis when both nurse and patient so choose. The nurse by virtue of role is in a position to seek out the patient and to see him in a variety of places rather than waiting for him to come to her.

Another aspect of nursing that is essential with many patients is the nurse's ease in physical caring and doing for others. In this instance, the mother-surrogate role, spelled out by Peplau has particular relevance (6). In tending the patient physically, the nurse demonstrates how much she cares, but the anxiety and disapproval which the patient's mother may have conveyed to him in her caring is absent. Caring activities are vehicles for deepening the relationship; the nurse may find it is when she is giving physical care that the patient will discuss his real concerns. But the patient who has difficulty in what he views as intimacy with another person will have increased anxiety if the nurse is not clear about the differences between her professional and her social roles, and about her own needs. The nurse may have a need to be liked and accepted by patients. The clearer she is on how this need affects her behavior the more useful she will be. By consciously manipulating her own behavior she can help the patient find himself through the acceptance, learnings, and subsequent satisfactions of their relationship.

When the nurse is helping a patient express and resolve his dependency needs, it is essential that she be alert to minute changes in his responses. She addresses herself to the healthy aspects of the patient. As she watches, listens, and infers meaning, she is able to sense when he has made some movement which she then uses in helping him to gradually assume more responsibility for himself and lessen his need to continue his mentally ill behavior. If the nurse does not notice the change in behavior, she will continue to deal with the patient as if it had not occurred, and thus make it more difficult for him to sustain the improvement. A small change in behavior may be a big step for the patient, and if the nurse fails to sense it, the patient may become greatly discouraged.

The very subtle cues which may come from the patient, particularly in terms of any movement toward a higher level of functioning, are extremely important. Even a small amount of understanding will reinforce his healthy behavior and help him feel that he is not completely "crazy." Understanding the patient's communication makes the whole process of illness more rational and brings about a sharing experience which for the patient may be a unique event. Each experience of this kind gives him hope that other experiences like this can happen to him, that he isn't so different from others, that he can be understood.

One difficult aspect of the one-to-one relationship is the silent listening and observing that is necessary. This skill is not easy to acquire because the nurse often feels unsuccessful if she hasn't been able to get the patient to talk to her. But if she recognizes the importance of the nonverbal cues and develops her ability to observe them, she will uncover signs she previously would have ignored.

One essential aspect of therapy is reflection on the meaning of what the nurse sees or hears, reflection that encourages the patient to expand on it further. The nurse who jumps in to say something, or says the first thing that comes to her mind, will shut off the patient's flow of self-expression. If she can sustain her own tension and anxiety and respond thoughtfully to the patient's comments, she will often learn more about the patient's particular modes of behavior. She may find out what he is looking for in other people; themes or consistencies may become obvious; knowledge may be obtained, for example, about a phase of his development. Is he operating for the most part at an infantile level? If so, what might be done to help him move to the next level of development?

The one-to-one relationship allows the nurse to structure her interventions to include experiences geared toward helping the patient accomplish a particular developmental task. But, one-to-one therapy is not always feasible nor always desirable. Some patients respond better to group therapy, and for some nurses group work is their métier.

Working With Groups

Obviously, the important aspect in groups is the reaction of personalities on one another. There is stimulation and contagion of emotion from one patient to another, and correlation of one person's problems with those of others—of help particularly to those patients who find it hard to verbalize their difficulties.

Another value of a group experience for a patient may be a realization that his problems are not unique. This realization tends to dispel his guilt and sometimes even lessens the weight of his problem. In the group, the individual obtains support not only from the therapist but from other patients as well. A problem the nurse needs to keep aware of is that of competition among patients for attention from the therapist and for status in the group.

Sensitivity to the needs and tensions in the group is very important. A common error is to focus more on individual rather than on group interaction. Another is to fail to recognize the unofficial patient leader and channel his leadership into healthy rather than destructive patterns.

A therapist working with groups learns to verbalize the underlying feelings of the group only when they are near the surface and only when many group members share them. In other words, the feelings should be easily perceived. In general, probing questions are ruled out, both in individual and in group therapy. Patients will discuss the topics of importance to them when they are ready to do so. The responsibility to make choices and to institute change belongs to them.

Group therapy draws only part of its methodology, dynamics, and techniques from psychiatry; sources of knowledge about the particular ways in which groups operate, cultural and class values and configurations, and concepts of role come from sociology, social psychology, and anthropology. Such ideas as role complementarity and role set have relevance in individual therapy, but these ideas are even more significant in situations where there are multiple "others" to assume roles in relation to particular problem situations.

Although group interviews deal predominately with current problems—following the patient's leads—the therapist develops a sensitivity
to group themes, individual incongruities, topics around which the group
clusters, silences, and the direction which patients are taking. She notes
whether silences occur around specific topics or whether there are situational changes. Continued silence by some patients may mean that they
are too embarrassed or too ashamed for the group discussion. Their usual
patterns of withdrawal might be reinforced by the discussion. Sensitivity
to this behavior would lead the nurse to help plan subsequent individual
approaches.

This paper, focusing on psychotherapeutic function, is not meant to
imply any view of the nurse as omnipotent. Although she may work independently, there are, of course, times when she collaborates with
members of other disciplines. However, when and how she collaborates
is a subject for another paper.

The Milieu

In the third avenue of approach—the milieu—the nurse has the authority as well as the responsibility for creative action. Many authors
believe that the milieu is the most important treatment modality for psychiatric patients. In the first place, psychiatric patients often are not able
to express themselves in a traditional interview, and often are not able to
talk easily about many aspects of their lives. Second, improvements in the
milieu reach a greater number of patients than do others therapies. Third,
and probably most important, the patient lives in a situation 24 hours a
day, 7 days a week; the benefits of a few scheduled therapy hours often
can be undone, or at least not capitalized upon, by the social setting.

In examining and creating a therapeutic milieu, a philosophy of
psychotherapeutic nursing must first be developed and then implemented in the situation. For example, admission routines are a good place
to start. Frequently, the way a patient is treated on admission reinforces
his negative feelings about himself and about hospitals. The procedure
often is depersonalized, the patient's belongings are removed, and few
explanations are given. Good practice would be to see that he has
everything he needs, and to introduce him, regardless of his behavior, to
patients and personnel he is going to live with in his immediate area.

For example, a graduate student told about seeing, on her first day on a
psychiatric ward, a tall, thin, well-groomed young man pacing the long
hall. Occasionally, he would pause, look into the living room, but would
never enter. The student introduced herself to him; he told her his name

was Bob. Presently, another patient joined them, remarked upon her Boston accent, and spent a few moments in conversation. Soon Bob resumed his pacing. At lunchtime, the student asked one of the nurses to tell her about Bob. The nurse replied, "Who knows him? He has been here for three weeks but doesn't say very much and just seems to wander about the ward. He's a chronic schizophrenic."

Three days later, when the student returned to the ward, she was told that Bob was becoming catatonic, had been posturing, was not able to swallow, and consequently had not eaten. He had been given sodium amytal and had been sleeping most of the afternoon. Following this report she saw him lying on the bed, unshaven and unkempt. She brought him a tray for supper and when she awakened him to eat, she noticed that he appeared dazed, frightened, and had tremors. In order to alleviate some of his fears, she forewarned him about all of her actions and told him that she would help him eat and remain with him. To her surprise, he ate all the food on the tray, but did not speak. Following supper, he stood up. The student asked him if he would like to walk in the hall; he responded by turning toward the door. He was unsteady, so she offered to hold his arm. They walked into the hall and the first words he said were, "Have you been to Boston lately?" Obviously, he remembered her.

She spent most of the evening pacing the hall with him. His verbalization was autistic for the most part. At one point, he told her he was frightened and he took her hand in his as they paced. An undergraduate nursing student relieved her for dinner and coffee break. Bob went to bed at 10:00 P.M. after the graduate student had told him she would return in two days. The night staff discussed Bob and his feelings of depersonalization as evidenced by some of his activities. When the student returned two days later, she found that Bob had been eating and that members of the staff, especially the nursing students, were taking turns pacing with him in the hall. When the graduate student began walking with Bob again, he was walking with a shuffling gait but shortly changed to a normal gait. At times, he was confused, but he told her about his brothers and sisters, and some of his interests. He was initiating conversation, not merely responding to the nurse's questions.

The staff nurse assigned to the patient was amazed at the change in his behavior and said, "His medication must finally be working." But the student said she thought the interpersonal attention he had been receiving might well be related to the change, pointing out that at the beginning of the week he was alone most of the time and no one had seemed to know anything about him (7).

This example illustrates a patient's awareness of events at times when he does not seem to know what is going on, the overlapping nature of the one-to-one and milieu approaches, and the contagious effect of one person's behavior on another. In this case, it was the nursing student who picked up the behavior of the graduate student. Sometimes, a nurse's behavior will be reflected by patients on the unit who, when they see a patient is treated, may also begin to behave toward the patient in similar ways. In fact, patients, like other people, are influenced as much by the nurse's behavior as by what she says.

In implementing a psychotherapeutic philosophy, another area to examine is that of communications. Are there opportunities for staff and patients to meet formally and informally? And for personnel to share information, both verbal and written? Is the ward routine so arranged that nurses can devote time to listening to patients and to each other? Does the setting allow for exploiting life issues? For example, is it possible for interveiws to be held when necessary and when indicated rather than only at prescribed hours during the day?

The direction of communication and the way decisions are made is another index of the philosophy of care. If the patient is to benefit from the milieu, he must participate in it so that his behavior actually influences what is going on. The same principle holds for the optimum functioning of all levels of nursing personnel. Personnel who are involved in decision making have an investment in the policies they have helped to frame.

Program, policies, and routines should insure that the patient is protected from traumatic handling by any personnel associated with the unit. In addition, there must be gratification divorced from consideration of whether the patient deserves it or not. Patients need gratification as part of their treatment; they don't win it on the basis of good behavior. Tolerance of symptoms and leeway for regression is necessary within the treatment environment, but protective interference by the staff at the moment when it is necessary to protect the patient from his own guilt, anxiety, or depression, or to protect other patients, is also a part of effective milieu therapy.

A patient may not be able to handle a permissive environment, especially at the beginning of hospitalization. Acceptance of him, his problems, and his symptoms may make him anxious. In this instance, patients and personnel need to recognize the difference between acceptance of symptoms and indifference or permissive enjoyment of problem behavior. Accepting a patient does not mean approval of everything he does. Approval of negative feelings may, in fact, be a hindrance rather than a help. The patient group, itself, will indicate over and over to individual patients the concept of permissiveness and acceptance that really exists. And the patient will sense this from the nurse's responses to him and from what he observes of her acceptance of other patients.

A treatment milieu also has rules or limits—rules for social and for

physical behavior that are really necessary, rules that are clearly understood and carefully observed. First of all, dangerous, aggressive behavior
against self and others obviously cannot be permitted. Some forms of obscene language and some forms of acting out also may be too seductive
under certain circumstances. Judiciously planned, rules, limits, or
routines will help to increase a patient's sence of security.

Routines should be part of the design, however, rather than a
challenge to patients to behave in ways which would then call out reward,
punishment, acceptance, or rejection on the part of the personnel.
Whatever the rules, let them be few, explicit, and understood by staff as
well as by patients. Nothing is more attractive to patients than testing
limits, especially with new staff.

Creative manipulation of the milieu is an exciting aspect of psychotherapeutic nursing. It suggest an infinite variety of work roles with
personnel and patients, and poses a fruitful arena for nursing research.

Summary

The role of the nurse as a therapeutic agent has been identified, using
three overlapping avenues of approach—the one-to-one relationship, the
group relationship, and the milieu. The philosophic frame of reference
has been that the patient has become ill as a result of the experience he
has had in living. His illness then can be influenced, interrupted, or altered by what other people do, to and with him. Behind a patient's rejecting behavior is potential for warmth and responsive behavior. This
potential can be reached through persistence in offering the patient a
responsive and respectful relationship.

Bibliography

1. Joint Commission on Mental Illness and Health. *Action for Mental
    Health*, Final report. New York, Basic Books, 1971.

2. **Schwartz, M. S. and Shockley, Emmy L.**, *Nurse and the Mental
    Patient*. Science Editions, John Wiley and Sons, New York, 1966,
    (Paperback) Introduction.

3. **Fagin, Claire M.** *Study for Desirable Functions and Qualifications
    for Psychiatric Nurses*. New York, National League for Nursing,
    1953. (Mimeographed)

4. **Sullivan, H. S.** *Conceptions of Modern Psychiatry.* Washington, D.C., William Alanson White Psychiatric Foundation, 1947, p. 6.

5. **Bruce, Sylvia J.** Adolescence, delinquent and distressed. *Nurs. Outlook* 8:499–501, Sept. 1960.

6. **Peplau, Hildegarde E.** Principles of psychiatric nursing. In *American Handbook of Psychiatry,* ed. by Silvano Arieti, New York, Basic Books, 1959, Vol. 2, pp. 1840–1856.

7. **Davidites, Rose Marie.** (Unpublished paper)

7 NURSE/ PATIENT PEER PRACTICE

Mary Bayer, B.S.N., R.N.

Patty Brandner, M.S., R.N.

AS CONSUMERS BECOME MORE CONCERNED ABOUT THE HIGH cost and inconvenience of illness, more knowledgeable about medical and health care, and insistent on making decisions in their own health care, they are seeking new answers to such basic human problems and new ways to meet their health needs.

Meanwhile, the health system hierarchy is struggling to maintain authority over the consumer. We believe that nursing should withdraw from this effort and join forces with consumers to achieve a more enhancing health care system.

Before the client can feel a true partnership with nursing, however, a major change must occur: Nurses must not only acknowledge clients' rights to have intelligence, but also encourage them to use it! That is one of the fundamentals of what we call peer practice in nursing. The patient here is a peer; one abandons the old stance of the doctor as "father," the nurse as "mother," and the patient/client as "child."

We believe an alternate attitude begins with the nurse's concept of her-or himself as a unique, never duplicated-in-the-past-present-future member of the human species; the holistic approach is applied to the nurse as well as to the client. The ongoing task of the nurse is to understand how her own human system functions and to be responsible for its integrity. With this awareness, she does not have to be afraid of becoming "emotionally involved" with clients nor of using them to gratify her personal needs.

Further, the nurse values her own time and that of others; she does not waste it. She recognizes that cooperation in peer relationships uses life energy more productively than do the competitive ways that characterize our present health care system. Maintaining authority and/or servility requires energy. That energy can be used more efficaciously to promote health for the relatively short time life offers each human being.

From this basic respect for life comes the recognition that each person has "health," which includes the ability to solve the problems of living; that each person is in control of her or his life-behavior; that each has a background of personal interactions, socialization, and education that he uses to make behavior choices. Survival in our society requires a complex of skills for problem-solving; nurses recognize those skills as a component of "health" and, working in a peer relationship with the clients, "diagnose" the clients' strengths, their "healthy" behaviors.

As the nurse and the client discover the healthy strengths together—the nurse bringing her special knowledge to the process and the client contributing his own uniqueness and survival ability—the two can pool choices for further health enhancement. The nurse can offer choices only from her experience and knowledge; the client can accept or reject those choices only as they fit his own health needs. At all times during the interaction, the client's intellect is engaged in the problem-solving process.

We outline problem-solving steps this way to each client:

1. Identifying *one* problem
2. Discovering and listing the choices for a solution
3. Exploring of the consequences of each choice
4. Making the choice

When nurse and client pool choices, the client has a greater variety from which to choose. When professional colleagues also are invited to offer their suggestions, the client has a still greater chance to make health-supportive decisions.

To help the client to a clearer understanding of peer nursing practice, we explain how the human system operates. We describe how the four major facets of each human being—physical, emotional, social and intellectual—are integrated into a unique system and the primary need is to maintain the system's integrity.

That primary function is often masked because every culture assigns roles to its members according to age, sex, race, educational, and economic levels, and the like. Nonetheless, the human system continues struggling, either awarely or unawarely, to maintain a balance among its component facets to survive.

We recognize that, because every client has existed within his own system for as long as he has lived, he is the "resident expert" on himself. Not only does that client know more about himself than does any other person, but he also knows how he has integrated his own human system to survive until now. In today's health care system, this vital information is seldom elicited.

In the peer practice of nursing, the nurse's role is to help clarify the manner in which each client responds to assaults on his unique human system. Then, working as peers and using a problem-solving approach, the two can identify and evaluate the choices available. Once all of the possible choices are laid out and probable consequences of each are determined, the client chooses the solution which appears to be the most self-enhancing.

Bringing the client's intellect as well as emotions into the therapeutic interaction provides the base for his future successful problem-solving. The nurse supports the client's past problem-solving (by which, after all, he has survived to that moment) and recognizes that professional help has been sought because the individual's usual pattern of problem solving is not appropriate for the current situation.

While the nurse is responding to the system or problem, she also strengthens the client's healthy behaviors and facets by calling attention to them. Most clients are responding to one or more assaults to their systems, and the nurse's role is to help the client deal with the effects of the assault and to serve as a consultant while the client attempts to re-integrate his human system. As consultants, we find that it is helpful to share examples of ways in which various facets can respond to assaults.

Assaults on the System

We note that no matter on which facet or facets an assault occurs, the categories of choices remain virtually the same. Some of the choices may appear bizarre in view of the seemingly insignificant assault but, because of the complexity of each human system, a choice that is possible for one person may be totally inappropriate for another. For example, in Maine where the winters are long and severe, often a body is found in the spring with a suicide note beside it saying, "I just couldn't take one more snow storm this year." To someone in Florida, that might seem an insane response to a spring snow storm. But the people of Maine understand.

PHYSICAL ASSAULTS   An assault to the physical facet might be a cut finger. The primary response is physical: bleeding. A secondary response follows quickly, one that seems to be integrative, representing simultaneous responses from the other facets. At the physical level there may be continued bleeding, perhaps an increase in pulse and respirations. Emotionally there may be anger, disgust, fear. The intellect may register pain and begin evaluating the severity of the injury. At the same time the social facet may be concerned over spilling blood onto a friend's new rug.

Once these responses are integrated, the individual automatically begins problem-solving either with past patterns of response or by aware use of the intellect. The choices for dealing with the cut finger might include ignoring it, helping oneself, turning to another for assistance—or possibly getting drunk, popping a pill, or even committing suicide. In the case of a cut finger, most persons probably consider that the best choice would be to cleanse the wound and apply a bandage; some might rush off to the family doctor.

EMOTIONAL ASSAULTS   As mental health nurse-therapists, we have been testing our peer nursing theory as we interact with so-called "emotionally disturbed" clients. We discuss the physical, emotional, social, and intellectual responses with each client as part of our nursing intervention. We express the view that each person is responding in the most enhancing ways of which he is aware at that time. We perceive this as individual behavior to preserve the integrity of the human system. We don't label clients "sick"; we talk about "protective skills" or "behavior choices" rather than about "defense mechanisms." We point out immediately that we want to discuss the "good things about you" for assessment of healths and strengths with which we, client and nurse, can work.

During the first interaction, we identify behavior responses as "choices" by which the client tries to preserve his human system. Reviewing the problem-solving process, we identify additional choices: "going crazy," "getting sick," drinking, running away, ignoring, attempting suicide, and so on. Many of these choices are ones that the client may have made in the past.

Many of our clients have been in traditional therapy before reaching us and have believed their "craziness" to be outside their control. They feel frightened and desperate, directed by forces outside themselves. They express surprise, recognition, and relief when they hear that we consider their behavior of their own choosing and that there are other choices they can make. With hope, often eagerness, clients examine solutions for health that the therapist can offer, but which only the clients can know will be enhancing in their situations.

With our clients we explore the responses of the human system to assaults on the emotional component. Take a verbal insult as an example. The primary response is emotional, usually in the form of hurt feelings or embarrassment. The secondary response involves all facets: flushed face, increased pulse; anger at the assailant and/or self; and asking self "why" or remembering previous insults: "be nice," "don't show anger," "what will my friends think."

The problem-solving choices are many: running away, ignoring (by stuffing the feelings back down), confronting and clarifying, getting drunk, taking drugs, fighting back, and so on. Individuals limited in response patterns and ability to conceptualize consequences realistically will often respond with the same choice regardless of the severity of the assault. Those who are aware of a wide range of choices, as well as the probable consequences of each, will usually choose a solution appropriate to the situation, with little energy lost in the selection process.

Intellectual Assaults

Hospitalized persons, because of their vulnerability, are particularly susceptible to intellectual assault, which often occurs when staff members talk about him in jargon he cannot understand. The covert message to the patient is "There, there, darlin. You relax and *we'll* decide what is to be done."

The primary response of the assaulted intellect is often "I'm too stupid to understand." The secondary responses appear simultaneously throughout the system: flushed face and tensed muscles; anger, fear, frustration, shame; "It isn't right to question a doctor's judgment"; "They know better than I do."

Again, the same choices are available, but where a person is at the mercy of others (as hospitalized patients can feel), the choices often take more subtle forms: stuffing feelings back down, regressing to a more dependent state (described in nursing notes as "cooperative" "no complaints") or displacing the feelings onto "safer" people than those who have charge of the individual's health situation.

SOCIAL ASSAULTS   Persons who would rather look after themselves, but who are forced to seek outside help, frequently perceive social assaults. When a patient enters the system on his own two feet and then is requested to replace street clothes with a hospital gown and hop into bed immediately, he may consider this an assault. The primary response takes place within the *social* facet: "I must look ridiculous in this get-up" or "People don't go to bed when they feel OK." The secondary, integrated responses might be blushing, tensed muscles; embarrassment, frustration, apprehension, anger; "Better cover up my bare legs"; "What would my friend think of me now?"; "I must be sicker than I thought" or memory of previous hospitalizations.

Although patients have been known to gather up their clothes and take off at this point, most will internalize their feelings by verbalizing their anxiety in a joking way (so as not to risk disapproval from the staff) or by ventilating to friends and family.

In each case, a primary response occurs at the facet under assault; followed by secondary responses at all facets. The intellect integrates the various responses and either awarely or unawarely proceeds into a problem-solving sequence in order to restore equilibrium to the system. We help clients to become aware of this process and together engage intellects to examine choices and consequences.

As consequences of behavior choices are explored, the nurse discusses with the client the concept that past choices were made because a limited range may have been seen at the time or the individual chose the least threatening, therefore the most protective, of those choices seemingly available. The nurse encourages the client to accept past choices, even those with self-destructive consequences as "protective skills" by which the individual kept alive until a wider range of choices was available and more self and social understanding had been gained.

Understanding the Consequences

When persons realize that past choices were made from a need to protect their survival in a hostile, unchangeable environment; that these choices are considered "skills" since the human system did survive; and that behavior is in the control of the individual, then feelings of guilt, self-blame, shame, frustration, and fear can be relinquished. The knowledge that each human system is in control of its own behavior frees the individual from self-defeating energy use.

Then, working in a peer relationship, the client and therapist each contribute from their unique human systems, and the probable consequences of each choice can be predicted. For example, running away can offer temporary relief, but often involves facing the problem again at a later date, possibly in another form. Stuffing feelings back down may work at the moment, but usually results in displacement of anger onto others or in eventual depression or psychosomatic illness. Potentially self-destructive choices such as getting drunk, taking drugs, getting physically and/or mentally ill are often made without self-knowledge, from patterns necessary for survival in childhood which have been carried into adult life. They may give temporary respite but usually lead to more serious problems than the immediate one. Suicide means death, loss of control, no chance to change one's mind in favor of another choice.

Such choices as confronting or expressing one's honest feelings may lead to further assault, rejection of the other, or they may open a path of communication by which effects of the assault can be remedied. Self-help can sometimes solve the problem; other times it provides only temporary relief. Turning to others can resolve a problem, but at other times it can lead to dependency.

When each choice and its probable consequence has been examined, the client can decide which appears most suitable, knowing that at any time, he can choose again or return to a more familiar, comfortable response pattern. A system that is generally in a state of equilibrium can usually regain its balance without much effort.

However, repeated assaults to a particular facet or simultaneous and/or frequent assaults on several components can quickly weaken the system, confuse the integration of responses, and mask correct identification of the problem(s). By understanding the basic responses to assaults, we can quickly separate out the various problems and help the client identify priorities. When the client has chosen which problem to attack first, we view together the available choices and carry out the problem-solving process.

In peer practice, the primary focus is on helping clients to learn how they have solved problems in the past and to call this "health"; on presenting a wider variety of available choices; on considering the consequences of each choice; and on continuing our support of whatever decision they make. We have found that, as we support the health and strength the client presents, the client's knowledge, self-reliance and self-esteem are increased to the point at which future need for health care services is significantly lessened.

In a society in which traditional authority figures are coming under constant attack, we suggest that nursing recognize that each human system has an intellect—one that has kept that human being intact and functioning until our services have been sought, that will continue to integrate that human being long after our services are no longer necessary. As peers, nurse and client can collaborate to strengthen the client's potential for self-direction, knowledge, maintenance of health and prevention of illness.

THE PSYCHIATRIC NURSE AS OUTPATIENT PSYCHOTHERAPIST

Beth Ann Moscato, B.S.N., R.N.

NURSING LITERATURE REFLECTS THE TREND TO FOCUS NURSING therapy primarily on dependent individuals in need of supportive therapy. June Mellow, who pioneered in the use of the nurse as therapist, coined "nursing therapy" as a term to denote an approach to the treatment of acute schizophrenia. Two parts of the treatment approach include:

1. An experiential order with therapeutic emphasis on meeting immediate patient needs, followed by,
2. An investigative therapy with emphasis on techniques from psychoanalytically oriented psychotherapy after the acute period was resolved.[1] Mellow was first to give nurses permission to be the major therapist in individual cases, where the nurse's role is viewed as "a contribution in its own right rather than an extension of the therapeutic arm of a particular psychiatrist."[2] Nursing therapy has evolved as a specialized area of psychiatric nursing to the present time.

It is generally recognized and provision made for nurse therapists to develop caseloads of clients in inpatient settings.[3-5] As nurses expanded roles in outpatient services, their functions have included: arrangements for aftercare, provision for home visits, supervision of activities in day-care programs, and supportive therapy with chronic clients. This supportive therapy may be assigned to the nurse so that the other professionals

Reproduced, with permission, from *Journal of Psychiatric Nursing and Mental Health Services*, September-October 1975. (Figure 1 which appeared in the original article has been omitted in this reprint.)

(psychiatrist, social worker, psychologist) may devote more time to the greater number of acutely ill clients who have more favorable diagnoses.[6]

This gravitation toward supportive relationships with chronic clients may result from colleague pressure, from an academic background stressing the medical-disease entity model, and from the general stereotyping of nurses as women, who are caretakers on the job as well as in the home. Psychotherapy dealing with regressed schizophrenic clients has been conceptualized by nurses as "the art of good mothering."[7] It is recognized that "good mothering" is essential for normal growth toward physical, social, and emotional interdependence. It appears essential, however, for the nurse to increase psychotherapeutic skills, experience, and theoretical expertise well beyond a framework of "good mothering." Thus, the nurse may better prove competency in individual, group, and family therapy to herself, her professional colleagues, and clients.

In researching utilization of nurses in United States outpatient clinics, Reres found that nurses' functions include: part-time clinic receptionist, assistance in physical exams and somatic treatments, administration of medications, making home visits, and therapy sessions. While over two thirds of the nurses serve as therapist and/or counselor in regularly scheduled client interviews with supervision, only one third of the nurses were actively participating in group psychotherapy as leaders or co-leaders.[8]

In private practice where the nurse's role is barely defined and legally without precedent, nurses have also been involved in systematic desensitization with phobic clients. It is surprising to note that homicidal, suicidal, or severely "acting out" clients are at times not assigned to the nurse therapist in private practice.[9-10] This presents a dichotomy, since one traditional function of inpatient nursing is to "special" or closely supervise these clients. It is also noteworthy that a study by Meldman suggests that nurse psychotherapists in private practice can provide the same level of client satisfaction as provided by doctors.[11]

Nurses have sporadically gained permission to be psychotherapists and are a potential source of man-power in outpatient facilities.[12, 13] I believe that nurses can do individual, group, and family psychotherapy on an outpatient basis within the provisions of the present state laws. A brief description of my specific roles as an outpatient psychotherapist may serve to support this general statement.

Functions of an
Outpatient Nurse Therapist

I was formerly employed on the adolescent unit of a large, urban, psychiatric, teaching, and research hospital. When the staff revised the adolescent treatment program to form an adolescent outpatient service, I was able to transfer to this service as a collaborative member of an interdisciplinary team (psychiatrist, psychologist, social worker, students from varied disciplines). Two points were emphasized in justifying the creation of the nurse therapist position to the administration. First, the nurse can utilize a unique background in elementary medicine, physiology, and pharmacology, coupled with a strong foundation in humanities in collaborative relationships to increase services to clients. Second, it was established that minimum academic requirements would be baccalaureate nursing preparation or extensive clinical psychiatric and public health nursing experience. Continued education was considered vital.

The following functions evolved during the one and a half year's experience as a nurse therapist. Functions are described from most time-consuming to least time-consuming roles.

1. *Primary therapist in individual psychotherapy.* Both short-term crisis oriented therapy and long-term therapy were utilized. The caseload consisted primarily of adolescents from thirteen through eighteen years of age. The following case summary exemplifies one long-term therapeutic relationship and may serve to illustrate various nurse therapist functions:

Holly was a sixteen-year-old female referred to the outpatient service due to self-destructive behavior and poor self-image. Holly would injure her arms and legs when angry, so that her limbs were often immobilized by casts and bandages. She contracted for therapy sessions three times per week over a six-month period.

Focus of the sessions was to increase awareness and ownership of body parts in the following manner: Holly would choose a body part to look at, describe in detail, exercise, and/or touch during the session. She was encouraged to discuss her feelings and attitudes concerning this body part. As she became comfortable with this body part, she would sketch this onto an ongoing picture of herself. Holly worked hard to complete her "body image" picture. The amount of intentional and accidental bodily injury decreased consistently throughout Holly's therapy.

---

2. *Telephone screening interviewer.* Clients were screened via phone to establish initial rapport while supplying information concerning available services.

3. *Social history interviewer.* Each team member was responsible for one outpatient diagnostic intake weekly. This included the formulation of an overall treatment plan with the psychiatric staff. The therapist participating in the initial evaluation generally carried out the recommended therapy with the individuals and/or family.

4. *Family therapist.* Family therapy was primarily short-term therapy with both male and female therapists among all available family members.

5. *Group therapist for outpatients.* This involved the formation of a women's group for mothers with a history of multiple divorces. Holly's mother was invited, but refused to participate in the group. Focus included learning to give and receive support from other women in non-competitive interrelationships.

6. *Health educator.* Health education was employed during therapy with clients having specific diseases or health concerns, especially in areas relating to human sexuality (anatomy & physiology, venereal disease, unwanted pregnancy).

7. *Liaison between outpatient and other community facilities.* These included the Visiting Nurses Association, school systems, and residential homes when placement was the issue. At times, therapy sessions took place at a local medical hospital as one client had surgery and as another mended from an unsuccessful suicide attempt.

Therapy with Holly (refer to function No. 1) exemplifies the liaison function:

Holly initially developed many somatic complaints which decreased school attendance, as she began to explore her body image. Frequent communication with the school nurse resulted in supportive, but firm insistence that Holly remain in the school health clinic when ill, rather than abruptly return home. Later during therapy, Holly considered residential placement. Holly was accompanied on tours of two local facilities to discuss this possibility with residential staff.

---

8. *Administration of medication.* This traditional nursing task involved the least amount of time, where few clients received weekly phenothiazine injections. Other clients were supervised concerning prescribed oral medications in collaboration with the psychiatrist.

The above functions represent roles developed in one particular out-patient setting. Additional functions may also include assessment by home visits, involvement in community education programs, and partici-pation in suicide prevention and crisis intervention services.

Guidelines for
Implementation

Concrete guidelines in terms of supervision, support, and self-explora-tion are recommended for implementation by the nurse as outpatient psychotherapist. These guidelines appear essential in developing credi-bility to self and colleagues in settings which traditionally sanction only inpatient psychiatric nursing.

1. *Provision for Supervision.* Mellow identified the following functions of a supervisor in relation to the trainee: a teaching function for the transmission of learnable techniques and attitudes; a supportive function for difficulties inherent and/or imposed on the thera-peutic relationship; and an analytic function to increase the trainee's awareness of how he or she affects the therapeutic rela-tionship and outcome.[14] Two types of supervision are beneficial to enhance therapeutic expertise, intradisciplinary and interdisci-plinary.

Intradisciplinary supervision of some clients was arranged on a weekly basis with a clinical specialist in nursing, while interdisciplinary supervi-sion with other clients was obtained from a clinical psychologist and member of the adolescent outpatient team. Supervision utilized process recordings, use of videotape and tape recordings, didactic instruction, and referral to specific clinical readings. In general, neurotic behavior dy-namics became the focus of supervisory sessions with the psychologist, whereas psychotic behavior dynamics evolved as the emphasis of the clinical specialist in nursing. Arrangements for supervision from both male and female professionals from different disciplines prove most effec-tive in teaching, supporting, and analyzing therapist-client relationships.

2. *Provision for Support.* Two types of support are useful in establishing the position of nurse therapist, administrative support and colleague support. Administrative support was obtained by an initial formal proposal justifying the nurse therapist position cou-pled with strong support from the medical director of the adolescent service. Administrative support is essential if the posi-tion is to be permanently budgeted and maintained by financial resources.

Colleague team support was available as the role of nurse therapist evolved, with frequent informal discussions concerning therapeutic processes and techniques. Support from nursing peers was questionable. There was an alienation that evolved from developing alternative professional roles and interests. This is in keeping with Glover's observation that the nurse therapist may be considered an outsider in her own profession. In breaking barriers into allied disciplines, the nurse may lose identity with her own discipline.[15] One solution to this problem was the formation of a literature review club to explore pertinent psychiatric nursing issues and to provide peer support through literature exploration.

3. *Provision for Self-Exploration (self-growth).* Nurses may provide for continued personal growth by experiencing personal psychotherapy themselves, by creating or joining seminars of fellow therapists, and by participating in workshops and ongoing training seminars in various therapies, such as Gestalt, Transactional Analysis, and Bioenergetics. An exposure to various therapies, techniques, and therapists broadens perspective, adding depth and creativity in psychotherapeutic work.

In addition to these major guidelines, further recommendations may prove beneficial:

1. Nurses interested in developing as psychotherapists need to seek out appropriate intradisciplinary and interdisciplinary role models to facilitate professional growth.

2. Nurses interested in developing as psychotherapists may form an assoication of nurse therapists to increase peer support, and to exchange knowledge in psychotherapeutices. This group may also serve as spokesman in establishing credibility of the nurse therapist to other disciplines.

3. Nurses interested in developing as psychotherapists may read, explore, and react to contemporary female/male issues, since sexual stereotyping is inherent in the nursing role, especially in any therapeutic relationship.

In summary, although nursing therapy has predominantly reflected treatment within inpatient settings, specific functions of an outpatient nurse therapist have been identified. Concrete guidelines in terms of supervision, support, and self-exploration were delineated for implementation of the nurse as outpatient therapist. It is felt that nurses can establish credibility and further develop innovative psychiatric nursing practice in outpatient services.

Bibliography

1. **Mellow, June:** *Professional Identity?* A paper presented at the American Nurses Association Regional Clinical Conferences at Atlanta, Georgia, Nov. 5, 1969 and Minneapolis, Minnesota, Nov. 17, 1969.

2. *Ibid.*

3. **Stern Melvin,** et al.: Training nurses to be therapists on a psychiatric inpatient service. *Hospital and Community Psychiatry* 23:7 (July) 1972.

4. **Gedan, Sharon,** et al.: The nurse-therapist: A staff nurse position which emphasizes clinical practice. *Journal of Psychiatric Nursing and Mental Health Services* 11:1 (Jan.-Feb.) 1973.

5. **Graff, Harold,** et al.: Nurses as multiple therapists. *Journal of Psychiatric Nursing & Mental Health Services* 11:1 (Jan.-Feb.) 1973.

6. **Tool, Ben and Boyts, Harold:** The nurse-therapist. *Hospital and Community Psychiatry* 23:7 (July) 1972.

7. **Hyde, Maida:** Psychotherapy as mothering. *Perspectives in Psychiatric Care* VII; 2 (March-April) 1970.

8. **Reres, Mary:** A survey of the nurses' role in psychiatric out-patient clinics of America. *Community Mental Health Journal* 5:5, 1969.

9. **Hatchinson, Sally:** The psychiatric nurse therapist in private practice. *Journal of Psychiatric Nursing and Mental Health Services* 10:4 (July-August) 1972.

10. **Meldman, M.J.,** et al.: Nurse psychotherapist in a private practice. *American Journal of Nursing* 69:11 (Nov.) 1969.

11. **Meldman, M.J.,** et al.: Patient responses to nurse-psychotherapists. *American Journal of Nursing* 71:6 (June) 1971.

12. **Glover, B. H.:** A new nurse therapist. *American Journal of Nursing* 67:5 (May) 1967.

13. **Graziano, Anthony:** Mental health, psychotherapy, and the new psychotherapist. *Journal of Psychiatric Nursing and Mental Health Services* 7:2 (March-April) 1969.

14. **Mellow, June:** Nursing therapy. *American Journal of Nursing* 68:11 (November) 1968.

15. **Glover B.H.:** A new nurse therapist. *American Journal of Nursing* 67:5 (May) 1967.

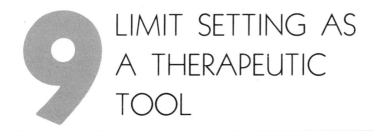

LIMIT SETTING AS A THERAPEUTIC TOOL

Glee Gamble Lyon,

B.S., M.N., R.N.

THE SETTING IS A DAY ROOM OF A state mental hospital. A cute, young, dark-haired student nurse is sitting talking with a tall, slender, nineteen-year old boy with hippie style hair and long sideburns.

PATIENT: I'm uncomfortable. I think I'll take my clothes off.

STUDENT NURSE: How will that make you comfortable, John?

PATIENT: I'll feel free. I can talk better when I feel free.

STUDENT NURSE: I don't understand. How does taking your clothes off make you feel free to talk?

PATIENT: I don't know—I guess it's my hang-up.

STUDENT NURSE: John, what do think will happen if you take off your clothes?

PATIENT: They always put me in the short hall.

STUDENT NURSE: Do you think you'll feel free to talk in there?

(The patient does not answer, but walks off. The student nurse remains seated in the day room. Shortly the patient returns with no clothes on.)

PATIENT: There, now I can talk. Am I embarrassing you?

STUDENT NURSE: Yes, you are. I'm afraid I don't understand how this helps you to talk.

Reproduced, with permission, from *Journal of Psychiatric Nursing and Mental Health Services*, November-December, 1970.

(At this point an attendent intervenes and puts John in his own room in short hall. The student nurse returns a little later—the patient is in his room with his clothes still off.)

STUDENT NURSE: John I'm leaving now, and I won't be back until Monday, but I'd like to talk with you again.

PATIENT: OK

STUDENT NURSE:ᐧ   But I cannot talk to you unless you keep your clothes on, OK?

PATIENT: OK, that's fine.

This student, as many new people entering the field of mental health, was attempting to show her acceptance of the patient, as well as her very nonjudgmental attitude. The first two principles stressed were: *accept the patient as he is,* and *focus on the patient's feelings.* New personnel in a psychiatric setting often find what appears to be a very permissive atmosphere. However, this acceptance and permissiveness needs to be limited. *That the patient feels the way he does is accepted, that he has a right to feel that way is accepted, but limits are established beyond which acting out his feelings is not allowed.*

Often a patient "asks" for limits, or tests out his unclear understanding of what is expected and accepted behavior. In the above example John really wanted external help in controlling his behavior. The next week he was with the same student nurse:

PATIENT: I think I'll take my clothes off.

STUDENT NURSE: No, John, you'll have to leave your clothes on, or I can't stay and talk with you.

PATIENT: Oh, OK. (His anxiety decreases and he spends a half hour talking with the student nurse.)

Why there is a need for limits

The need for limits is closely related to the feelings of security and trust. Everyone has the basic need to feel secure, to have a sense of assurance and predictability about himself and his environment. When this feeling does not exist, much of his behavior is motivated by the need for security.

The feelings of security are learned. In the process of growing up, children try to find security by attempting to control and direct parental authority, and in so doing go through many periods of anxiety.[1] If the parents are themselves secure, able to respond to the child's behavior with consistency and predictability, and able to encourage the child to be independent in his behavior according to his capabilities and judgment, the child accepts the restrictions, and through this guidance learns to control his own behavior. Each time the child gains mastery over one more area of his life he receives not only parental approval, but (more importantly) the increased feelings of security and of self-worth in knowing that he can handle himself and his behavior in a growing number of situations.[2]

However, if the parents are constantly anxious and unpredictable, the child is faced with the impossible situation of trying to find security in a desperate struggle where the rules are constantly changing. The child reacts by giving up the struggle and spends the rest of his life acting out roles that he thinks will gain approval, while constantly carrying a burden of anxious, angry and frustrated feelings.[3]

The person who comes to the mental hospital is usually experiencing insecurity. He is often overwhelmed by the amount of anxiety with which he has to deal, overpowered to the point that he cannot function adequately in his daily living. In order to relieve the anxiety the patient does something; he often feels compelled to do something without understanding why he is doing it—it is his way of trying to deal with the lack of security, his attempt to gain mastery over himself and his environment. It is intended to relieve his anxiety, but often this acting out behavior brings further loss of control, loss of self esteem and more anxiety.

The hospital setting and the nurse-patient relationship must both offer the patient a structure that is secure, consistent and that communicates what is expected behavior. Within this structure, the patient may experience what he may not have had earlier, an atmosphere that will allow freedom to try out and learn new ways of behaving. Limit setting is one aspect of the nurse-patient relationship which helps the patient to reduce his anxiety, enabling him to reestablish himself and to function on a more acceptable level. This new level of functioning will bring new responses (approval instead of disapproval) from those around him. He can then use these different responses to change his concept of himself, to learn new behaviors, to manage his own life, and to experience success in areas in which he was not successful before.

Types of behavior needing limits

Limits are established for the broad categories of acting out behavior and manipulative behavior. *Acting out* is behavior in which the patient is responding to a present situation as if it were a past situation, seeking gratification of unconscious impulses or desires.[4] Acting out might include behavior which is potentially harmful to the patient or to others, and behavior which in a particular situation is socially unacceptable, such as nudity or sexual misconduct. *Manipulative behavior* is a process by which one person influences another to function according to his needs without regard for the other person's needs.[5] This behavior might include gift giving, flattery, or asking for special favors.

Definition and Purpose of limit setting

Limit setting is a process through which someone in authority determines temporary and artificial ego boundaries for another person. Determining for the patient the boundaries of acceptable behavior provides protection for the patient and others, provides security, decreases the patient's anxiety, and provides a reality contact between the person and his environment. The limit forms a framework within which the person is freer to function more adequately, to learn new behaviors, and is thus able to develop his self identity and to raise his self esteem.

Steps and Techniques in setting limits

IDENTIFY THE NEED FOR THE LIMIT   In any situation the need for limits must be considered within the context of the particular situation and patient. The nurse's use of rational authority in setting limits is based on her knowledge and understanding of the dynamics of the patient's behavior. The more capable the nurse is in understanding and interpreting the meaning of the patient's behavior, the more likely she will be able to establish both realistic and meaningful limits for the patient. For example, a nurse who interpreted a patient's slow, systematic way of getting dressed as a way of manipulating her, and preventing her from moving on to her other duties, tried to set limits on the patient's "unnecessary" and time-consuming actions, which resulted in an increase in the patient's anxiety. Another nurse, aware that this was the patient's compulsive ritual and his way to give structure and security to his environment, not only found no need to try to stop the behavior but was able to remain with the patient very patiently and to facilitate a relaxed atmosphere in which the patient could carry out his ritual and, therefore, reduce his anxiety.

In every situation the nurse needs to ask herself, "Why do limits need to be set? What is the patient trying to say with his behavior at this time? And what about this person's personality structure and resulting behavior makes it necessary to take over his ego function temporarily? And furthermore, does this limit lead to growth for the person?"[6]

In answering the above questions about the patient in relation to limit setting, the nurse must also ask and seek answers about herself. She needs to look at her own feelings about limits, about the particular patient and his behavior. She needs to ask herself, "Is the limit for my own comfort or is it because it meets some need of the patient? Is what's being done really limit setting or is it punishment?"[7]

Just as too hasty a judgment and setting of limits might be a serious misuse of rational authority, the nurse's failure to identify the need and to set limits can also deprive the patient of needed guidance and learning experiences. Sometimes in the process of building a relationship, the nurse is afraid that she will spoil a good relationship if she sets limits. She does not set limits for fear the patient will interpret the limit as her rejection of him, or she is afraid that the patient in return might reject her. Or the nurse may rationalize that the patient has suffered enough and she does not want to add any further hardship or hurt by setting limits on the patient's behavior. The nurse's own feelings and attitudes toward authority and limits need to be explored so that they do not interfere with her ability to evaluate the situation, recognize the need, and be able to establish effective limits.

COMMUNICATE EXPECTED BEHAVIOR   In many situations before a limit is definitely stated, the nurse communicates expected behavior in the particular situation to the patient, which gives the patient a structure within which he can operate. This might be done through a nonverbal motion such as indicating "no" with a shake of the head, or the nurse's motioning for the patient to leave a room. In effect, in communicating expected behavior the nurse forewarns the patient that a limit will be set if the expected behavior is not followed. For example, "It is time for you to take your medicine," or "Make your bed," or "This is a time for you to talk about yourself," communicate to the patient what is expected of him at a given time.

STATE THE LIMIT   After the need for the limits has been identified and, if indicating the expected behavior did not precipitate the necessary behavior, the nurse needs to inform the patient exactly what the limit is. The limit is stated clearly as a statement of fact and is not presented as advice, bribery, or punishment. It tells the patient specifically what he is to do, or specifically what he must not do in the situation.

When stating what is unacceptable behavior and putting a limit on it, the nurse needs to also offer a substitute—a behavior that is acceptable. For example, a patient who was continuously asking a student about her personal life was told: "We are not to talk about me and my life outside the hospital. We can talk about what you did today . . . tell me what you did in the OT metal shop." Or, after stating the limit, the nurse can offer the patient a choice of alternative behaviors. "You cannot hit Mr. W. You can tell me how you feel about Mr. W., or you can go run in the gym."

The best limit is total, not partial, so that the boundaries are very clear. A patient was banging a board loudly on the table. The staff member said, "You are not to make so much noise; you can bang a little but don't make too much noise." The patient was left without any clear criterion with which to judge the boundaries so he continued to bang, becoming increasingly louder until he found out what was meant by "too much noise."

The limit should be stated firmly with the nurse's conviction and belief in · the value of the limit reflected in her voice, which increases the patient's security in knowing the limit is meant and will be carried out. If she is not sure about the limit, or what to do in the situation, the nurse should not do anything until she has further thought through the situation and her own feelings. If the nurse is ambivalent toward the limit, her uncertainty might challenge the patient to argue against the limit, or to test it.

There is some disagreement about whether to warn the patient of the consequences, or of what he can expect if the limit is tested or if he continues the inappropriate behavior. Often the statements of consequences act as threats—or invitations—to repeat the behavior, as: "If you do it once more. . ." , the patient tends to not hear the "if you" and hears only "do it once more" and sometimes interprets it as "she expects me to do it once more." The warning of the consequences can serve as a challenge and "to do it once more" to retain his self esteem and show himself as not a weakling, or someone who is afraid.[8]

In other situations, the explanation of consequences is of therapeutic value, for it presents the patient with responsibility for the effects or results of his behavior. Within the limit-setting situation the patient is encouraged to look at his own behavior and the resulting consequences, and to then make a choice or decision about his behavior. For example, a patient was told "you are expected to go to school each day; if you don't you will be restricted from the next hospital extracurricular activity." In understanding the expected behavior and the resulting effect, the patient was given the opportunity to govern his own behavior, to learn how to postpone immediate pleasure for future gratification, and thus to act more responsibly.

HELP THE PATIENT UNDERSTAND THE REASON FOR THE LIMIT   To increase the therapeutic and learning value of the situation the person needs to understand the limit. The nurse tells the patient as clearly, simply, and concretely as possible the reason for the limit. The amount of explanation varies according to the situation and to the patient's need and ability to understand. For example, a patient who refused her medicine and was to receive an injection was told: "The Doctor ordered this medicine, he thinks it will help you feel better." Even if the person is unable to accept the limit at first, he will be less likely to misinterpret the nurse's motives if a brief explanation is given.

ENFORCE THE LIMIT   To be effective, the limit must be one that can be realistically enforced or put into effect if the patient tests it. If there is no way to enforce the limit, then there is no point in setting the limit in the first place. A patient was told that she was to clean her room. After several attempts to make the patient clean her room, including locking her in her room with the needed supplies, the patient was told if she did not clean her room she would not eat. By this time the patient had accepted the challenge and remained more stubborn than the staff until the staff, unable to enforce the limit beyond several missed meals, allowed the patient to eat without the room being cleaned. The limit and the consequences of not following it were not enforceable; thus the limit was useless.

To be effective the limit must be realistic and reasonable; in addition, the consequences should be related to the limit. In the last example, an effective limit would be: "You are to clean your room. Until it is clean, you are restricted to your room." This limit is not only enforceable, but it presents the patient with a choice, to clean her room and be able to join in the other ward activities, or to not clean her room and suffer the consequences of wallowing in the messiness of her room, deprived of any activities going on outside of her room.

Limit setting has a cause and effect relationship; if the limit is not followed then another action will be initiated by the staff member. For example: A patient was told to get off the top of a table; when he did not, the limit was enforced by the necessary staff members physically removing him from the top of the table. When it is necessary to enforce the limit, it is done quickly and with a sense of conviction and sureness on part of staff. If the patient has exceeded the limit or not followed the restriction, this is not the time to be drawn into long discussions of the fairness of the limit—or even to give further explanation. When a patient exceeds a limit, it causes him anxiety; if the nurse talks too much or is hesitant to act to enforce the limit, it conveys to the patient some uncertainty and weakness at a time when he needs most to know that his environment will provide security and that he can lean on the others for support and strength.

HELP THE PATIENT VERBALIZE HIS FEELINGS ABOUT THE LIMIT   To prevent the patient from accepting limits docilely and without questioning, as though he had nothing to say and no control over what is happening to him, the nurse or staff member needs to help the person express his feelings about the limit. When the staff member encourages the patient to say what he feels, acceptance is conveyed to the person. This also helps to involve the person more in the total limit-setting process, helping the patient to better evaluate reality and to judge rational controls. If the patient is unable to express how he feels about the restriction, the staff member can verbalize to the patient what she believes he is feeling as, "I wonder if you were angry with me this morning when I told you not to leave the ward."

Often it is not appropriate to help the patient to verbalize feelings right at the time that the limit is being set. However, after the limit has been enforced and the patient is less anxious, the patient should be given the opportunity to better understand the limit and to verbalize feelings. This might be within an hour, or maybe not even until the next day; however, the important thing is that the nurse does approach the patient to discuss the total limit setting situation, giving him the opportunity to integrate it into his total life experiences.

EVALUATE THE LIMIT   Effective limits should make the patient more secure, for he knows what others expect of him, what behaviors he can and cannot do, and what others will do in relation to him. The setting of a limit often communicates that the nurse does care and is interested, that she will stop a behavior which would later make the patient feel ashamed or embarrassed. For example, when a patient entered the day room hall exposed, the nurse told her to button her blouse. The patient would not, and the nurse did it for the patient although the latter vehemently protested. The next day the patient apologized for her behavior and thanked the nurse. As in this situation, although a limit is needed, it does not mean the patient will readily accept the restriction.

The patient's initial behavioral response cannot always be used to evaluate the effectiveness of a limit. The patient may need to question rational authorities' interest and conviction in himself and in the limit by testing it to see if the staff person really means what he says and can be relied upon to follow through and actually supply the boundaries indicated by the limit. The patient needs to know that he can count on the boundaries, and his continued—or even increased—acting-out behavior is calculated to test the boundary for its strength and reliability before accepting rational controls. If the patient interprets a limit as someone in authority trying to control him, and to leave him powerless, his behavior will also probably be in the direction opposite that of the limit. He might resort to even greater acting out or regressive behavior in an attempt to decrease the overwhelming feeling of powerlessness and anxiety. Knowing a patient's previous experience with authority figures and limits often helps in understanding the patient's behavior. However, in many situations it is difficult to evaluate whether the limit itself is not approrpiate or whether the behavior is just the initial reaction to the new experience of rational control. If the limit is reevaluated and then continued with consistency, the patient's behavior over a longer period of time should serve as a measurement of the effectiveness of the limit.

The evaluation of the limit needs to be continuous; limits are not established for an indefinite period of time. As the limit is gradually internalized and used by the patient in the management of his own behavior, staff must relinquish their own external controls and return the responsibility for control to the patient.

These then are the basic steps involved in setting limits. Because each patient in each situation is different, limit setting needs to be flexible within this basic framework. Each limit-setting situation will vary in terms of how many of these actual steps are necessary and the order and emphasis placed on each step. In addition to using the principles and techniques already indicated in each step, one aspect that must prevail over the total limit setting situation is consistency.

CONSISTENCY   Consistency is necessary in order for the limit-setting process to be effective. This consistency must be present in the individual authority figure. When a staff member states the limit, she must then be consistent in her attitude and actions, communicating the same thing nonverbally that her works are communicating. She must be consistent over a period of time. If she has put a limit on a particular behavior, she must enforce it each time; not overlook it because she is tired, or because it is easier than causing a "scene" when there are visitors on the ward.

There must also be consistency among all the staff members who have contact with the person. It is necessary for the staff to both understand and accept the particular limit. If there is not consistency on the part of all the staff members, the patient will usually respond with increased anxiety and behavior which is more "out of control." A ward setting where inconsistency thrives can easily result in the patient playing one part of the staff against the other with a breakdown in staff working relationships and the patient's growing distrust of the staff's ability to use rational authority to help him control his behavior.

Two examples of limit setting

The types of situations within a nurse-patient relationship requiring limit setting are innumerable. However, two types of situations which seem to be particularly difficult are those in which the patient tries to deal with his feelings about the nurse and their relationship through inappropriate behavior which has a sexual connotation or through a gift-giving behavior.

Within a nurse-patient relationship, the patient often has difficulty expressing his feelings for the nurse, and his attempt to communicate positive feelings often results in inappropriate behavior. This is particularly true in a situation where a nurse works with a patient of the opposite sex.

PATIENT: Is it OK I sit here? I mean I wouldn't want to take you away from Gary (another patient). I mean, after all, he loves you, and I love you too, but you're too good to love. I mean I love you like a nurse.

(The patient is talking very fast and moving his hand over the nurse's hand, which is in her lap.)

STUDENT NURSE: (Picking up his hand and moving it away.) Eric, I don't want you to hold my hand. It makes me uncomfortable to have people touch me—and this is not the behavior a nurse and patient should show.

PATIENT: (Pause; then he touches the student nurse's knee)

STUDENT NURSE: I told you I don't want to be touched.

PATIENT: (Pulls hand back very fast) Oh, that's right—you're too good to be touched. I wouldn't want to touch you. I'm sorry. I won't touch you again, but that doesn't mean I can't look at you. (The patient becomes increasingly restless and very shortly gets up and leaves.)

In this situation, although the nurse set a limit on the patient's behavior and the behavior stopped, the patient's anxiety did not decrease and he had to leave the situation.

A patient's behavior, in this case putting his hands on the student nurse, in other situations trying to kiss the nurse, is his way of communicating his caring for and liking the person who is working with him. Although the behavior is not appropriate, only to limit the behavior blocks the patient's attempt to communicate his feelings—and leaves his anxiety increasing with no outlet. The nurse must assume, if he knew a healthier way to express his feelings, he would have used it. So in addition to limiting the inappropriate behavior, she needs to either help him communicate verbally or to seek validation of her understanding of what he is trying to communicate. She also needs to tell what is appropriate behavior. For example:

NURSE: You can't hold me or kiss me, but I think you want to show me you care; I'm glad you like me, but I wish you would tell me—how you feel.

The nurse accepts the patient's positive feelings toward her, but not his mode of communicating; and helps him learn a healthier way to deal with his feelings.

Gift giving is another behavior through which a patient may try to communicate; it may be to show appreciation, to seek closeness, to gain favor, to attempt to manipulate the relationship of that of a friend or servant, or to bribe for some future favor. By accepting the gift, the nurse communicates that she understands the meaning of the patient's gift giving and that there is no need for the patient to verbalize the meaning. In this way she may be approving and reinforcing a patient's problematic or pathological behavior.[9] Sometimes the nurse accepts the gift to meet her own needs to be liked or appreciated.

Gift giving requires limit setting; yet, if the nurse rejects the gift, the patient and the nurse often feel that the patient himself is being rejected. The nurse's intervention must reject the gift and set limits on that form of communicating while accepting the patient and providing a more healthy way to communicate feelings.

PATIENT: (Handing the nurse a bottle of hand lotion) Here, I have something for you.

NURSE: Oh, Mrs. P, I can't accept this but I'd like to sit here and talk with you.

Although she rejected the gift, she did not reject the patient but stayed to talk over the situation with the patient. After they were seated, Mrs. P. put away the hand lotion and brought out a tube of lipstick.

PATIENT: Here—you'd like this better anyway.

NURSE: No, Mrs. P, but you seem to want to give me something.

PATIENT: Yes—you're a nice girl—here.
(Looking in her purse)

NURSE: I wonder how you feel when I say I don't want you to give me anything.

PATIENT: I guess you don't want my gifts. (Looking very rejected, returns to looking in her purse)

NURSE: No, I don't want to accept your gifts and I won't be giving you any gifts—but we both can share lots of things—our feelings and ideas when we spend time and talk.

PATIENT: I guess I'd like that. (smiling, closes purse)

After the nurse indicated another way of accepting and sharing with the patient-spending time and talking-and put limits on gift giving in their relationship, only once more did she attempt to give; this time to share food. However, the gift giving did continue between this patient and other people. In many of these situations the nurse had an opportunity to help the patient look at her behavior, express her feelings, and explore the desire ("I want other people to like me and to do things for me") behind the behavior. The patient and nurse were then able to do some problem-solving and help the patient to learn some new ways to meet her need for acceptance.

In any limit-setting situation, controlling inappropriate behavior is only one of the goals and only the beginning of the therapeutic value. The very process involved in setting limits provides many opportunities for the nurse to help the patient meet his other basic needs—the need for physical safety, for security, for acceptance, for self esteem; and to develop the abilities to assess, to evaluate, and to problem solve, as well as the ability to change. Once the patient gains control over his behavior he is able to make use of other therapeutic processes that can further influence his path toward growth and health.

References

1. Holmes, Marguerite J., and Werner, Jean A., *Psychiatric Nursing in a Therapeutic Community* (New York: The Macmillan Company, 1966), p. 44.
2. Borel, Jack C., "Security as a Motivation of Human Behavior," *Archives of General Psychiatry* 10:107, February, 1964.
3. Borel, pp. 106–107.
4. Edwin, Lawrence Abt., and Weissman, Stuart L. (editors), *Acting Out, Theoretical and Clinical Aspects,* (New York: Grune and Stratton, Inc., 1965), pp. 3, 40–41.

5. Kumler, Fern R., "An Interpersonal Interpretation of Manipulation," *Some Clinical Approaches to Psychiatric Nursing;* Burd. Shirley and Marshall, Margaret A. (editors) (New York: The Macmillan Company, 1963), p. 116.
6. Holmes, p. 51.
7. Holmes, p. 50.
8. Ginott Haim G., *Between Parent and Child,* (New York: The Macmillan Company, 1965), p. 53.
9. Clark, Janice, "The Patient's Gift," *Some Clinical Approaches to Psychiatric Nursing,* Burd, Shirley and Marshall, Margaret A. (editors) pp. 91–92.

Bibliography

Cohen, Raquel and Grinspoon, Lester, "Limit Setting as a Corrective Ego Experience," *Archives of General Psychiatry,* 8:74-79, January, 1963.

Wolf, Nancy Anderson, "Setting Reasonable Limits on Behavior," *The American Journal of Nursing,* 62:104-106, March, 1962.

10 COMMUNICATION THROUGH ROLE PLAYING

Patricia R. Underwood

M.A., R.N.

TAKE A NURSE WHO GREW UP IN THE little New England town in which her family lived for generations. Put her to work in a big-city hospital in the Middle West. Give her a patient from the Southwest, of immigrant parentage. That nurse is likely to run into communication barriers that make providing adequate care more than a little difficult. But role playing can serve her well in breaking down those barriers.

Role playing might best be defined as a learning experience in which the nurse and the patient act out a situation, either past or expected, as if it were really happening. They might act out a discussion the patient has already had with a family member or a job interview the patient is anticipating. The situation to be acted out depends on the needs of the patient. I found it valuable in working with Mary.

Mary was a 20-year-old, unskilled factory worker with nine years of education, a history of immature acting-out behavior, and limited communication with her family. She had immigrated to the United States 11 years ago.

I saw Mary shortly after her admission to a residential home for unwed mothers, angry, frightened, unable to adjust to the residential center. After several meetings with her, I found she thought there was something wrong with her or her unborn baby. Our discussion revealed an underlying fear of doctors and nurses based on a few unhappy encounters. She was unable to ask questions of the doctor or nurse and left each antepartal examination frightened and certain she was ill. To help her overcome her fears, I tried role playing.

MARY: *I have an itch down here.* (She indicated the pubic area).

NURSE: *That is something the doctor should know.*

MARY: *You know I can't tell him.*

NURSE: *Let's try. I'll be the doctor and you be you. O.K., tell me.*

MARY: *I have an itch down here.* (She laughs and blushes.) *That sounds funny. What do you call this?*

NURSE: *It's the pubic area.*

MARY: *I have an itch in—on—which is it?* (laughs)

NURSE: *Try "around."*

MARY: *I have an itch around the pubic area.*

DOCTOR: (as played by the nurse): *How long have you had it?*

MARY (relaxing): *About two weeks.*

DOCTOR: *Can you show me exactly where it is?*

MARY: *Right here.*

NURSE: *Good, that's it. You'll be able to talk to the doctor and tell him how you feel.*

MARY: *Hey, it's not too hard once you know what to say.*

Mary had numerous other questions about her pregnancy that had been on her mind for weeks, questions that could easily have been answered by the nurse. But role playing with less complicated questions helped her to learn to express herself more directly. Over the weeks we worked on more difficult areas until she was able to talk to the doctor with ease. Her sense of well-being increased as her self-confidence increased, and this encouraged her to try talking more directly not only with me and the physician, but also with other staff members and with patients in the residence.

Mary had difficulty in communicating with her family and rarely disagreed or openly resisted decisions they made. She simply did not comply with decisions she did not like. That usually got her into trouble. Although she did not really want to relinquish her child, Mary agreed with her family's decision that she should. She said her family made her depressed. Believing they did not understand her, she felt angry and resentful toward her family. However, she did not recognize the anger she felt. Again role playing helped.

MARY: *I wish they would quit asking about what I'm going to do and then saying what I have to do.*

NURSE: *That must make you angry.*

MARY: *No! I just feel low.*

NURSE: *What do you do when they start telling you?*

MARY: *Nothing, just listen.*

NURSE: *What would you like to do?*

MARY: *I don't know.*

NURSE: *Let's role play. I'll be your brother Joe and you be you.* (I had seen the brother once, and Mary had talked about him quite often. Even if the nurse doesn't know the person she is playing, the situation will build as one gets into it.)

JOE: *Well, Mary, what have you decided? Have you seen the adoption lady? You should begin to plan.*

MARY: *Just shut up! I don't want to plan anything. I don't know what to do.*

JOE: *Why are you yelling at me? I asked you a simple question.*

MARY: *Nag, nag, nag. That's all you ever do. I hate you and I'm tired of it all.* (The patient looked at me bewildered.) *What did I say?*

NURSE: *You seemed to be saying what you felt. You're pretty upset with your brother who is pushing you.*

MARY: *But I don't hate him. He has been good to me.*

NURSE: *It's all right to be angry. You can love and hate at the same time.*

MARY: *I shouldn't have said that.*

NURSE: *It was the way you were feeling.*

MARY: *But that would just make him mad at me.*

NURSE: *What might you say that would get the point across without making him angry? I'll be Joe again.*

JOE: *Well, what are you going to do? You should be thinking about what to do with the baby.*

MARY: (looking straight at me, speaking with a calm, confident voice): *I don't know. I haven't decided. When I do, I will tell you.*

JOE: *O.K., Mary. As long as you're thinking about it.*

NURSE: *That's it. There is nothing left to say. Now you be your brother, and I'll be you, Mary.*

We exchanged roles and repeated that conversation. Mary had the same feeling I had had: She had made a final statement that left no room for further questioning. Mary then used this approach with her brother. He responded by telling her to let him know what she decided. He did not question her further. Shortly thereafter, Mary was able to begin to work on her feelings about the child she was expecting and to decide what she was going to do.

Mary's sister planned a large church wedding the month following Mary's due delivery date. Mary wanted very much to be in the wedding; however, her family felt she would not be well enough. Although Mary knew otherwise because of her antepartal classes, she did not assert herself, but went along with the family's decision. She was hurt and felt the family did not want her. She said she really didn't care about the wedding, but as the date drew near and plans were being made, she finally admitted that she cared very much but didn't know how to tell her sister. Role playing helped her decide how to express herself after she had decided what needed to be said. I played Mary while she played her sister, Lynn.

MARY: *(as played by the nurse): Lynn, I have been thinking, and I really want to be in the wedding.*

LYNN: *But you won't be well enough.*

MARY: *Yes, I will. The baby is due a month before the wedding, and I know from my classes that I will be fine in about two weeks.*

LYNN: *How will we ever get a dress for you? When will you be able to be fitted?*

MARY: *I get discharged four days after the baby is born, and I can go then.*

LYNN: *How will I know what kind of dress to get?*

MARY: *Well, it is your wedding, and you know what you want. You and mother know what I like. I really just want to be in the wedding.*

LYNN: *What will we say to the relatives if you don't get there? If the baby is late?*

MARY: *I can have the flu, or something.*

That sounds like a question and answer session, but it allowed Mary, by playing her sister, to ask a lot of questions about what she herself was thinking that she had been unable to ask before. We then discussed the questions and answers until she felt she could answer anything her sister might ask. She left the session feeling that she could talk to her sister and that she could also take part in the wedding.

The actual encounter with her sister was much easier than she had anticipated. Lynn agreed immediately and was very pleased that Mary had asked to be in her wedding; she had believed Mary was not interested. Thus, when some of her fears had been acted out in role playing, Mary was able to discuss the matter and discover that her sister wanted her in the wedding as much as she wanted to take part.

As the delivery date approached, Mary began to think about being discharged from the residential center and returning home and to work. We used role playing to clarify her feelings regarding what to say if she met someone who was a patient with her in the residence; what to say if Aunt Sally remarked that she was fat; how to tell her mother that she wanted to use contraceptives, and how to ask the doctor for contraceptives; how to obtain information about enrolling in a school of beauty culture rather than returning to the factory to work.

When the baby was about seven days overdue, Mary began to feel helpless and depressed. She cried, was despondent and unable to talk about her feelings. Her anger seemed to be directed toward the baby and herself. She berated the unborn child and would then feel guilty and still more depressed. I tried a different version of role playing.

MARY: (looking at her abdomen): *You stupid thing. Why don't you come out? I hate you. You are seven days late, and you just sit there.*

NURSE: *If the baby could talk to you, what would he say?*

MARY: (after some hesitation, surprised at the question, responding in an angry voice): *It's not my fault. I didn't put me here; you did. I don't know why you yell at me. I'd like to get out too.*

NURSE: *The baby seems angry too.*

MARY: *Why shouldn't he be. He's right! I put him there. It's all my fault. God is punishing me.*

That allowed the whole area of punishment to surface, and Mary could talk about fears previously expressed only in tears and berating of the baby. She could recognize that the anger she felt was actually toward herself rather than the child. She was able to verbalize rather than internalize her anger.

The foregoing are only a few examples of how effective role playing can be. It allowed me to utilize rather than overlook basic differences—in this instance socioeconomic differences. I could work at the educational level of the patient without embarrassing her. On the other hand, Mary got immediate satisfaction, quick results. Role playing added action to the interview sessions, and Mary felt she was getting something done, not "just talking." And it opened areas that might otherwise have remained closed to both the nurse and the patient.

As with any other interpersonal technique, role playing is not appropriate for every situation. It can, however, be a very simple and effective tool for improving communications, understanding, and treatment.

Bibliography

Corsini, R. J., and Cardone, Samuel. *Role Playing in Psychotherapy: a Manuel.* Chicago, Ill. Adline Publishing Co., 1966.

Edwards, G. Role-playing theory vs. clinical psychiatry. *Int.J.Psychiat.* 3:203-205, Mar. 1967.

Gould, R.E.Dr. Strangeclass: or how I stopped worrying· about the theory and began treating the blue-collar worker. *Amer.J.Orthopsychiat.* 37:78-86. Jan. 1967.

Hersch. C. Mental-health services and the poor. *Psychiatry* 29:236-245, Aug. 1966.

Riessman, Frank. Role-playing and the lower socio-economic group. *Group Psychother.* 17(1):36-48. 1964.

———. and others. *Mental Health of the Poor.* New York. The Free Press of Glencoe, 1964.

Suchman, E. A. Social patterns of illness and medical care. *J. Health Hum. Behav.* 6:2-16. Spring 1965.

11 "WHERE DID YOU GROW UP?"

Lois Davitz, Ph.D., R.N.

LUIS RODRIGUEZ APPEARED REGULARLY FOR HIS SCHEDULED APPOINTMENTS at the store-front community mental health clinic. Although he came on time, he resisted the therapist's attempts to discuss his problems. He sat slumped in a chair during the whole forty-five minute sessions. Long hair fell to his shoulders, and his eyes remained partially closed as he concentrated on playing an elaborately decorated guitar.

At the close of the fourth session, Miss Lawson, a psychiatric nurse, pointedly asked him why he bothered to come if he didn't want to talk about his problems. Mr. Rodriguez responded by playing a number of chords and then replied, "Why the hell do we do anything in life?"

"We do things for different reasons. I assume you came here because you wanted help."

"Are you serious?"

"Yes, I am serious."

"Kid, you have lots to learn. Time, what's time? Talk, what's talk? What the hell does talking get you in life?"

"Through talking we can resolve problems, or at least try to."

"Where did you grow up?"

"In the city, Mr. Rodriguez."

"Baby, so did I." Mr. Rodriguez leaned over and patted Miss Lawson on the knee. "But, baby, I got a feeling that you and me sat on different front stoops."

"May I ask why you are coming?"

"You mean you don't know? The police, baby. The police. This is going to help me, they said. I need therapy. I need to get adjusted. I need to find myself. Twenty-nine, and I got to find myself. Baby, there are times

Reprinted from Lois Jean Davitz, *The Psychiatric Patient: Case Histories*, pp. 135–154. Copyright ©1971 by Springer Publishing Company, Inc., New York. Used by permission.

when I know who I am. There are times when I know exactly what it means to be Luis Rodriguez. Those times are in my mind, baby. You don't forget those times."

"Why don't you tell me about them."

Mr. Rodriguez stopped playing his guitar and laughed.

"You're serious?" he said. "You really mean that?"

"Certainly, I mean that."

"You won't corner me. You think I want a second charge against me? I want to be free, baby, free.[1]

"I can't see how telling me about those times you truly felt yourself has anything to do with these charges you're talking about."

"She's for real," said Rodriguez, picking up his guitar and playing softly. "You're for real. You're really something. You know, you're kind of cute. I didn't know there were any like you around anymore. You're a cute kid. You get paid, don't you, whether I talk or not?"

"That isn't the point."

"What difference does it make if I sit here or some other slob?"

"The difference is, Mr. Rodriguez, that I'm here to help. I can't help you if you don't talk and won't cooperate."

"Get off it, kid."

"There's nothing to get off. You're trying to escape from talking. Your body is here, Mr. Rodriguez, but that is only part of you."

"Who says my mind isn't here? It's here all right. The mind goes along with the body. Remember? They go together."

"Why have you come."

"Didn't anyone tell you?"

"I'd like to hear it from you."

"The police."

"You mentioned the police, but I want to know why *you* want to come here."[2]

"I don't want to do anything, baby. I want to live free. You get the idea—free!"

"Yes."

---

[1] In a very real sense, Mr. Rodriguez is asking the therapist to participate in a deception: If he shows up for his therapy appointment, the police won't bother him. This places the therapist in an extraordinarily difficult position and, understandably, she is showing her impatience. However, at this point, rather than belabor the issue of his not talking, it might be more helpful to focus on the deception itself.

[2] The therapist assumes the patient has come because of emotional distress or because he wants relief from some symptons, and she thus expects him to discuss psychological problems. The patient, however, views the situation quite differently, and the difference in their expectations blocks communication.

"Yes what?"

"Go on."

"I've been talking, baby. You're the one who isn't listening."

"I am listening."

"Listen, I'm talking." Mr. Rodriguez smiled. His hands moved quickly over the strings. "You listening? You hear now, don't you?"

"I'm afraid, Mr. Rodriguez, that there is a difference between talking and telling me how you feel and playing the guitar."

"You're for real," said Mr. Rodriguez, leaning his head back against the wall. "You're real, kid. Real." His beaded headband slipped over his forehead and covered his eyes. "I'm talking. You get the message? I am talking loud and clear. Listen. Is it coming through, baby?"[3]

The clinic consisted of a large store with the interior sectioned into cubicles for therapists to see patients. Plasterboard partitions gave the illusion of privacy. The central area of the store contained a row of folding chairs for patients and families, several desks, filing cabinets, and bookshelves.

Patients waiting to be seen sat quietly. An infant whimpered; an older child dragged a toy car along the wall, admiring the scratches made by the metal wheels; a policeman held an adolescent by the wrist; therapists spoke to new patients; a secretary and two volunteer assistants answered telephones.

The area surrounding the clinic was heavily populated with tenements, stores, new buildings, and decaying structures scheduled for demolition. A music store next to the clinic had rigged up a street amplifying system and popular tunes blared to a background accompaniment of automobile horns, fire engine, police, and ambulance sirens. Within the clinic, Mr. Rodriguez played his own melodies, occasionally swinging his head to toss his long hair away from his eyes.

Mr. Rodriguez had been referred to the clinic by a member of the local Narcotics Squad. He had been charged with possession of drugs but the charges were dismissed for lack of evidence. Luis Rodriguez was encouraged to get psychiatric help, so he had voluntarily applied to the clinic and had been assigned to Miss Lawson.[4]

Twenty-three years of age, Miss Lawson, a graduate of a diploma school of nursing, had completed her baccalaureate degree and was currently enrolled in a graduate program leading to a master's degree in psy-

---

[3]But of course all of us express our feelings in many ways other than talking.

[4]The word "voluntary" obviously must be interpreted carefully. From the patient's point of view, he probably had little choice in the matter.

chiatric nursing. As part of her clinical field experience, she worked one day a week at the store-front clinic. Mr. Rodriguez was one of three patients in her case load.

"I'm a gutter kid growing old. Who are you?" Mr. Rodriguez asked her at the next meeting.

"I'm a nurse, Mr. Rodriguez, a psychiatric nurse."

"Ever been a gutter kid?"

"Why do you ask?"

"For the simple reason that what the hell do you know what it is like?[5]

"Know exactly what?"

"This is a bloody bore," replied Mr. Rodriguez, leaning over and playing his guitar. He refused to speak for the rest of the period.

Miss Lawson was admittedly surprised when he showed up for the next meeting at the exact time scheduled. She had discussed his reluctance to communicate with her supervisor. It was felt that Miss Lawson should not try to compel Mr. Rodriguez to open up, but listen to his guitar playing and perhaps try to lead into his problems through a discussion of his music.

"Perhaps you'd like to tell me something about your guitar playing?" Miss Lawson asked him at the opening of the next session.

"What do you want to know?"

"Anything you'd like to tell me."

"Is this part of your act?"

"There isn't any act."

"Come on off it," he told her. "You want me to put the guitar down and open up. I wasn't born yesterday. I've been around—a helluva lot more than you have. Remember?"

"Remember what, Mr. Rodriguez?"

He put down his guitar, slipping the strap off his shoulder. Leaning over the desk, he asked, "What do you want to know? Tell me, baby. You want my life history in forty-five minutes? It's a long story—a long continued story—kind of like a TV serial. Sometimes the strip goes frontwards with me. Now, baby, it's going backwards, up and down. See," he clapped his hands. "Interference, shadows, blocks. That's the

---

[5]Perhaps this is also part of the patient's resistance to therapy, yet there may be a good deal of validity in his question. Surely a therapist doesn't have to live through all of a patient's experiences in order to empathically understand him. But social and cultural differences between people can indeed make communication and mutual understanding exceedingly difficult. As a first step in resolving such difficulties, it is important to understand the possible differences and appreciate their significance rather than make believe that they don't count.

static in the air. No antenna up. You got to turn me on before I talk. You got to find me, baby. Like the poet said," Mr. Rodriguez recited, *"Deja tu mundo, y sueña conmigo."* [6]

"Would you care to translate that for me?"

"It doesn't translate too well," said Mr. Rodriguez, picking up his guitar and beginning to play again.

"That's a very lovely song you're playing, Mr. Rodriguez. Do you write your own music?"

"You like it?"

"Yes, very much. I believe you have real talent."

"Thanks," said Mr. Rodriguez sarcastically.

"I really meant what I said. Have you considered studying music?"

"Damn it," he shouted, "You don't need teachers. It comes from inside. Did you know that? Did you know that you don't have to go to school for everything? I suppose not. You're not the type. You're the kind who goes to school for sex. Let yourself go, Miss Lawson. Relax kid, relax. You're uptight. You're sitting there frozen. Afraid?"

He reached out and took her hand. "What are you afraid of? Don't pull back. Easy now, easy."

Miss Lawson attempted to free her hand.

"Don't you like that?"

"Let go of my hand, Mr. Rodriguez."

"After you answer, kid. Don't you like it? Perhaps just a little?"

"You're going to let go of my hand."

"Go ahead. Take your hand away. I'm not stopping you."

Miss Lawson pulled her hand back.

"Rough on you?"

"What do you mean?"

"You know what I mean. You kind of liked it."

"We're here to talk about your problems, Mr. Rodriguez."

"Still on that," he laughed. "Sure. I get the idea. You're here to give me advice."

"As a nurse, yes."

"Then why in the hell don't you dress like one?"

Miss Lawson stood up and went to open the door to the room.

"Not bad from the back—and from the front either. Come on, sit down. I get the message. I won't try anything. What do you want to know? I'll play the game. I don't want to get you in any kind of trouble. Though between you and me, I'd try wearing something one size larger—

---

[6]Mr. Rodriguez is obviously bright and verbally facile, and he uses his talents to fence with the therapist.

just for kicks. There's an old Spanish proverb. I forgot you don't speak Spanish. I'll tell it to you anyway. Listen." Mr. Rodriguez played a musical background to his words. "*Tu eres mariposa aleteadora. Yo soy un hombre total.*"

At the next session, Miss Lawson asked Mr. Rodriguez to sit in a chair she had placed on the other side of the desk. She sat behind the desk.

"Not taking any chances," he told her.

"How did the week go?"

"Same as usual."

"What do you do?"

"Live."

"Are you working?"

"Me?"

"Yes."

"Sure, I work."

"Would you like to tell me about what you do?"[7]

"I'm trying to improve my pool game. There's a shot I haven't been able to make. I thought of doing some library work."

"Mr. Rodriguez, we won't get anywhere unless you try to let me help you. What are some problems you have faced? What disturbs you?"

"I told you, kid, a pool shot. You see, there's this one shot I've been trying to make. Every time I go for it, my fingers get sweaty and I miss."

"Where do you play?"

"In a pool hall."

"Where do you sleep at night?"

"Now we're beginning to move."

"I just wanted to know if you are living with your family. Do you live alone? Are your parents in this country?"

"What parents?"

"Are they living?"

"My mother died when I was five."

"And your father?"

---

[7]Rather than pay attention to the meaning of his behavior in their sessions together. Miss Lawson continues to repeat that she and the patient are supposed to talk about his problems. Mr. Rodriguez tries to define the relationship in social-sexual terms, and finally, as if to underscore the differences between them, he ends the session with a quotation in Spanish. He talks, but in a language Miss Lawson cannot understand. Given the patient's defenses, motives for coming to the clinic, and his talent for manipulating the situation, there is perhaps little that one can reasonably hope to achieve in a brief period. Nevertheless, instead of repeating that a patient should talk about his problems, it might be more helpful in the long run to focus directly on Mr. Rodriguez's immediate behavior and attempt to achieve some understanding of it.

"He's a lottery salesman in a hill town in Puerto Rico."

"Have you seen him recently?"

"He came up last month."

"Is he still here?"

"No. He went back on a plane last week. You know those planes—little birdies in the sky, where dreams come from. I put him on the plane," said Mr. Rodriguez. "That goddamn bundle of bones without his teeth. He has no teeth. His gums are raw and rough. You ever see rough and red raw gums? I hadn't seen him since I was twelve when he brought me up and left me here. Let him go home. Let him go home to live on his dream of a winning number. Can you imagine selling scraps of paper for a whole lifetime?" Mr. Rodriguez pulled out a lottery ticket from his pocket.

"A dream of a number. He was always going to win. He's sixty-nine and he's still going to win. Someday, he told me, his number is going to come in and he's going to have the right ticket. For the one whole week that he was here he went crazy without his numbers. He couldn't control his hands. They're used to holding numbers. A whole week without numbers and he was slobbering like a baby. Couldn't wait to get home."

"Did he come up to visit you?"

"You want the truth?"

"Yes."

"He came up because he was going to die and he was alone in the town."

"Why did you let him go back?"

"For a last chance at a winning number. He's lived for his system. I used to believe that he had a system. I asked him to tell it to me. Fat chance. He went home with his damn system."

"Our time is just about up, Mr. Rodriguez."

"You doing anything tonight?"[8]

"I don't accept personal invitations."

"Why not?"

"I'm here to see you in the clinic, Mr. Rodriguez, as a patient."

"Cut the Rodriguez bit. Luis is the name."

"Alright, Luis. I will see you here next week."

"How about tonight?"

"No."

"You'd like to, wouldn't you?" There's a lot more to tell. Wouldn't you like to hear?"

---

[8]Mr. Rodriguez's invitation is an attempt to change the nature of their relationship, and once again, rather than repeat what the patient already knows, it might have been more useful to focus on the psychological meaning of his behavior and its consequences in terms of their relationship.

"We can begin right where we left off next week in the clinic."

"It won't wait."

"Yes, I think it can, Luis. You can tell me next week."

Mr. Rodriguez put his guitar in its cover. He put on a suede fringed jacket.

"You didn't ask what happened to my father."

"What happened, Luis?"

"He didn't get off the plane alive. I knew he was dying. That's why I made sure he got on that plane. I didn't want him here with me. Get it? I knew he held a winning number—the one number that counts in life— and I didn't want to be around when he cashed in on the stakes. Pretty lousy of me, wasn't it? Rushed him off to that plane. Got him on and all the time I knew what was going on. Maybe tomorrow night? Are you free tomorrow night?" he asked.

Mr. Rodriguez did not come for his next appointment. Miss Lawson waited for him, and after the time had passed, she asked the secretary to telephone his home. A call was made, and the secretary was told that no one by the name of Luis Rodriguez had ever lived there. The receiver was slammed down.

Miss Lawson tried herself later that morning, and a young male voice admitted knowing Luis but insisted that he hadn't seen him in some time and refused to give any further information. Miss Lawson wrote a letter to Luis, and the letter was returned to the clinic with a scrawled note to the effect that the party was unknown. Miss Lawson decided to wait another week to see if Luis would keep his scheduled appointment. He did not appear.

Concerned about him, Miss Lawson talked about the case with her supervisor, Mrs. Danelle, and the clinic director, Mrs. Engle. She explained that Luis had been so regular that his unexplained absence concerned her. She wondered if something had happened and felt a responsibility to check on his whereabouts.

"You can't go chasing patients in their homes," said Mrs. Engle.

"It's not a matter of chasing. Luis simply isn't like that. He was a most intelligent, serious young man. He really wanted to be helped. I felt that. I felt him reaching out and that's exactly why I am bothered. He would come if something hadn't happened to prevent him. We took on the case and we should see it through."[9]

"Now wait a minute. We take on cases here in the clinic. But we're

[9]In the light of her previous experience with Mr. Rodriguez, the statement "He really wanted to be helped" appears to reflect some distortion. Mr. Rodriguez may indeed want help, but Miss Lawson's statement leads one to consider the possible counter-transference feelings of the therapist for the patient.

only indirectly responsible for the people when they are on the streets. We help; we try to help them but we can't go ordering other peoples' lives around," said Mrs. Engle.

"I don't want to order his life. That's absurd. You mean if a patient stops coming without any warning, we just let the case drop? That isn't right."

"What isn't right.?"

"That we stop our responsibility at the front door. People live outside of those doors, Mrs. Engle. They have lives elsewhere. Yes, we're one small part of their lives, but sometimes the smaller bits can make the difference."

"How was Luis with you?" asked Mrs. Danelle.

"Responsive."

"Did he tell you anything about himself?"

"He was beginning to. I will say the first few weeks I couldn't get him to say anything. He did resist. I waited it out. And then the last meeting he opened up, or started to."

"What did he tell you?"

"About his father, his life. He might have some guilt feelings about his father. I don't know. He said he hadn't seen his father since he was twelve. His mother died when he was five. He's lived his whole life here alone."

"Did he say that?"

"No, but I gather he didn't have much of a home life. He's wandering. He said he's trying to find himself. He's twenty-nine and he seems much younger, I think. He's so lost."

"Did he tell you he felt lost?"

"Yes and no. One thing I know is that he didn't want to leave our interviews. He asked me to see him outside of the clinic."

"What did you say?" asked Mrs. Danelle.

"I told him that was impossible."

"How did he take it?"

"He didn't do anything, but that is why I am upset. He had been so silent; then he opened up and told me a few things, and I said I couldn't see him outside the clinic. What worries me is that he didn't understand my explanation and he might interpret my not wanting to see him as a rejection of him personally."[10]

She continued saying that she really thought it right to contact him and

---

[10]At this point, problems of counter-transference are apparent as Miss Lawson's concern seems to be over-determined and her reactions influenced to a large extent by her own feelings. This does not mean that therapists should not be realistically concerned about their patients or that their concern stops at the office door. But one must carefully distinguish between reality-based concern and reactions that stem largely from the therapist's own feelings and conflicts.

to explain that she wanted to see him in the clinic and could even arrange to see him more than once a week if that was necessary, but that she could not see him outside of the clinic.

"I feel so up in the air about him," she told the supervisor and the director. "It just ended. It doesn't seem right. I mean, we were beginning to talk. He's not just any kind of beatnik from the street. He's quite a sensitive young man. He plays the guitar magnificently. I was impressed. I've tried taking guitar lessons, so I have some idea about how good he is. And he has a fantastic literary knowledge. He loves to quote poetry. He really needs some help, and I do feel worried."

Mrs. Engle said that Miss Lawson might have communicated more than professional involvement with Luis. "Remember how he might see it," explained Mrs. Danelle. "You're an attractive young woman; he's an appealing young man. I wonder if this is what's bothering you."

"That wasn't the case at all," insisted Miss Lawson. "I won't say he wasn't attractive, but the relationship *was* definitely a professional one on my part—certainly that and nothing more."

Miss Lawson said she might make one more effort to reach him by letter. "If he returns to the clinic," Mrs. Danelle said, "he must be assigned to another therapist."

That afternoon Miss Lawson wrote a brief, formal note to Luis, inquiring about his welfare and suggesting that he continue coming to the clinic. She personally delivered the letter to his home address, which was several blocks away from the clinic. An elderly woman answered the doorbell and took the letter. Although she spoke little English, she was able to tell Miss Lawson that Luis was sick and in Depester Hospital. She asked Miss Lawson why she wanted to see Luis.

"He's no good. You'll be hurt," she warned Miss Lawson.

"I'm not here on a personal call." Miss Lawson tried to explain her position, but the woman shook her head and slammed the door.

Three weeks after Luis Rodriguez's last clinic visit, he telephoned Miss Lawson and asked her if she would come and visit him in Depester Hospital. The large hospital complex included both the medical and psychiatric facilities that served the various community mental health clinics, half-way houses, and other social agencies.

That afternoon Miss Lawson went to the hospital and spoke to Mr. Gordon, an attendant who worked on the tenth floor ward where Mr. Rodriguez had been placed. She explained that she had been seeing Mr. Rodriguez at a store-front clinic and had recently learned that he had been hospitalized.

"There, too," commented Mr. Gordon.

"What do you mean?"

"You know much about Luis?"

"Some. He told me a few things about his background."

"Don't tell me," said Mr. Gordon. "I can hear him. Down and out Luis. Poor misundstood Luis. If only his mother had loved him, life would have been different. What else did he tell you?"

"That he was from Puerto Rico and about his father. He's had a difficult life, Mr. Gordon. It's not been an easy way for Luis. He's a very sensitive young man."

"Don't tell me how sensitive he is. We all know Luis. He's one of our regular old patients. You can count on Luis. He's been in and out of here, oh, I'd say, going on ten years. Ten years, young lady. And when he isn't around here we know Luis is over telling his sob story at some other clinic. What line did he hand you? The one about being an actor?"

"No."

"I know, don't tell me. He gave you the musician line."

"He does play the guitar."

"Luis doesn't play the guitar. He's an unrecognized star if you listen to him. If he only had money; if he only had time; if he only had a teacher, he would be great. There's one thing Luis forgets, and that is you need talent."

"He has talent, Mr. Gordon. I've heard him play. He's got a great deal of potential talent."

"You know anything really about guitar playing? I bet not. Luis is third rate. I think things are beginning to catch up on him. When did you last see him?"

"Three weeks ago?"

"Was he shooting up then?"

"Luis wasn't on narcotics, Mr. Gordon."

"Now Luis wouldn't do that sort of thing. Maybe he was clean when you saw him. That's not the way he came in here. He's on his way. We'll keep him awhile and then let him out. Luis will be back pushing. I told him, though, we weren't going to take his pals coming in here passing the stuff. We had our hands full last time he was here. His gang was in here selling to everybody the minute our back was turned."

"If you can't do anything here for him, why aren't you referring him somewhere so he can get help? Luis wants and needs help."

"Reform him? You didn't know Luis too long, did you?"

"I said refer him and maybe reform him. He only came to the clinic for a few months. He was just beginning to open up and then he stopped coming."

"I know his line. He needed you. You were the one who really understood him. You had true feelings. You could see what he was trying to express. Come on, what else did he hand you."

"Nothing else, Mr. Gordon, I believed him. He's had a difficult life."

"You believed him? You couldn't see through him? You mean you really believed his line? A hard life. You know what his hard life has been—mugging for purses on Sylvester Street—little old ladies. A hard life. Two kids, one's four and the other's three—a hard life. I got the two mothers coming here every week ready to kill him. A hard life. Listen, what did you say your name was—Miss Lawson, that guy has never worked a day in his life. He's lived off the streets, off people like you. I don't mean we shouldn't help him. I don't mean that at all. But this soft sister bit—weeping for Luis, who would steal you last dime—I don't think that's the way. He's been no angel here. You want to see him? He's playing pool. He's pretty mad now because we won't let him have his guitar.[11]

"Why not? The guitar meant so much to him."

"Because if something happens to the guitar the city gets sued for personal property being damaged. You should see the lawsuits we got from patients."

Luis was playing pool at a table in front of the elevators. Two attendants were seated opposite the elevator doors watching to see that patients did not leave the floor.

Luis continued to shoot pool. He walked around the table and said to Miss Lawson, "Got a cigarette?"

"No."

"Nice to see you."

"How have you been, Luis?"

"Fine. What else?"

"I wondered why you didn't show up for your appointments?"

"Now you know."

"You will get good care here."

"Sure. Miss me?"

"We wondered what happened."

"This is it, kid. This is it baby—the real thing."

"That's a good shot, Luis."

"Good shot, but the wrong one for this game. Say, you got any pull around here?"

"You don't need any pull. You just have to be straight, Luis. What is it you want?"

---

[11]Mr. Gordon's reaction is in dramatic contrast to Miss Lawson's, and one is tempted to evaluate his view as more realistic than hers. Yet in his own way, Mr. Gordon's countertransference problems are as evident as those of Miss Lawson. One emphasizes strengths and the other emphasizes weaknesses. Both, of course, are right: Luis is indeed bright and sensitive, and he probably is also psychopathic. But both, too, are wrong insofar as the narrowness of their views has distorted the total picture. In any case, neither unrealistic optimism nor total pessimism is likely to be very helpful to the patient.

Luis walked over to her. "My guitar. You got to tell them. I need my guitar. See my fingers." He fluttered his fingers. "They're crying, baby, crying. You ever see crying fingers? I got to have it. You be a good baby. Get it for me. I don't forget favors. I'm coming out in a few weeks. Will you be doing anything? Just where we left off. How about it?" said Luis, hunching his shoulders. He grinned at Miss Lawson while he plucked an imaginary guitar, his shoulders swaying, his left foot in a hospital slipper tapping a steady rhythm.

12 OPERANT CONDITIONING IN CHRONIC ILLNESS

Roy S. Fowler, Ph.D.

Wilbert E. Fordyce, Ph.D.

Rosemarian Berni, B.S., R.N.

THE WAY STAFF GIVE ATTENTION TO PATIENTS IS as powerful as medicine and should be planned as carefully. When sick behaviors are rewarded, patients can be predicted to display sick behaviors. On the other hand, rewarding well behaviors can be expected to help patients drop sick behaviors. We have demonstrated that applying operant conditioning to chronically ill patients does indeed increase the behaviors that are rewarded.

Operant conditioning is especially important with the chronically ill, because long-term care presents patients with many opportunities for learning. Traditionally, too, nurses and other care-taking persons may be tempted, particularly when there are staff shortages, to give the most attention to the patient who makes the most noise. Many patients prefer negative attention to having very little attention.

In applying operant conditioning in a chronic-disease facility, we found that the most useful principles were:

Behavior is largely a function of its consequences.

Behavior which is followed by positive or rewarding consequences will tend to be maintained or to increase in rate.

Behavior which is followed by neutral consequences will tend to diminish or drop out altogether.

Without the patient or staff being aware that it is happening, staff can train a patient to become sick or to slow his progress. The experience of Mrs. S. is an example, not only of this, but of a change that brought healthier responses.

Relearning To Walk

Mrs. S. was a licensed practical nurse, 33 years old. She had partial paralysis of the legs and with this paraparesis, chronic neurodermatitis. Because of skin breakdown in the ischial areas, she had come to the hospital for plastic surgery. She had been bed bound postoperatively for some time when the physician prescribed ambulation, starting with the patient's walking between parallel bars.

On attempting to walk between the bars, she became dizzy and faint. The physician then prescribed starting her ambulation program with the tilt table. She soon could tolerate having the table tilted 50° for 30 minutes. Four weeks later, however, she could tolerate no more than 60°, becoming faint when tilted beyond that angle.

At that point, the psychologists evaluated the behavior of Mrs. S. and those treating her. The routine was for the physical therapist with an aide to place Mrs. S. on the table, while interacting freely with her. She slowly raised the tilt table until the angle was close to that of the previous day. Then, keeping the patient under observation, she left the patient's side to carry out other duties.

Typically, after a few minutes, Mrs. S. would complain of feeling dizzy and faint. The therapist would immediately return, lower her gradually, measure her blood pressure, and reassure her that she was all right. When Mrs. S. was calmed, the procedure was again repeated, with the therapist departing as soon as the patient was stabilized in her tilted position.

Obviously, the therapist's presence and attention were contingent on the patient's complaints of discomfort. Also, Mrs. S.'s complaints always resulted in her being moved into the more comfortable horizontal position. The therapist ignored any desirable movement toward the upright position. In the graph of Mrs. S.'s progress, the period in which she was rewarded for complaints is labeled contingency A (Graph I).

We suggested a change, making rewards dependent on progress, which is labeled contingency B on the same graph. The therapist was asked to remain at the side of Mrs. S. throughout her movement toward the upright, interacting with her naturally.

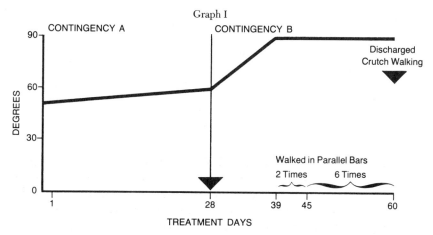

MRS. S.'s TOLERANCE of elevation on a tilt table improved with operant conditioning. Until day 28, the therapist was attentive only when Mrs. S. complained of faintness (contingency A). In contingency B, the therapist's reward of her presence depended on progress.

As soon as Mrs. S. complained of discomfort and dizziness, she could again be lowered to the horizontal. The therapist was then to measure her blood pressure and minister to her as much as necessary, while remaining as matter-of-fact and socially neutral as practical.

The therapist was then to depart from the side of the patient. When the patient indicated she was again ready to approach the vertical, the therapist was to return to her side and continue the social interaction.

Eleven days after the contingency change, Mrs. S. achieved a vertical position, no longer needed the tilt table, and walked two lengths between the parallel bars without discomfort or dizziness. Fifteen days later, Mrs. S. was crutch walking and was discharged soon after.

Assuring Fluid Intake

Most patients who have injured spinal cords are told that they should drink enough fluid to insure approximately 2,500 cc. of urine output. The traditional teaching has been to explain the importance of fluids in preventing genitourinary infections and calculi. Such patients on physical medicine and rehabilitation services are reminded periodically, and a record is kept of their intake and output.

Patients find that drinking so much fluid is not an easy habit to establish, and many do not achieve the goal. When that happens, the nurse reports to the physician that the output of urine is low or that the urine is extremely concentrated.

Ordinarily, the staff then try anew to impress upon the patient the importance of fluids. Sometimes the campaign is effective, but often the records indicate the patient drinks less, not more. The staff may then take this as a personal challenge and renew their exhortations. The patient receives more attention for not drinking than he is likely to receive for drinking.

If one were to apply operant principles in treating this problem, one would reverse the contingencies. This reversal is being done in the following manner.

The nurse gives the patient a clipboard or notebook, which he keeps with him at all times to record his daily intake. This record is made public, in the form of either a daily note on the clipboard or a graphic record. Treatment staff is responsive to any increase in drinking and nonresponsive to decreases. They call attention to the increases and praise the patient, saying that drinking this much fluid is not easy. Decreases are simply not commented upon. Mrs. N.'s story illustrates the effectiveness of such a program of behavior conditioning.

Mrs. N., a 37-year-old, paraplegic housewife, had a long history of poor self-care and frequent medical complications. She had been repeatedly advised to drink at least 3,000 cc. of fluid a day, but her records indicated a gradual decline in drinking (Graph II).

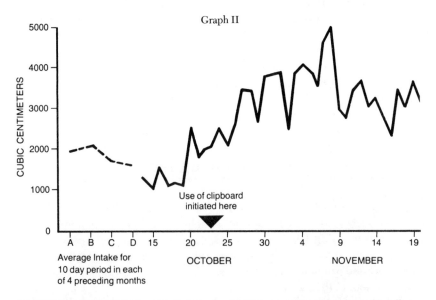

Graph II

NAGGING LOWERED Mrs. N.'s fluid intake. Staff began on Oct. 23 to praise her efforts, to publicly display her records of accomplishment in forcing fluids, and to ignore lapses. In three days, she was drinking the prescribed 3000 cc. and she maintained a good fluid intake.

The more attention her malperformance received the more her performance declined. On the graph, points A, B, C, and D represent 10-day samples of Mrs. N.'s drinking record, drawn from the four months immediately preceding a program based on operant principles.

On October 23, the psychologist gave her a clipboard and instructed her in its use. Her increased fluid intake is obvious. At the time of discharge, she was still drinking, on the average, 3,000 cc.

A Bad Back

Another patient had chronic back trouble for more than 20 years. At age 66, Mrs. W., a bookkeeper, suffered from postmenopausal osteoporosis with multiple compression fractures of the vertebra. Although she had possessed a prescribed back brace for many years, she had steadfastly refused to wear it, claiming it restricted her motions and caused much discomfort.

She had been in the hospital several weeks before she was admitted to the rehabilitation program. Here, in spite of (or perhaps because of) recommendations to wear the brace, she had refused to do so. Her chart indicated that for the two weeks preceding a program of operant conditioning, the longest period she had worn the brace was one-half hour at a time.

In the conditioning program, she was requested to record in a small notebook each time she put on and took off the brace. For the first several days, the psychologist in a brief daily session added the total minutes she wore the brace. These totals were then transcribed onto a graph and placed on the bulletin board beside her bed.

By the end of the first week, the psychologist turned the recording entirely over to Mrs. W. Staff on rounds and nurses throughout the day checked her graphic records. They praised her appropriately for increased tolerance of the brace. For any declines in tolerance, they simply made no response. As can be seen in Graph III, shortly after the treatment began, Mrs. W. was discharged.

When she was discharged, the psychologist gave her a supply of graph paper and asked her to continue recording. When she came to the hospital once a week for a brief recheck, the psychologist transcribed her week's record to a permanent record.

She became proud of her records and spontaneously displayed them to anyone who showed the slightest interest. The public health nurse who was instructed in the program and who made routine home visits verified our impression that her records were quite faithful and accurate reports.

Graph III

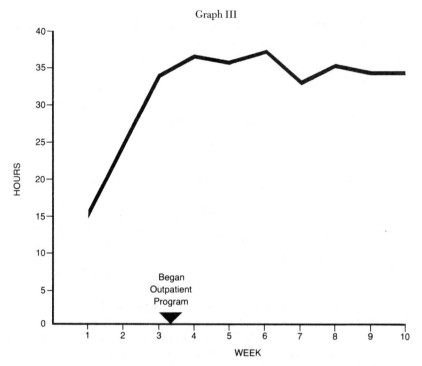

OPERANT CONDITIONING more than doubled the hours Mrs. W. wore a back brace. Started on the rehabilitation unit, the program was carried out chiefly through the OPD service.

In each of these three cases, the patient was receiving ample professional attention and responsiveness which, however, had come to be contingent upon sick behavior by the patient. At the same time, well behaviors that were low in frequency, and low in strength failed to receive appropriate attention and social responsiveness. It was only after a shift in contingencies, allowing the patients to receive attention for well behavior, that their performances changed dramatically.

It is important to realize that these principles can be applied without ignoring or neglecting patients. A distinction can be made between ignoring certain patient behaviors and being socially nonresponsive to a patient. A person can be treated adequately while providing minimal social interaction, when to withhold socializing is considered vital to improving the patient's performance, as long as the program assures attention to the patient for well behavior. To respond as positively to sick behavior as to well behavior is to risk teaching the patient to be sick.

13 STRATEGIES FOR INTERVIEWING IN LANGUAGE AND THOUGHT DISORDERS

Janet Kroah, M.S., R.N.

ANYONE WHO WORKS WITH A SCHIZOPHRENIC PERSON SOONER or later experiences bafflement. It may seem that both you and he are talking about the same subject and yet as the exchange continues it becomes clearer to you that neither is understanding what the other is saying. As a therapeutic person you know that both the therapist and the client must understand what this individual is trying to communicate if you are to help him overcome the obstacles that prevent him from becoming a functioning member of the community. As Cameron has suggested, it is easy to conclude that even though your communication is not always clear, the primary difficulty lies with this other individual; that something has gone wrong with the schizophrenic person's machinery of communication, although it is difficult to pinpoint the trouble. The client arrives at conclusions that you cannot share, by logical methods that you cannot follow. He uses words in a way that you cannot understand.[1]

In order to classify and thus move toward clarification of the language and thought of the schizophrenic individual, this paper will include three foci. Initially, some theories explaining the language and thought process of the schizophrenic will be reviewed, forms of the schizophrenic's speech will be identified and illustrated, and finally strategies that the therapeutic person might use to intervene in the language and thought disorder will be suggested.

Reprinted, with permission, from *Journal of Psychiatric Nursing and Mental Health Services*, Vol. 12, No. 2, 1974.

Some Theories About the Language and Thought of the Schizophrenic

Sullivan says that the young child uses "private language" and at some point undergoes revision because the child discovers that he is better able to get what he wants from the adult if he uses their language.[2] Throughout life language is largely an instrument for getting what we want. Generally, according to Sullivan, this is obtaining satisfaction and preserving a feeling of personal security. Sullivan concludes that most children learn to use language more to preserve security than to obtain satisfaction.[2]

The schizophrenic individual uses language primarily because of an extreme need for personal security. The individual who becomes schizophrenic is one who early in his life has had many, repeated traumatic experiences which generate a continuing insecurity. In accommodating these experiences, and in an attempt to gain personal security, he uses language exclusively for counteracting his feelings of insecurity among other people. Thus he uses words as protective mantles or shields rather than as a means of communication. What further compounds the difficulty between the schizophrenic person and someone else is that the former has not learned to consensually validate, or to use language as a device for checking up on things.[2]

Miscommunication leads to increased anxiety on the part of the "listener." This increased anxiety is felt by the schizophrenic individual. He in turn gets more anxious, needs more security, but gets more "schizophrenic" in the process. In other words, the initial use of language to gain security becomes, later on, a way of perpetuating his insecurity, and thus the language becomes more problematic as its use to counteract continuing insecurity escalates and becomes more widespread.

Haley presents his explanation of what happens to the schizophrenic individual when he attempts to relate to another person but miscommunicates instead. Haley indicates that when any two persons meet each other for the first time and begin to establish a relationship, any range of behavior is possible. As they define the relationship they work out what type of communicative behavior is to take place in this relationship. They decide what is and what is not to take place. In this way the relationship is mutually defined by the presence or absence of messages interchanged between two people. Messages are not always verbal. Tonal qualities or bodily movement (away or toward) also convey a message.[3]

When assessing the schizophrenic individual's difficulty in getting into a relationship, Haley indicates that this person has been in an extremely

dangerous or painful, or disorienting family situation in which it was impossible for him to attain a positive health relationship. Thus when he encounters a therapeutic person, he tries many language maneuvers to
avoid defining the relationship. Haley says that he may do this in any one
of four ways: (1) the individual can deny that he communicated something, "The voices told me," "God is speaking through me," "It's the alcohol or drugs that made me say that"; (2) he may deny that something
was communicated; "I don't remember saying that" or "You don't understand what I said"; (3) he can deny that he was communicating to another
person, simply that he was talking to himself; or (4) he can deny what he
says is said in this situation by labeling his statements as referring to some
other time or place, "My parents treated me badly before and will
probably when I go home."[3]

Thus, Haley is suggesting that because talking "straight" would be too
threatening or because he has never learned to do so, that when the
schizophrenic person gets into any interpersonal setting he tries to avoid
defining the relationship and in so doing his language sounds "crazy,"
illogical or autistic.

Another theorist, Kasanin, has described the development of the
thought process. First what Kasanin describes and defines as the normal
thought process will be presented and then how he sees the thought
process in the schizophrenic.

Kasanin defines three stages in the normal development of thought:
physiognomic thinking, concrete thinking, and abstract thinking. In the
first state the child animates an object, and projects his ego into it (when a
child plays with a chair and calls it a horse). He then advances to the level
of literal or concrete thinking. At this point, when the child says table or
chair, he does not mean table or chair in general, but the particular table
or chair which is in his house, or belongs to him. The third state, abstract
thinking, usually occurs after the individual has acquired formal or informal education.[4]

After testing the levels of thought that the schizophrenic individual obtains, Kasanin's conclusion was that the schizophrenic has a reduction in
abstract thinking and that his thought process was at a more concrete,
realistic, matter-of-fact stage which had a personal rather than a universal
value.[4]

There would seem then to be a relationship between both Sullivan's
and Haley's ideas about the highly personal language of the schizophrenic
and Kasanin's ideas about the personal concrete level of thought process
that schizophrenic individuals exhibit.

One may then wonder if one process, language, affects the other
process, thought? Whorf says that it does. He proposes that all higher

levels of thinking are dependent on language, and that the structure of language a person habitually uses influences the manner in which he understands his environment and behaves with respect to it.[5]

Forms of Schizophrenic Speech

After having reviewed some theorists' explanations of the language and thought process of the schizophrenic person, I will now identify some patterns in the schizophrenic's language.

Concrete rather than abstract. A colleague of mine related an incident which is a good example of this. She had just met this person and told him her name and then said "Give me your name." The person responded by saying "No, I need mine. You have your own."

The schizophrenic's language contains many private meanings as evidenced in neologisms or symbolism.

Perseveration of sounds. "The Purple Paulist" priests pushed, pulled, and provoked parishioners, poorly, piously, and proportionate to propriety."

Coded mechanisms. For example, in *I Never Promised You a Rose Garden*, Land of Ur, Mapmaking, and list making.

Mixed "C"s. Frequently the language of the schizophrenic gives evidence of his confusion when the person mixes the command, context, and content.

Word salads. Scattering, prototaxis, circumstantiality.

Variants of Language and Thought Disorders and Strategies of Intervention

Initially I mentioned that if the nurse (or other therapeutic person) is to help the schizophrenic individual become a functioning member of society, she must make every effort to understand his language and help him become understandable to others. This is no easy task. But these are strategies that you can use to help him communicate in a clearer manner. The strategies that I will talk about are based on Sullivan's, Haley's Kasanin's, and Whorf's ideas which have been applied to psychotherapeutic nursing by Peplau. Peplau firmly believes that the corrective language the nurse uses will directly affect the language of the schizophrenic individual. In turn this will have a positive effect on his thought processes and behavior.[8]

It should be pointed out that change does not occur overnight. The nurse may use a strategy over and over again before the language of the schizophrenic individual changes, but it will change.

Now, to make things clearer, I will focus on variants of language and thought disorders, describe each, and show interventions appropriate to each that either my students or myself have had with schizophrenic individuals.

Scattering

Mr. W.'s initial session was characterized by scattering or "looseness of associations," prototaxis and parataxic associations. However, what I want you to listen for is the scattering. After the nurse had introduced herself and told the patient why she was there, he said:

P: Insemination, Rugers—The State University. If you are outside for inquire, I won't lie for you. I will lie in bed for you. Age, money, worry about war, government circumstance and his son, kerchief, nice hair-do, oh is good hair-do, Irma.

N: Who is Irma?

P: Might be our own daughter?

N: Who is Irma to you?

P: Can you think? Strong good features. I will shrink for her. I will solve Germany's problems.

The patient's initial response seems scattered, although there are other elements present. It is quite difficult to determine what he is talking about. This is the function of scattering. The hearer will not understand and may become disoriented. Anxiety increases scattering. In this instance the nurse told the patient that she would be seeing him twice a week for 15 weeks. This fact alone tends to increase anxiety on the basis that most schizophrenic patients do not expect such attention. Thus one strategy of intervention has to do with anxiety reduction. If the anxiety is reduced the scattering will also be alleviated in some degree.

A second strategy based upon the assumption that the focus of the patient's attention is more likely to be sustained on the last thing in the scatter sequence, is to ask about the last word or phrase. In this instance when the nurse asked, "Who is Irma," he gave an answer (distorted) but did not scatter. After the second question, "Who is Irma to you," the patient began to scatter again.

The first few sessions were characterized by scattering. However, the nurse continued using the same strategy of exploring or focusing on the last thing the patient said or occasionally she would interrupt his string of associations by saying: "Before you go on, tell me more about X." By the sixth session, it seemed that the patient had begun to feel more "safe" in the relationship, could sustain a focus, and the security derived from these two newly generated behaviors obviated the former language usage   . called scattering.

Improvement in the patient's language behavior is illustrated by the following data from the sixth session.

N: Tell me one thing that has happened since I was here two days ago.

P: I took a shower today. We had a Christmas party. Ice cream, cake. They put the curtains up.

N: When was the Christmas Party?

P: Yesterday.

N: What was one thing you did at the party.

P: I ate, sang songs.

In this excerpt, when the nurse asked for one thing, the patient gave her two or three answers. The nurse then explored the one which she thought had the most interpersonal content. The patient was able to offer a brief description of the party. This was a noticeable difference from the first few sessions.

Circumstantiality

When the patient uses a language pattern called circumstantiality, there is usually an idea or event that he wants to talk about, but finds the material too threatening to his self-system. He is in conflict about this and goes around the problem attempting to reduce his anxiety and to lose you, the hearer.

A patient in a Community Mental Health Center that I have been seeing in individual therapy opened the session a few weeks ago like this:

P: Mothers shouldn't take sides. I don't think it's right that mothers favor one son over another. It's not fair. My brother's coming home this weekend. I should be able to also. Dr. X said I could go home.

N: What are you trying to say Mr. P.

P: Mothers shouldn't take sides.

N: But what's the issue?

P: (angry) She said I couldn't come home this weekend 'cause my brother is.

Then I focused on the actual incident that occurred and the patient's thoughts and feelings about not going home.

When the patient is being circumstantial, that is, talking around the issues, the nurse must abstract the theme or decode what the patient is saying and help him get to the main idea and stick to it. Strategies like: Describe one time your mother took sides; What are you trying to say? What's the point you are trying to make? What's the issue? force the patient to stop being circumstantial and begin dealing with the anxiety also. Once the issue is apparent, further exploration of the patient's thoughts, feelings, and actions is necessary.

Idiosyncratic Language

Another aspect of a schizophrenic individual language usage and thought process that can be extremely difficult to understand is symbolism or idiosyncratic wording. When you hear this language being used it is necessary for you to decode this language in order to understand what the patient is saying.

Umland defines decoding as the process of reclassifying key symbols in a sentence by using synonyms to a given word to rephrase the sentence to show its meaning.[8] To further clarify what I mean I will decode a proverb: "When the cat's away, the mice will play." (1) Pick out the key symbols in the proverb ("cat's," "away," "mice will play"); (2) list synonyms for each of the words (*Note*: Do not impart sex where there is none. Do not change the tense of the verb. Do not add value judgments):

When the cat's   away   the mice   will play.
        authority gone   subordinate will have fun.
        superior absent   inferior   will frolic.

Now translate the decoded proverb: "When superiors are absent the inferiors will frolic" or "When authority is gone the subordinates will have fun." Now let's do the same process with a patient's symbolic data. One of the nurses was working with a paranoid woman who said: "The *witch is going to try me* because *they say I am a war mongerer.* You are a war mongerer, you are going to have a witches trial." Synonyms for the italicized words (in order of appearance) are:

female	judge	female	I'm bad.
mother	question	mother	I'm wrong.
nurse	punish(?)	nurse	
person		person	

The decoded message becomes, "What person punished you because she said you did something wrong?" Now what the patient seems to be saying is a lot clearer than her initial symbolism. The second half of the message the patient gives to the nurse is also threatening (?) her and subsequently the nurse was going to be punished, by whom is not clear. After the nurse decoded the message, she recognized that she had been pushing the patient too hard to make a decision about staying in or leaving the hospital. The nurse then began to deal with this issue with the patient who was indeed angry at her. Now the nurse did not ask the patient what female had punished her because the patient's anger with the nurse was very apparent. The nurse first focused on the patient's anger toward her. After the patient has sufficiently dealt with her angry feelings towards the nurse, then the initial message can be decoded and dealt with (who in the past had punished the patient because she thought the patient was wrong).

There are times when it is not always necessary to go through this process to decode symbolic or idiosyncratic language the patient uses. If you have been working with a patient in therapy for a time and have a fairly good idea of what the symbolic language represents, you may interpret what you hear and then validate your perceptions with the patient. I'd like to explain how I did this with a 15-year-old patient I am presently seeing in therapy.

During the first five sessions Barbara had been describing her life style, her friends and problems with parents. I thought I had a fairly good idea of her thoughts on these topics. She opened the sixth session with the following words: "Last night as I lay awake in bed I sent a rocket off to chip away at something that's around the world."

N: What do you think is around the world?

P: I put a glass ball around the world two weeks ago when I was tripping. I planted rockets around the world and set them off at night to chip away at this glass ball so I won't suffocate now. Last night I knocked a big chunk off but man came and replaced part of it.

N: I wonder if you put the glass ball around the world for protection?

P: I'm afraid I'm going to die. I keep seeing a coffin close in on me. I can't sleep. I get up and have peppermint tea with my father. I'd like to go away where nurses and doctors can check up on me to be sure I'm alright. I'm afraid I'm going crazy. I'm losing control of my thoughts.

N: Are you saying that two weeks ago you wanted someone to protect you and help you control what was happening?

P: Yes. Another girl went on the trip with me and I couldn't leave her—she got scared. I had to spend all my time with her—no one helped me.

N: So you created something artificial to help you (a fantasy). Now something has happened within the last two weeks that you feel trapped or alone.

P: No one is helping me. My father listens at night. I'm losing control of my thoughts. I'm afraid I'm going crazy.

As a strategy, when you hear indefinite pronouns ask the patient whom he means. For example: Who are you talking about? What is her name? Who is we? Name one person. By forcing the individual to present real names, the therapist gets the patient to think more particularly about specific people and his relationship with them. The therapist needs to influence the person to think in terms of relations and connections and not to incorporate others in a roundabout way.

Overgeneralizations

Frequently, what you will often hear from a patient is not a description of an experience or observation of the situation (raw data), but a conclusion he has already formed about an experience or situation. (The nurses don't like me around here, Mary is jealous of me.)

When an individual draws conclusions the next step is some behavioral pattern in response to this conclusion. What has usually happened with the hospitalized patient is that his conclusions about his experience can get him to adopt behavioral patterns that society labels as deviant or sick.

Thus when an individual makes assertions or draws conclusions without giving the description or raw data, the hearer cannot check the validity or accuracy of the incident. An example is global vagueness: everything happened today, everybody hates me around here. The strategy for encountering this is to: (1) ask for an example of one thing, what's one thing that happened?; or (2) cast doubt—Everything? Everybody?

Erroneous Misclassification of Experience

An individual, instead of describing, classifies a situation or draws a conclusion. An example: "Mary is jealous of me." The strategy: Where did you get that idea? Tell me one time you thought that Mary was jealous of you.

By using the various strategies suggested you are forcing the individual to be specific. You also are assisting him to recover, review and recheck instances from which he drew the conclusion. The therapist cannot validate the patient's perception unless she knows all the facts.

Non-Actual Experience

The individual most likely to exhibit this type of language and thought disorder is the obsessive-compulsive or someone who is guilt-ridden. The problem with the non-actual experience is that it has never really occurred and time is spent in talking about what hasn't happened unless she intervenes.

Examples of this are: (1) *Future* oriented: I will do it tomorrow; (2) *If* oriented: If I could get out of this situation; (3) *Negative* oriented: I don't think I can do that; (4) *Compulsive* oriented: I should go home.

The most obvious strategy the nurse uses in this type of language and thought disorder is to get the patient to say what he *did* do today, or the reality is he can't get out of this situation and what *is* he going to do about it *now*. One other strategy that is useful for the compulsive oriented patient is to say: Who *said* you should go home?

Now, I might point out that there is a great deal of anxiety and psychotic behavior occurring in Barbara. Thus, I did not decode a lot of what she said. Primarily because during this session I did not know how much stress she could handle and I heard the message that she felt alone and was fearful of losing control. Thus to prevent any more psychotic material from coming into awareness I only decoded what the glass ball represented to her. This was enough to get her talking about what she perceived happening to her then.

The following variants of language and thought disorders occur frequently in patients as well as in people who are not labeled patients.

Automatic Knowing

In automatic knowing the individual assumes that the therapist knows what he means or is thinking without his having to tell her. There is a quality of mind reading and taking for granted that the hearer knows what the user is thinking without any data. With the constant use of this problematic language the individual begins to think others know about him without any information. This is a major problem you may hear with a paranoid patient. Expressions like: *you know* how it is; *you see* how it is, indicate this disorder.

Strategy: No, I don't know. What are you assuming I know? Tell me what you want me to know. I don't know how it is, tell me.

Inability to Name Referents to Pronouns

Psychiatric patients use pronouns to conceal themselves from others and to hide information that is being conveyed. Eventually they lose the ability to recall names and thus never deal with people on an individual basis. The identity of the people to whom the pronouns refer are lost and communication is ultimately hampered. Example: they did it to me; she said so; we went downtown.

I have talked about seven variants of language and thought disorders that have already been defined in literature. I think it is extremely important for nurses to continue observing patients' communication patterns, to compile these observations and from them develop appropriate strategies.

Summary

In this paper I have attempted to clarify the communication patterns of the schizophrenic person by looking at various theorists' descriptions of the language and thought process and by identifying and illustrating specific forms of schizophrenic's speech. I hope to build on your therapeutic communication by suggesting strategies to intervene in the language of the schizophrenic individual.

References

1. Cameron N: Experimental analysis of schizophrenic thinking. *In* Kasanin JS (ed): Language and Thought in Schizophrenia. New York, W.W. Norton and Company, 1944, p. 50.
2. Sullivan HS: The Language of Schizophrenic. *In* Kasanin JS (ed): Language and Thought in Schizophrenia. New York, W.W. Norton and Company, 1944, pp. 4-7.
3. Haley J: Strategies of Psychotherapy. New York, Grune and Stratton, 1963 pp. 6-8, 89-90.
4. Kasanin JS: The disturbance of conceptual thinking in schizophrenia. *In* Kasanin JS (ed): Language and Thought in Schizophrenia. New York, W.W. Norton and Company, 1944, pp. 41-43.
5. Whorf B, Carroll JB (eds): Language, Thought, and Reality. Cambridge, Massachusetts, M.I.T. Press, 1956.
6. Peplau H: Psychotherapeutic strategies. *In* Perspectives in Psychiatric Care VI(6):264-270, 1968.
7. Peplau H: Steps in the Causation of Anxiety. New Brunswick, New Jersey, Rutgers—The State University (unpublished papers).
8. Umland T: A Manual for the Evaluation and Development of Intellectual Competence. New Brunswick, New Jersey, Rutgers—The State University, 1961, p. 14 (unpublished papers).

14

THE HALLUCINA-
TING PATIENT
AND NURSING
INTERVENTION

Sylvia T. Schwartzman, M.S., R.N.

A BEHAVIOR PATTERN WHICH I HAVE OBSERVED IN
working with mentally ill persons that seems especially problematic is
that exhibited by the hallucinating patient. From various observations it
appears that nursing staff, other professional personnel and para-
professionals find it difficult to work with the hallucinating patient and
sometimes quite frustrating. It was this that spurred me to investigate the
hallucinatory process more in depth. Furthermore, the fact that an
hallucination is the form that dissociated material of the self has taken and
hence is representative of a partial psychological death of the individual's
self-system, perhaps as a last-ditch mechanism against actual physical self-
annihilation, has intrigued me for a number of years.

The mental anguish that many acutely hallucinating people display
compelled me to make an in-depth analysis and appraisal of this process to
find answers to the following questions: Why does the person manifest
hallucinatory behavior? What need(s) does this behavior serve for the individual? What does the patient mean by this behavior? What is the
nurse's role in relationship to this behavior? In this way, it is hoped that
this paper will transmit a notion of hallucinatory behavior and the nursing
intervention required to effect a well integrated plan of care for the
patient. There will be examples of nurse-patient encounters cited from
my own professional experiences which will serve to illustrate various

Reproduced, with permission, from *Journal of Psychiatric Nursing and Mental Health
Services*, November-December 1975.

points. In no way will the identity of the patient be made directly so as to insure anonymity and respect the confidentiality of the patient.

In order to try to make some sense of the hallucinatory process and its significance for the patient, it is first necessary to define an hallucination. Gravenkemper states:

. . . an hallucination is an inner experience expressed as though it were an outer event. It arises out of the dissociated motivations of the self-system and is an uncanny, yet real, experience for the person.[1:186]

To know what is meant by "dissociated motivations of the self-system," one must first gain some understanding of the self-system itself. As Sullivan has viewed it, the self-system originates from early childhood in which the child becomes aware of himself through the appraisals of the significant others in his life. The child comes to internalize these appraisals accorded him into a formulation of self—the self-system. This development involves beginning personifications of "me" as the good-me, the bad-me, and the not-me.[2:161]

. . . The good-me is the personification that organizes experience in which satisfactions have been enhanced by rewarding increments of tenderness, which come to the infant because the mothering one is pleased with the way things are going; therefore, and to that extent, she is free, and moves toward expressing tender appreciation of the infant. Good-me, as it ultimately develops, is the ordinary topic of discussion about "I." Bad-me, on the other hand, is the beginning personification which organizes experience in which increasing degrees of anxiety are associated with behavior involving the mothering one in its more or less clearly prehended interpersonal setting . . . with increasing tenseness and increasingly evident forbidding on the part of the mother.[2:162]

Sullivan continues to state that:

. . . For the expression of all things in the personality other than those which were approved and disapproved by the parent and other significant persons, the self refuses awareness . . . It does not accord awareness, it does not notice; and these impulses, desires, and needs come to exist disassociated from self, or dissociated. When they are expressed, their expression is not noticed by the person.[3:21]

This essentially is the not-me, which develops out of experiences with significant others that have been fraught with intense anxiety. This overwhelming experience of anxiety prevented the developing individual from developing any grasp of or making any sense out of the particular circumstances which dictated the experience of this intense anxiety.

. . . Thus while the self-system excludes from awareness clear evidence of a dissociated motivational system, that which is dissociated is represented in awareness by some group of ideas or thoughts which are marked uncannily with utter foreignness—they have nothing to do with oneself.[2:361]

H. S. Sullivan posits that the next step in this sequence is the actual occurrence of the hallucination, which the individual perceives as deriving outside himself, alien to himself and engendering feelings of terror, hatefulness, fear or something like this.

Before I can cite examples of an encounter with the patient demonstrating hallucinatory behavior, it is necessary first to provide a brief background history of the selected patient before the reader will be able to grasp the significance of the hallucinatory behavior for the patient. The patient was a twenty-nine-year-old, Caucasian woman, henceforth designated as P.(for "patient"). She was diagnosed as "acute schizophrenic." She was born of Catholic parents and was one of five children. At the age of two it was noted that her father had inflicted beatings upon her. Because there were marital difficulties between the parents and because of the father's frequent abandonment, the mother placed P., then a child of eight years, into an orphan home for approximately five years to be cared for by religious sisters. The patient stated that these nuns showed her many injustices. For example, she had recollection of their forcing her to eat her own vomitus on an occasion when she refused to do

more work than some of the other girls in the home and she became upset
to her stomach as a result. The patient was returned to her natural home
at the age of thirteen, and recalled that living there was intolerable. That
is, she had to assume a great deal of the work around the house and there
were many ill-feelings among family members. She completed school to
the eighth grade, began drinking and engaging in sexually promiscuous
activities thereafter. She was married at the age of seventeen, "to get
away from home." She married a manual laborer, who was alcoholic.
They had six children, but, the paternity of the children was questionable.

The patient characterized her marital life as "beautiful at first"—approximately for the first two years—but later, as the husband subjected
her to many abuses, she became more unhappy. When he began to
engage in extramarital relationships, she believed he no longer cared for
her but was only exploiting her. She then resorted to drinking and engaging in her own extramarital affairs for outlets to her feelings. Because of
her various acting-out behaviors, the children were not being adequately
cared for and as a result, all six of them were taken from the patient and
her husband and placed in different foster homes by the court. The
patient was twenty-six years of age at this time. Shortly after the place-
ments, the patient made a suicide attempt, without success, by drowning.
As a result of this attempt, she was hospitalized for a period of six months
of continuous treatment followed by her release and readmission approximately one year later for a second suicide attempt.

It was during this second hospitalization that I met P. who was very
verbal throughout meetings but her main manner of relating was quite
psychotic. That is, she related auditory hallucinations, which she had continually been experiencing for two months prior to hospitalization. P. related that the voices were "a thousand of my voice. I can't fight them anymore." If one looks at P.'s above brief developmental history sketch, it
becomes apparent that she experienced early in her life:

. . . a self which arose through derogatory experience, hostility
toward the child, disapproval, dissatisfaction with the child, then
this self more or less like a microscope tends to preclude one's learning anything better, to cause one's continuing to feel a sort of limitation in oneself, and while this cannot be expressed clearly, while the
child or the adult that came from the child does not express openly
self-depreciatory trends, he does have a depreciatory attitude
toward everyone else, and this really represents a depreciatory attitude toward the self.[3:23]

Thus, P., with early childhood rejections and injustices by parents—her father beat her; she was placed in an orphan home; she stated that her mother neither held nor cuddled her much as a child; her father called her a "tramp" and "bum" as she got older; neither parent came to visit her while she was hospitalized; and later injustices inflicted by her husband—she became one of, " . . . those people with chronically low self-esteem who have advantage taken of them, and who may later go on to plunge into the bad waking dream of schizophrenia attendant with all its uncanny emotions of awe, dread, loathing, and horror."[2 : 359]

An example of P.'s early dealing with anxiety, precipitated by her separation from her family at the age of eight to go to an orphan home, is that she began to have "visions" at that time of the Blessed Virgin Mary and God whom she related were "the only ones I have been close to." On a superficial glance one might be inclined to label these visions as part of the normal fantasy life of a child. And yet, because of the abrupt development of the visions approximating the separation of the patient from her family, and the extreme detail with which she described them—for example, the physical attire and characteristics of the Blessed Virgin Mother were identical with the patient's own mother and the God figure was her father's chronological age—the visions appeared to be more than merely childhood fantasy. Rather, the visions seemed reminiscent of Phase I in the development of an hallucinatory process as outlined by Janice Clack in "An Interpersonal Technique for Handling Hallucinations." In this Phase I, the person first experiences mounting stress and severe anxiety (for P. this was separation anxiety), loneliness (for P. this was rejection by her parents both physically and emotionally). The patient then willingly and wittingly focuses on certain personal thoughts (in this case, P. focused on the holy figures) that to some degree are comforting. These figures seemed to represent substitute parents for the eight-year-old girl who had been separated from her own biological parents.

Apparently, the patient did not re-experience any more "visions" after being returned to her natural home until the time just prior to hospitalization but, of course, the available information of this is limited and at best subject to speculation. I have given this brief account of an early experience to point out: (1) the extreme vulnerability of this patient's self-system by virtue of her past history to future evolution or predisposition to an hallucinatory experience—actually, a schizophrenic process; (2) a way in which this individual attempted to deal with mounting anxiety in her earlier years; and so provide the reader with some indication of her ego functioning.

In adult life P. apparently was finding it more difficult to deal with her rising anxiety so that by the time I met her she was blatantly hallucinating. She exhibited flight of ideas—mostly of religious, sexual, and aggressive themes. She stated the voices told her to "do all sorts of awful things." An example she gave was "to roast my children; put my bottom in God's and the Virgin Mother's faces; urinate in people's mouths," and engage in assorted sexual activities. She stated, "I'm no lesbian, don't be afraid of me." Thus, as the unconscious feelings and thoughts which the self-system tends to keep dissociated are recalled—the hallucinations— the individual experiences renewed anxiety and much psychic pain as demonstrated by the content of the hallucinations cited.

Sometimes P. would cock her head to one side and assume the "listening attitude" that Clack describes in Phase II of the hallucinatory process. Another characteristic of this Phase II which P. demonstrated was P.'s attempt to place distance between herself and the hallucinatory phenomena by projecting the experience outward as if the sounds were coming from another person or place. For example, as P.'s anxiety increased when I was touching on material too emotionally laden for P. to deal with at that time, she stated "Oh, they just told me to pee in your mouth. My golden mind (she saw this as her healthy mind) would never tell me to do that. I'm sick of this disgusting mind!" Here she has projected the hallucinatory phenomena outward as not belonging to her being. She assumes possession of the "golden mind" as part of her former real self as opposed to not assuming possession of "this disgusting mind," which is dissociated and separate from her.

Another indication that P. was in Phase II of the hallucinatory process occurred when she related that two months before, when the hallucinations had first begun, the voices were "friendly." That is, she experienced thoughts that were "happy—of the holy people and not dirty." She also (two months before) had more control over focal awareness of these thoughts. That is, she was better able to control them stating, "I'd think of pleasant thoughts or sing happy songs instead to fight them, but now they're getting bad and harder to fight!" Thus, the nature of the hallucinations was changing and becoming more controlling, indicative of Phase III described by Janice Clack. It must be added that P. did not advance further into the various remaining phases as a result of the therapeutic relationship she and I had developed. P. seemed to want to exercise and/or regain control of herself. She had not given up forming or wanting to form satisfying relationships with real people in favor of the hallucinations—unlike some of the more chronically institutionalized patients one sees lining the walls of state hospitals today. In fact, two episodes during the course of P.'s hospitalization—one episode in which she eloped from the hospital, went to a tavern, was picked up by two men, and then submitted to sexual advances; and the other episode in which she left the hospital with a fellow patient to get inebriated at a local tavern—although demonstrating the inappropriateness of P.'s actions and her apparent lack of ego controls also revealed that on both occasions the patient went out to have "fun" and "try to lose the voices," as she related. One can interpret this behavior as Sidney Levine does in *The Meaning of Despair*, " . . . Many patients seek relief from depression by acting out sexual impulses."[5:371] There seems to be a parallel here between Levine's statement and the patient, who attempted to seek relief from the constant bantering, persecutory, and accusatory voices by engaging in rather tenuous relationships with others.

If one looks at P.'s life in operational terms to understand the evolution of the hallucinatory experience, first the patient probably had feelings and thoughts that were disapproved of by significant others in her life resulting in the formation of the bad-me personification. These negative standards and appraisals were next incorporated by the patient. Sometime later in her life she experienced one of these disapproved feelings causing a rise in her anxiety level to severe proportions. If she could not handle the anxiety via healthy security mechanisms, pathological ones came into play. When the mechanisms worked effectively she was free from the disapproved occurrence, thought, or feeling in that it had been adequately banned from awareness with a subsequent decrease in anxiety. But, gradually, the dissociated content continued to appear in disguised forms—that is, hallucinations.[6:138]

For the purpose of example, I would now ask the reader to focus back into the childhood of P. when she was two years of age upon the occasions of her father beating her. Hypothetically, this two-year-old child probably expressed anger by perhaps hitting back, kicking, saying "No" to him. Now, it must be remembered that shortly after this, the father abandoned his wife and children. The departure probably engendered a great deal of anxiety and guilt in the child, for her unconscious wish to kill father, in her child's mind, had been attained. Hence, any future expression of hostile feelings, actions, or thoughts—which seemingly had been so destructive and overpowering to effect father's disappearance and/or death—became forbidden and never ventilated or displayed directly by P. because of their potential for devastation.

Whenever feelings of anger toward parents, husband, or children entered awareness in the adult P., anxiety and guilt concomitantly arose and her usual methods of coping with the anxiety: (1) confession of her wrongdoings/thoughts to an authority confessor figure; (2) repression; (3) substitution of happy, pleasant, unrelated thoughts and feelings for the anxiety-provoking ones; and (4) fabrication of fantasies—no longer proved effective in decreasing the anxiety such that, hallucinations ensued.

Furthermore, "a hallucinating patient is generally unaware of the dissociated, disintegrating, unconscious material. When it bursts through into awareness, it produces anxiety; it seems foreign; it is 'not-me.' "[4:17] A most fitting example of this from interaction with P. occurred in relation to an hallucination she was experiencing in which she was "told" that she had inflicted harm upon her children. Whereupon, after relating this to me, she immediately added, "I would never do those things to my children. I would kill myself first. I love my children. It's *them* voices!" One could say the voices were representative of a rigid, punishing superego. P. seemed to have had little opportunity to freely express her feelings towards the significant others in her life as evidenced by the parents' use of physical rather than verbal discipline meted out to P. during the course of her life. It is noteworthy that whenever I interpreted or labeled an affectual display, which the patient exhibited when talking about her parents and which obviously was fraught with much hostility, as "anger" the patient immediately denied this threatening interpretation but would ask immediately afterward, "Do you get angry with your parents?" This response is reminiscent of a child who seeks and tests for the reassurance of a parent for possession of hostile feelings. At times I had the impression that P. was asking for permission to safely express these pent-up feelings of hostility without fear of condemnation or retaliation by me.

It is most significant to comment that P. could not differentiate thought content of the auditory hallucinations from actions and oftentimes she would believe that the hallucinations were facts and had meaning for her in reality. But, since she was convinced that the hallucinations were not-me, she could not be held responsible for her "evil thoughts/actions/feelings." One can see then that the voices were of social significance to P. in that she dissociated the voices from belonging to herself and so she became socially inculpable of any enactment of the voices' demands. For example, if the voices told her, "You are a whore," and the patient then proceeded to engage in endless promiscuous activity, she might, for awhile at least, believe she had no responsibility for her actions but rather the voices, which she perceived as external to herself, would be the culprits.

Another social function that the hallucinatory behavior served for P. was to ward off loneliness. From the "visions" experienced at the age of eight and in adulthood where the patient heard the holy voices "singing songs to me" two months prior to hospitalization, it appears that the hallucinations provided her with a fantasy world of "loving" others away from her world of loneliness where she described herself as "starved for love." The patient described two other visual hallucinations she experienced prior to entering the hospital. One was of a "holy man with a bald head and a kind face who kissed me" and another of a "man burned in the fires of hell who came to give me comfort"—which, by their described loving and comforting natures, one must seriously consider the need for contact and tenderness. That is, for P. these hallucinations served a need for interpersonal intimacy. Therefore, this woman, who as a child was lonely and resorted to substitute satisfactions in fantasy did not fully as an adult, " . . . despite the pressures of socialization and acculturation . . . sufficiently learn to discriminate between realistic phenomena and the products of (her) own living fantasy."[7: 4]

As evidenced from the brief developmental history presented earlier, P. probably experienced loneliness which in a Sullivanian sense can be described as an extremely uncomfortable experience connected with an insufficient discharge of the need for human closeness. For Sullivan, real loneliness in infancy appears as a need for contact. P. stated that her mother rarely cuddled or held her but was too busy with the other children. Might not this early deprivation of maternal tenderness have planted the seed of loneliness within this patient? According to Sullivan, in childhood the need extends to adult participation in activities. As previously stated, the patient's father was frequently out of the home and the mother was "busy" and likely not free to engage with the patient in any expressive play activities so that P. was deprived of learning . . . "how to express emotions by successes and failures in escaping anxiety or in increasing euphoria; in various kinds of manual play in which one learns coordination, and so on; and finally in verbal play—the pleasure giving use of the components of verbal play speech which gradually move over into the consensual validation of speech."[2:261]

After the orphanage experience, P. reportedly quit school, started to drink, and began engaging in sexually acting-out behavior. In these ways the patient seemed to have been attempting to satisfy the need, of which Sullivan speaks, for an interpersonal relatedness with a fellow human being to gain a sense of personal satisfaction and security. That is, not having had her need for contact and freedom from interpersonal loneliness ever met from infancy onward, the patient resorted during her teen-age years to socially unacceptable ways, knowing little else. Her unbearable need for interpersonal intimacy culminated in her marriage, but the need was met only momentarily until the time her husband became abusive and unfaithful to her. The children provided her with some comfort but only sporadically because the patient was such a deprived child herself, who saw her children as "my dollies that I used to play with." The patient's later extramarital relationships plus the two elopements from the hospital represent her reaching out to anyone—strangers—and anything—alcohol—in an attempt to search out a loving, caring relationship that would provide her with safety from loneliness despite how transient the relationship. By these examples, one can see that loneliness played an important role in the genesis of P.'s mental disorder.

When Sullivan points out that people will even resort to any anxiety arousing experiences in an effort to escape from loneliness, even though anxiety itself is an emotional experience against which people fight, as a rule with every defense at their disposal, one can perhaps see parallels with P. whose hallucinations, at least early in their development, served as defenses against loneliness! The hallucinations not only have social significance for the patient but also dynamic significance as well.

When one examines P.'s hallucinations in a dynamic context, it becomes apparent that they contain elements of a triple wish as Freud had posited. There is the pleasure-seeking, libidinous wish; an aggressive wish exists and; an undoing of the erotic/aggressive components as expressed by a punishment component. The content of most of P.'s hallucinations consisted of primary process (Id) preoccupations where the voices told her to engage in all kinds of sexual pleasures with others so that, here the voices served to fulfill an unconscious libidinous wish. The hallucination in which the patient was told to "urinate in people's mouths," illustrates one way in which the hallucination is symptomatic of an unconscious aggressive wish. The patient related this very hallucination during a meeting immediately after I had attempted to structure the patient's activity, which was not in accordance with her wants at the moment. This demonstrated P.'s attempt to tell me in the language of "schizophrenese" that she was angry with me and not in agreement. The patient could only relate such "forbidden" feelings via the hallucination and not on a more direct communication level. In like fashion she could only tolerate talking lucidly about her parents for brief intervals and then would say that the voices told her to put "my bottom in God and the Blessed Virgin Mary's faces." This translated communication meant that P. was telling her parents, as signified by God and the Virgin Mother, to kiss her *derriere*—a most aggressive wish indeed! The hallucinations, centered on harming her children, are also a reflection of her aggressive wishes toward them. Once her husband could not come to visit her because, "He had to see the kids in the homes. The kids are more important to him than me. No one gives a damn for me!" This example provides some indication of the aggressive competitiveness she had felt with her children for her husband's attention.

The hallucination is symptomatic of a third wish as well—that of undoing the erotic/aggressive components through punishment. This was displayed in the example just cited in that, after P. expressed that her children were more important to her husband than herself, she experienced increased anxiety as evidenced by her outward restlessness as well as by the content of the voices. The voices then said she was not a good mother to her children and that the children were better off without her. The patient then stated that she believed the children were more important than herself and that her husband *should* be visiting them instead of her. Thus, one can see how an hallucination can consist of a punishment component as well. It is interesting to note that P. perceived the later developed and more "disgusting" hallucinations as punishments for her "sins," and for her entire life stating, "I was born to be punished; my life's been so rotten that I think God chose some people to suffer all their lives with no love." These statements are representative of the patient's need for self-punishment. And, an interesting side note to this is that, according to Sandor Rado, self-punishment is a way of winning love. "It is an expiatory act, a plea for forgiveness for the attack of rage (that is, aggressive wishes harbored toward significant others) in order to reconcile with the mother, toward whom the depressed person is still resentful for the deprivations suffered from the mother."[8:98] So, in a way, when P. stated, "God chose some people to suffer all their lives with no love," she was speaking of herself and the self-punishing aspect of the hallucinations is, in Rado's terms, a means of achieving love from the mothering one. Thus, the hallucinatory behavior pattern is a manifestation of a person's mental suffering and indicates often times a desperate need for help.

With these understandings of the social and dynamic significance of the behavior for the individual and the possible developmental processes contributing to the person's utilizing such problematic behavior, what then is the nurse's role in relation to the patient's behavior? Gravenkemper cites:

. . . The patient who hallucinates has a strong need to believe in the reality of the hallucination . . . The patient will not begin to doubt the reality of the hallucination until the need that the hallucination is fulfilling has begun to be met in some other way. To discover the purpose of the hallucination and to satisfy the need in another way are the functions of the nurse . . . .[1:186]

Arteberry adds:

. . . The need may be for dependence or to be rejected, or it may be a more personalized need such as for reassurance, self-esteem, acceptance. The nurse should be alert to these cues of needs, and should provide for means to meet them, if meeting them seems to be the therapeutic goal.[9:35]

For the nursing intervention then, the nurse must first know the purpose(s) which the hallucinatory process serves for the patient. That is, she must know the need(s) the hallucinations meet before she can satisfy the need(s) in other ways. In the case of P. the need was to escape from loneliness and rejection and to obtain some degree of interpersonal intimacy. With this understanding then, the first step in working with the patient is to begin establishing an interpersonal relationship with her. In this way, the nurse's "love" toward the patient as exemplified by the nurse's "recognition of the patient as a total being (hallucinations and all) with acceptance and no strings attached,"[10:165] would help the patient escape from loneliness, the subjective state of illness most productive of psychic pain. In such a relationship, the patient would be given the opportunity to begin to develop trust and closeness with the nurse in her capacity as a benevolent, non-punishing authority figure. But, the nurse must be cautioned not to encourage too much dependency of the patient upon her, especially where the patient's ego strengths are tenuous as in the schizophrenic and the patient may strive to engage in therapy beyond the need for such intervention.

Once the patient is provided with a reliable relationship with the nurse, he may no longer need to burst through the particular dissociated material, which the hallucination arouses, because, the patient will have "lost" the hallucination in favor of more interpersonal and more reality-based situations. With the hallucinating patient, the nurse requires an understanding of interpersonal techniques she can use in handling the hallucinations. Foremost, the nurse should recognize and acknowledge the feeling (affectual) tone behind the patient's experience of the voices—to the patient directly—in order to convey to the patient her understanding for what it must be like to be hearing voices, seeing visions, feeling crawling objects, and so forth. For example, when P. related she was hearing "a thousand of my voice," the nurse, after also noting the panicked expression on the patient's face and her agitated, restless body movements, should say, "I can see you are frightened by the voices you seem to be hearing so I will stay with you now."

Secondly, the nurse should be alert to not only the verbal but also the non-verbal cues (for example, the patient moving his lips, or placing his head to the side as though listening intently) that the patient is experiencing hallucinations. In this way, the nurse can use such observations to elicit the patient's descriptions of the hallucination. The rationale for this nursing measure is based on the guiding principle t..at, "whenever the patient is anxious, the nurse assists the patient with the recognition and naming of the anxiety in order to initiate the patient's learning and/or problem solving."[11: 311] The hallucination is an example of a dissociated perception by the patient of his own anxiety so that, by questioning the patient and eliciting observation and description of the hallucination, the nurse helps to bring this aspect of the situation into the patient's perceptual range. As in the case of P., by encouraging description of the hallucination in its fullest context—the thoughts, feelings, and actions attendant with it—the nurse can help the patient to differentiate between thought, feeling and action in reality. At times P. believed the hallucinations were fact, and she required frequent pointing out that the hallucinations did not necessarily have basis for her in reality.

Thirdly, as Grosicki and Harmonson point out, the nurse must present reality to the patient by simply pointing out to the patient that she, the nurse, does not experience the hallucination. In doing this, the nurse must be very careful not to deny the existence directly of the hallucinations since, for the patient, the "voices" are very real. The nurse must avoid conveying to the patient that she believes the voices are real or that she hears them too. She does this by using such terms as, "the voices *you* say *you* hear."[12] By so doing, the nurse refrains from entering into the psychotic process with the patient; nor does she reinforce the hallucination's reality for the patient. Rather, the nurse consensually validates what is real in her sensory awareness. In this way, according to Clack, doubt and question is raised regarding the reality of the hallucination without directly denying the patient of its reality. The nurse attempts to introduce her own reality in lieu of the reality which the hallucination has for the patient.

Fourthly, the nurse should provide protection when needed to prevent patient self-injury or injury to others in the environment if the hallucinations are accusing, frightening, or commanding the patient to harm himself or others.

Fifthly, as Grosicki and Harmonson further state, the nurse should respond verbally to anything that is real that the patient talks about in an effort to reinforce reality away from the hallucinatory experience. Another help for the nurse is to avoid non-verbal approaches such as shaking her head, gesturing with her hands that may add to the patient's hallucination. The nurse should ask the patient to let her know when the auditory or visual hallucinations intrude into his conversation with the nurse so the nurse can attempt to structure the conversation to some topic of interest to the patient in his immediate environment—that is, in reality. Another guide for the nurse is to help the patient focus on and identify current situations and/or people that evoke anxiety and lead to hallucinatory development. It is the nurse's task to identify the triggering mechanism of the hallucination if one indeed exists. Peplau comments:

. . . Counseling in nursing has to do with helping the patient to remember and to understand fully what is happening to him in the present situation, so that the experience can be integrated with rather than dissociated from other experiences in life.[13 : 64]

A good example of this with P. would be for the nurse to help the patient realize the connection between going home on weekends, outside the protective hospital setting, and coming back to the hospital on the following Monday with an increase in the hallucinations, which the patient described as "harder to fight when I'm home." It would be helpful for the nurse and the patient to consider this "differentness" in the intensity of the hallucinations whenever the patient was placed in the family situation with all its conflicts for her. By looking at the home environment with the patient, the nurse can help the patient identify anxiety-arousing situations, which are particularly bothersome and contribute to an increase in hallucinatory activity, and so help the patient seek alternative, less anxiety-provoking methods of dealing with these situations.

As the nurse continues to work with the hallucinating patient, she should gradually increase social interaction in the patient's environment. That is, by introducing others into the patient's interpersonal world by moving from one person (the nurse) to small group activities such as conversation groups, or games, such as cards, ping-pong, to interaction with larger numbers of people (patient government groups; and eventually perhaps some form of group therapy) as the patient is able to tolerate this, the nurse is, according to Clack, assisting the patient in increasing his interpersonal relationships and identifying other helpful means of satisfying his persistent needs for interpersonal closeness.

It is well for the nurse to remember that there may be and probably is more than one underlying problem deriving from a single need, as in P.'s case. Eventually the nurse in working with the patient may move to help the patient see the linkage between the hallucinatory experience and the need(s) that it serves. As Clack observes, the nurse and patient may discuss the outcomes of using the hallucination to meet the particular need, but the patient may not recognize all aspects of the hallucination so that some of the learning and self-integration involved in abandoning the hallucination are outside the patient's awareness.

Some other objectives the nurse must consider in working with the hallucinating patient but which are not directly related to dealing with the hallucinations *per se* are the following: (1) to provide greater alleviation of the hallucinations—that is, the anxiety—through prescribed dosages of medication in order to decrease this anxiety to workable levels which allow the patient to engage more psychotherapeutically with the nurse; (2) to consider the possibility of entering the patient into a group experience within the hospital and perhaps eventually on an outpatient basis, which would be conductive to the patient's forming new relationships to help replace overwhelming feelings of loneliness and gain new insights into self. In this way, the patient can gain group support, which if adequate, can lead to an increase in self-love and esteem by the patient and an elimination of the intense loneliness; (3) to enlist family cooperation into the patient's treatment plan. This would be accomplished by having meetings with the spouse primarily, and perhaps other family members in order to provide some educative measures regarding the patient's illness so they may come to understand the behavior more clearly. Eventually the patient and spouse may be involved in some form of counseling whereby lines of communication between them could be improved. In this way, continuity of treatment which originated in the hospital with the nurse could be effected into the home setting.

By way of summary, this paper has been concerned with a patient's problematic behavior pattern, namely hallucinations. The social and dynamic significance of the behavior for the individual have been explored and analyzed and a formulation of possible developmental processes influencing the patient to utilize hallucinations has been discussed. On the basis of these analyses, formulations for a psychiatric nursing treatment plan of intervention have been presented.

In conclusion, it is well to bear in mind that the schizophrenic patient, who is hallucinating, is striving to communicate in as clear and straightforward a way as he knows, the nature of his anxieties and experiences, despite how radically different they are from the nurse's, with speech content that is difficult to follow. Thus, with this understanding, it behooves us as nurses to intervene accordingly and "decode" the hallucinated messages and thereby assist in breaking into the third stage in the evolutionary cycle of a psychosis, as cited by R. D. Laing: Stage 1 = Good (me); Stage 2 = Bad (me); Stage 3 = Mad (not me).[10 : 131]

References

1. Gravenkemper, Katherine H.: "Hallucinations," *Some Clinical Approaches to Psychiatric Nursing*, edited by Shirley F. Burd and Margaret A. Marshall. New York: The Macmillan Company, 1963, pp. 184–188.

2. Sullivan, Harry Stack: *The Interpersonal Theory of Psychiatry.* New York: W. W. Norton and Company, 1953.
3. Sullivan, Harry Stack: *Conceptions of Modern Psychiatry.* New York: W. W. Norton and Company, 1953.
4. Clack, Janice: "An Interpersonal Technique for Handling Hallucinations," in Monograph No. 13, *Nursing Care of the Disoriented Patient.* New York: The American Nurses' Association, 1962, pp. 16–26.
5. Levine, Sidney: "Some Suggestions for Treating the Depressed Patient," in *The Meaning of Despair,* edited by Willard Gaylin. New York: Science House, Inc., 1968, pp. 353–386.
6. DeAugustinis, Jane: "Dissociation and Memory Gaps," *Some Clinical Approaches to Psychiatric Nursing,* edited by Shirley F. Burd and Margaret A. Marshall. New York: The Macmillan Company, 1963, pp. 137–142.
7. Fromm-Reichman, Frieda: "Loneliness," *Psychiatry,* XXII (1959), pp. 1–16.
8. Rado, Sandor: "Psychodynamics of Depression from the Etiologic Point of View," in *The Meaning of Despair,* edited by Willard Gaylin. New York: Science House, Inc., 1968, pp. 96–107.
9. Arteberry, Joan K.: "The Disturbed Communication of a Schizophrenic Patient," *Perspectives in Psychiatric Care,* III (1965), pp. 24–37.
10. Laing, R. D.: *The Divided Self.* Baltimore: Penguin Books, 1960.
11. Burd, Shirley F.: "Effects of Nursing Intervention in Anxiety of Patients," *Some Clinical Approaches to Psychiatric Nursing,* edited by Shirley F. Burd and Margaret A. Marshall. New York: The Macmillan Company, 1963, pp. 307–322.
12. Grosicki, Jeanette P. and Harmonson, Marguerite: "Nursing Action Guide: Hallucinations," *Journal of Psychiatric Nursing and Mental Health Services,* VII (May-June, 1969), pp. 133–135.
13. Peplau, Hildegard E.: *Interpersonal Relations in Nursing.* New York: G. P. Putnam's Sons, 1952.

15 COMMUNICATING WITH DEPRESSED PERSONS

Ardis R. Swanson, Ph.D., R.N.

SADNESS, HOPELESSNESS, DEJECTION, EMPTINESS, A
FEELING OF LOW self-esteem—these are the affective content of
depression. Readily communicated by body language and other non-
verbal behavior, their natural tendency is to drive others away. When the
helping person is alert to the content of the non-verbal communication,
he can be less put off by it, and can utilize it to detect a depressive state.

Depression is not neatly confined to "reactive depression," "manic-
depressive psychosis," or some other medical or psychiatric nosology.
Indeed, depressions appear in all areas of practice. On occasion we encounter an acute or crisis-type depression, but more often we see it in-
termingled with physical illness or complicating convalescence. If we
were more observant, we would detect its presence more readily and
recognize how often it inhibits full and meaningful living.

Therapeutic communication with depressed persons requires both a
theoretical and practical foundation. Depression originates as a loss—
whether an actual loss of a love object, or through emotional detachment
of the significant adult with whom an immediately gratifying communication might have existed. The treatment of depression includes the use of
one's self in communication, for it is through communication that the
depressed person can see more clearly his withdrawal from life, and can
begin to make investments in new relationships. Correction by interpersonal means requires that the helping person have a conceptualization of

From *Perspectives in Psychiatric Care*, Vol. XIII, No. 2, 1975, pp. 63–67. Reprinted with
permission from Nursing Publications, Inc., 194-B Kinderkamack Rd., Park Ridge, New
Jersey 07656.

the self-system, anxiety, hostility, manipulation, aversion to influence and gratification. Also, an awareness that characteristically the depressed person bids for help yet avoids it permits the helping person to deal more openly and constructively with feelings of manipulation and irritation provoked by the depressive.

Problematic Non-Verbal Messages

In an "affective" disorder, such as depression, the person feels inappropriately sad or dejected, low in self-esteem, bored, or empty. These feelings are readily and inadvertently communicated non-verbally through such signs as the tone of voice and body posture. Consequently, depressed persons are not the most comfortable people in the world to be around. When in the presence of a depressed person, one need not be surprised at suddenly feeling low, irritable, or somewhat hostile. Depressed persons do not stimulate a zest for living, nor imbue a spirit of loving kindness toward others. (Sullivan, 1956)

When depression is subtle, one's own feelings may be the first cue that the other person is depressed. The communication of depressed persons is therefore excellent in one sense; namely, the efficiency with which messages of dejection, hopelessness, or underlying anger get through to another. In lay terms, his actions speak louder than words. Even in silence the person "cannot *not* communicate," an axiom in communication theory. (Wazlawick, 1967).

Some persons are more susceptible or vulnerable than others to messages of depression. Depression in another often triggers one's own latent feelings of depression. This phenomenon can be truly problematic to health care personnel, and accounts for the inability of some to work with depressed persons. On the other hand, it is doubtful that any person is thoroughly immune to catching a bit of the feeling of a depressed person. Seeds of depression appear to be part of the human condition, and are readily planted in another.

Despite the knowledge that a great deal of communication occurs non-verbally, much of it remains at the periphery of our awareness. Some of the more obvious non-verbal cues one does observe in the depressed person are the slow movement (of the large joints, especially), poor posture, monotonous quality of the voice, and a somewhat non-mobile facial expression. Other messages which may escape direct verbal communication are fatigue and bodily aches and pains. Of course, these symptoms may have an organic cause, but it is also possible that they may mask a depression. (Chrzanowki, 1959)

Problematic Verbal Messages

Verbal and non-verbal messages are so interrelated that any attempt to single one out from the other is an artificial separation. Yet, it is useful to focus momentarily on the characteristic verbal content for its value in understanding and intervening in depression. Though illustrations in this article are drawn from my own experience with clients in a psychiatric-mental health setting, the same phenomena can be vividly observed in non-psychiatric settings. For example, there is a characteristic reduction in the person's total verbal output. The content expressed once may be repeated without really adding anything new. There is a noteworthy paucity of detail about people and interpersonal relationships. For example, one client told the story of his life in a few sweeping sentences. Then, when asked about the people at the home where he lived for several years, he could neither name a single person nor could he tell about his relations with anyone. Instead, he gave a few details of the physical environment and activities he engaged in. "I told you the whole story," he would say in irritation.

Another characteristic of depressed persons' communication is the appeal, sometimes overt, sometimes subtle, to do things for them or to act on their behalf. They present themselves as unable, or unworthy persons, but "you" could provide for them. To illustrate:

Mr. R was overt and extreme in his bids for help. Wanting to get certain information from his physician, who was on the ward every day, he made several bids in one hour for me to ask the doctor questions. "You, nurse, you could do it . . . you could ask . . . better than I." The persistence in attempting to maneuver the nurse into a do-for-me position was illustrated in his closing statement: "When I see you Friday you'll have talked to the doctor." His concept of himself as being "unable" persisted for some time, and his brief narrations remained largely unpeopled during the few months that he was on the ward.

Dynamics of the Verbal Messages

Both the reduction in verbal output and the bids for help can be understood in light of early life communication. A loss or failure in adult life, real or perceived, inflicts a wound to any human being, but the depth of reaction differs according to one's self-view. Self-view, in turn, depends largely on the way one was responded to and appraised as a child. If a child is consistently responded to, and if he has received an abundance of positive appraisals, he has a better self-view and is better equipped to deal with losses in later life. Depression after such a childhood, if it appears at all, is not critically deep or long lasting. However, if attempts to reach out to others are met with minimal response, in later life losses or failures tend to confirm the earlier position.

For the depressed person with the less fortunate childhood, to talk freely, to take initiative in actions, to have influence, and to be gratified is inconsistent with his self-view and tends to elicit anxiety. His self-view does not permit him to see himself as having something worth saying or possibly having influence. Over a period of time, this view would generate a good deal of anger, but who is *he* to get angry? The result is depression—with anger repressed but active through a kind of unconscious, seductive manipulativeness and stubbornness.

In the depressive's characteristic bidding for help lies a seeming paradox: when he is offered suggestions (or interpretations in a therapeutic relationship), his hedging response indicates an aversion to being influenced. In part, it is his low self-view that interferes. To accept therapeutic help requires him to accept a more positive assessment of himself. In part, it is a passive-aggressive way to manipulate others, to express wariness of possible ulterior motives of others toward him, and is indicative of repressed anger.

As Sullivan wrote (p. 296), attempts to explore grief-provoking ideas tend to be brushed aside or met with irritation or anger. The depressed person fears open communication and intimacy. Basically, he fears anger. Through the complicated mechanisms of introjection and projection, he has come to fear both destroying and being destroyed.

For example, one of my clients was inclined to say "Yes, I guess that's right" to interpretations, but her other verbalizations and behavior revealed her response was effective in prematurely closing the issue, giving her room to think and act as before, and to retain her same self-view. Clearly, a restrictive self-view and its related affects are not altered quickly. For instance, when depression does begin to lift, the person is not inclined to acknowledge it, or to allow himself or others any gratification from the change. (Crumb, 1964)

According to Ruesch (1959), certain conditions promote the development of the depressive character. Persons who experience considerable depression have not allowed themselves gratifications and pleasures of the moment; instead, satisfactions are extrapolated to the future.

If parents emphasize end results rather than the pleasure of the moment, ideals and conscience grow to the detriment of skill. Such parents attach more importance to having succeeded . . . than to the acquisition of skills. Therefore, the youngster learns to anticipate and to extrapolate. . . . The goal of action is projected more and more into the future and becomes progressively more difficult to attain.

Ungratified, the person is ambivalent about gratifying others. The depressive does unto others what he experiences as having been done unto him.

Dynamics of Depression

The dynamic elements in depression, according to Bonime (1966) are: 1) manipulativeness (covering so-called dependency), 2) aversion to influence, and 3) unwillingness to give gratification. Bonime also lists hostility and anxiety as additional dynamic elements. Ruesch (1959) attributes the hostility in the depressive to the lack of synchronization of codification, and the inevitable frustration. He explains that the original lack of synchronization between goals, actions, and gratifications leads to a lack of synchronization between the verbal and non-verbal systems. Consequently, the depressed person's verbal and non-verbal systems do not match, giving the impression of "falseness." He compares the frustration of the depressed person with the frustration of the aphasic person. Similar to the aphasic, the depressive cannot speak words (digital-verbal codes) that match the thoughts and feelings (analogic-non-verbal codes).

The frustration and anger underlying the behavior of depressed persons can be viewed from at least two perspectives: as a re-activation of the frustrations at a very early age (the psychoanalytic view), or as a product of the current depressive situation (psychoanalytic-interpersonal view). Both views are useful and compatible with one another.

THE PSYCHOANALYTIC VIEW.   The psychoanalytic view of depression has been described by Abraham (1924), Freud (1917), and Klein (1934). Abraham explained the psychogenesis of melancholia (depression) as the failure to retain the original love-object "round whom, his whole emotional life revolved." (1966) Withdrawal of libido (psychic drive or energy) from the love-object was accompanied by detachment from interest in all the external world. Both love and hate were directed toward the original love-object, and "unable either to achieve a complete love or any unyielding hatred, he succumbed to a feeling of hopelessness." In the years that followed, every failure in attaining or retaining a love-object "brought

with it a state of mind that was an exact replica of his primal parathymia
. . ." (p. 118)

Spitz (1946) and Bowlby (1960), some years later, began to report their
systematic studies of losses and separations in infancy which produced
"anaclitic depression." The losses and separations experienced by infants,
however, are not limited to the physical loss of the mothering one, nor are
they always so severe that they produce an anaclitic-type depression.

PSYCHOANALYTIC-INTERPERSONAL VIEWS: The frustration and anger
of depression can be further understood by viewing it in light of the
person's current depressive situation. A failure to receive emotional
responses from anyone significant, or a failure of significant others to accept the child's spontaneity, can also lead to a depressive lifestyle. In both
the original and current situation, the person has failed to get response to
efforts at reaching out. Whether it be caused by physical separation or
emotional detachment, anxiety is aroused and communication patterns
are disturbed. In the words of Pearce and Newton (1963), "the pathology
in depression is centrally located in gross intimidation about genuinely
experiencing that which one could feel clearly. . . ." (p. 275)

In a circular fashion, failure at communication evokes anxiety and fear;
the more anxiety and fear, the more failure in communication. The person no longer dares to communicate and ultimately even fears to feel.

Dynamics of Communication in Treatment

Pearce and Newton say that the individual needs a new experience in
interpersonal communication for releasing the bonds of feeling and "using
this as a basis for expanding the horizons further." The therapeutic
problem with a depressed person lies initially in helping him notice his
general emotional flatness. As stated earlier, directly confronting the
person with his behavior may be met with irritability and denial of the behavior. Nevertheless, open affective response to the demanding maneuvers of depression has been used effectively by some clinicians such as
Mabel Cohen, Frieda Fromm-Reichmann, and Edith Jacobson, to name a
few.

By provoking the therapist to irritation, the depressed patient converts
anger against himself into anger toward another; a step toward losing his
anger altogether. On another level, however, provoking the therapist
may then "legitimize" his own anger (which is actually irrational) and give
him rational reason to be angry at the therapist who, after all, is angry at
him! On still another level, the therapist transferentially represents the
object of the patient's anger.

However, if the therapist provokes a depressed person's repressed anger too much, he may severely frighten and overwhelm him. If the patient can be helped to discover that the therapist is not frightened or intimidated by his anger, the experience of outwardly directing anger is useful to him. (Reusch) For example, Mrs. W's anger was near the surface. Any remark that confronted her with her pathology would evoke denial and the expression of further hostility. While Mrs. W feared the expression of anger, nevertheless she expressed it occasionally. The therapist's unruffled response to her during these periods was a profoundly new experience: it was "safe" to express anger and to talk about it. Neither she nor the therapist had been destroyed by her anger, as she had fantasized.

Also, depressed persons talk about various longings and frustrations in their life experience with someone to whom it is "safe" to talk. Verbalizations can be expected to be brief and general at first. Questions may need to be posed that elicit detail. Future depressive episodes will be averted if the original situation that imposed them is thoroughly explored. Working through the problem is facilitated by talking about origins in the context of present re-enactments.

The psychotherapeutic course involves a constant exploration of the emotional and interpersonal context in which the patient fights against use of his capacities, fights to exploit the resources of the therapist and others, struggles by self-paralysis against the enhancement of others, and punitively, angrily and provocatively attacks those who frustrate his maneuvers. (Bonime, 1966 p. 253)

The depressed person can also be given help in matching his verbal and non-verbal systems, a problem described earlier. Communication, in the approaches described earlier, provided the *means* of reaching therapeutic ends. Communication is also a gratifying experience in itself. During depression the person greatly needs human company and communication, despite the lack of interest the person may seem to have for either. Spiegel (1959) wrote, "The person with depression experiences a diminished impulse toward communication and despairs of attaining it, though *he longs for it*. . . . Communication is not only a psychobiological means, it is also an end. . . . a process whose fulfillment brings its own gratification." (pp.939–48) The depressed person needs help to realize life inside himself, and to make new attachments or commitments to life outside himself which he can enjoy in the present.

Bibliography

Abraham, Karl, "A Short Study of the Development of the Libido, Viewed in the Light of Mental Disorder," London: Hogarth Press, 1942, p. 527 in *On Character and Libido Development*—Six Essays by Karl Abraham (ed. Bertram D. Lewin), New York: W. W. Norton, 1966.

Bonime, Walter, "On Depression," *Contemporary Psychoanalysis*, Vol. 2, No. 1, 1966, p. 49ff.

Bowlby, John, "Separation Anxiety," *International Journal of Psychoanalysis*, Vol. XLI, 1960, p. 89ff.

Chrzanowski, Gerald, "Neurasthenia and Hypochondriasis," *The American Handbook of Psychiatry*, Vol. I (ed. S. Arieti), New York: Basic Books, 1959, p. 258ff.

Crumb, Frederick W., "A Behavioral Pattern of Depressed Patients," *Perspectives in Psychiatric Care*, Vol. II, No. 4, 1964, p. 40.

Freud, Sigmund, "Mourning and Melancholia" (1917), reprinted in *The Standard Edition of the Complete Psychological Works of Sigmund Freud*, Vol. XIV, London: Hogarth Press & the Institute of Psychoanalysis, 1957, pp. 43–58.

Klein, Melanie, "Contributions to the Psycho-Genesis of the Manic-Depressive States," 1937, reprinted in *Contributions to Psycho-Analysis*, 1921–1945, London: Hogarth Press, 1948, pp. 282–338.

Pearce, Jane and Saul Newton, *The Conditions of Human Growth*, New York: Citadel Press, 1963, p. 275.

Ruesch, Jurgen, *Disturbed Communication*, New York: W. W. Norton, 1959, p. 140.

Spiegel, Rose, "Specific Problems of Communication," *American Handbook of Psychiatry*, Vol. I (ed. S. Arieti), New York: Basic Books, 1959, p. 909ff.

Spitz, Rene and K. M. Wolf, "Anaclitic Depression: an Inquiry into the Genesis of Psychotic Conditions in Early Childhood, *The*

Psychoanalytic Study of the Child, Vol. II, New York: International Universities Press, 1946, pp. 313–342.

Sullivan, Harry Stack, *Clinical Studies,* 1956, pp. 296–297.

Wazlawick, Paul et al., *Pragmatics of Human Communication,* New York: W. W. Norton & Co., 1967, p. 51.

16 GUIDELINES FOR INTERVENTION IN AGGRESSIVE BEHAVIOR

Barbara H. Nissley, M.A., R.N.
and Nellie Townes

MANAGEMENT OF A PATIENT WHO IS PHYSICALLY OUT of control is a difficult task and a frightening experience for nursing staff who are not prepared to handle such a situation. Instinctive responses are usually inadequate and can result in injury to the patient and/or staff. Knowing when and how to use physical restraint is important, but only one component of a comprehensive management plan. This paper presents four aspects of dealing with the aggressive patient: guidelines for prevention of loss of control, approaches to the patient prior to restraint, management of the patient after restraint, and the effects of a violent patient on the rest of the patient group.

Among the most important factors in the therapeutic management of a patient who is striking out at others or objects in the environment are understanding of the patient's need for external control and awareness of one's own feelings. In this kind of situation, the patient is very frightened or very angry and may seem unable to stop himself. He may not be oriented to who you are or where he is. There may seem to be no definite target for his rage if he is reacting to internal and external stimuli which are not obvious to others. For these reasons, those involved with his care must view the behavior objectively and not respond as though the hostility is a personal attack.

©1977 by Barbara H. Nissley and Nellie Townes. The paper was written for this text. The authors wish to acknowledge the contributions of Deana Williams and Thomas Krejci.

The most effective techniques—and the safest—for dealing with assaultive behavior are adequate forethought and preparation, which may eliminate the need for dealing with it at all. Sometimes patients erupt into physical rage suddenly and unexpectedly, but most of the time there is adequate warning. Nurses need to be able to recognize and respond to signs of escalating anxiety, fear and loss of control. A patient's anxiety and fear will usually be lessened when he senses that those caring for him will respond calmly but firmly to help him control his impulses. The occurrence of violent behavior can often be prevented if all staff members are prepared to respond according to guidelines such as those presented below.

Guidelines for Prevention of Loss of Control

It is important to trust one's own feelings and judgement regarding a patient's behavior. If a patient's verbal threat to strike out or other expression of fear and poor impulse control makes you uneasy and distrustful of his potential to harm himself or others, the chances are good that limits need to be imposed immediately. The patient's behavior may be a direct message that he is afraid he cannot control his behavior and needs controls imposed from the outside. This may be evidenced by tense pacing, kicking at objects, provoking arguments, or making statements like "I feel like I'm going to hit something or somebody."

Initial intervention should be a calm, slow, verbal approach such as "Why don't you hit the wall instead," or "You are obviously upset and I want you to come with me to your room where we can talk about it." You may want to suggest that the patient accompany you to the gym where he can release some of his energy physically with a punching bag.

Whoever is directly involved with the patient at the time should have the authority to impose necessary controls. Staff do not need permission to initiate decisive action and a patient need not be overtly destructive before you employ whatever measures of control are warranted by the patient's behavior. Removing the patient quickly from the immediate environment by escorting him to his room or the unlocked quiet/seclusion room may help to decrease stimulation and thereby decrease the intense anxiety he feels. A *prn* medication order may be indicated to allow administration of a tranquilizer according to nursing judgment. If you hesitate in order to check out your judgment with someone else, you may lose the opportunity to apply controls before injury has occurred.

Although verbal interventions should always be tried first, keep in mind that attempts to talk to the patient may increase rather than decrease his anxiety and agitation. Sometimes a patient will simply be more stimulated by your attempts to reason with or calm him. This may be no reflection on your ability to communicate effectively with patients in general, but means the approach will not work in this situation. A high level of emotional arousal (be it fear, anger, or other emotion) decreases a person's ability to think clearly and respond to logic and reason. While it is important to try to talk with the patient and encourage him to express his feelings verbally rather than acting on impulse, be prepared to use other measures if talking does not work.

The following could be suggested to the patient in an attempt to prevent further escalation of behavior. "You might feel some relief if you were able to tell me what's bothering you" or "I realize it is difficult for you to talk about your feelings but try to remember that I am here to help you, not to judge you." In some instances it might even be suggested that the patient scream or rip up a telephone book to alleviate intense emotion. This may not be the ideal mode for expression of feeling but it has obvious advantages over head-banging or striking out and can often be effective in releasing enough pent-up tension to allow the patient to verbalize more effectively.

A patient's resistance to and denial of need for control does not mean your decision to impose control is wrong. A patient may resist your authority at the moment of his rage only to tell you later he was actually relieved by your decisive action. It is important not to personalize sarcastic remarks such as "Well, look who's telling me what to do. You can't even get your own act together;" or "Who'd want to talk to you anyway? I want to see a doctor." Initiating limits despite the patient's verbal attacks is very important in indicating to the patient that you *are* competent and able to help him.

You must make the decisions in order to remain in control of the situation. If you hesitate, change your mind, and avoid taking action when there is time to prevent an untoward incident, the patient will make the decision for you. By this time, he is in control even though his behavior may be out of control. It can be a terribly frightening experience for a patient to realize that the staff he has been told are there to protect him seem afraid to intervene when he needs that protection most.

At all times remain aware of your own reactions to and feelings about the patient's behavior. Objectivity and being in touch with your own responses are necessary ingredients in making proper judgments and initiating appropriate treatment. If you remain in control of your own feelings and behavior, you will communicate this sense of control to the patient, and this may strengthen his impulse control. But, when efforts to calm the patient and prevent assaultive behavior fail, immediate action is needed to minimize the threat of injury and destruction of property. You will be able to respond more confidently and effectively if you have discussed and practiced means of physical restraint beforehand. In the next section, we describe methods we have found most effective for approaching and restraining physically aggressive patients.

Approaching and Restraining the Patient

The way in which you approach the patient is of utmost importance. First, remove your glasses, watch, and any jewelry that may cause injury or get broken. Remain calm, speak low and slowly, but firmly, and move slowly. Address the patient by name, introduce yourself, and state your intentions "I'm going to escort you to your room/the seclusion room now". Try to remember that your goal is to decrease stimulation and fear in the patient, who will be very sensitive to any anxiety and fear evident in your behavior.

Use the least number of staff possible for necessary control when initiating your approach so that the patient will not panic. It is helpful for one staff member to be the designated person who is in charge of the staff's approach to prevent confusion or delay. Make sure that all staff has coordinated their effort by brief discussion prior to any contact with the patient. Decide who will restrain the patient's right arm, right leg, etc. and make sure the path to the room of your destination is clear and the door open. Don't underestimate the strength of a patient who is acting on such intense emotion; four strong staff members may be required to subdue a hundred-pound woman.

If you are alone, do not stand face to face with the patient, as he can strike you more easily in that position. Instead, approach from the rear and attempt to put the patient on the floor for better control by getting him off balance. When you are approaching a patient who is in possession of a potential weapon, hold a mattress in front of you and back him into a corner, or throw a blanket over him to render him less dangerous.

When handling the patient, hold firmly at the joints such as elbows, shoulders, and knees for best control. To unlock a hand grip, start by disengaging the thumb. Be careful not to place any part of your own body close enough to the patient's mouth to get bitten. Do not back off once you have initiated an action, but block a swing if necessary and continue to hold on. When you are walking with a patient do not break stride, as the momentum helps your control. If he is attempting to strike out, walk the patient backwards rather than forwards so that he is off balance and cannot get force into his swing.

Do not respond to the patient's accusations that you are hurting him by breaking your grip. Determine the credibility of the complaint by evaluating your actions, but be aware that this is a common tactic to induce guilt so that you will let go. Remain aware of your own feelings so that your judgment is not impaired.

Management of the Patient After Restraint

If, as we do, you employ a Quiet/Seclusion Room for patients who are out of control, it is imperative that all staff have an opportunity to discuss their reactions and opinions regarding this treatment. Ability to act in the patient's best interest in this type of emergency will be greatly influenced by personal feelings. A Quiet Room is often seen as a method of punishment by both staff and patients due to its austerity and isolation. When used sparingly and appropriately, however, it is a therapeutic tool which reduces the input of stimuli from the environment, thereby decreasing emotional arousal and impulsivity in the patient and giving him a chance to regain internal controls. If at all possible, this should be explained to the patient in simple and relevant terms whenever you isolate him from his environment.

The next step is removal of all potentially dangerous items from the patient, including jewelry, hair accessories, glasses, belts, shoes, matches, pocket contents and anything concealed in the hands. A body search is advised only if warranted, but we strongly emphasize the need to be thorough. Many times staff members, due to their anxiety, don't notice matches or broken pieces of glass, only to have the patient harm himself while "protected" from his environment. The message that this conveys to the patient about our concern and ability to help is hardly a positive one.

Retreating from a room once you have placed the patient in it can be as hazardous as getting there in the first place. Instruct the patient to remain on the floor or against the wall. Be sure that all staff are coordinated in their movements and back out in unison. Do not leave one person behind in the room and do not allow the patient to get between you and the door. When you are all out, lock the door while butting it with your foot or body to prevent reopening by the patient.

During the time a patient is in Seclusion there are procedures that should be followed by all staff who are caring for him. First and foremost, never enter the room alone. Two or more people should always enter together. Remember to stay between the patient and the door at all times and leave in unison. Make frequent trips to the door of the room to check on the patient and prevent the other patients from loitering around the door. Visit the patient frequently to provide human contact and reality testing. Always announce your intentions when entering the room ("I'm going to take your blood pressure now") and introduce yourself anew each time if necessary. *Never* ignore the patient.

When choosing items to be used in caring for the patient, do not bring glass items into the room. When serving meals, use plastic trays, dishes, forks and spoons. Food should be cut, the bread buttered before entering and cold, not hot liquids provided. Do not leave harmful items alone with the patient and supervise use of all items, taking them out of the room when you leave. Sometimes, as when the patient is very psychotic, it may be necessary for the patient to remain in the Quiet Room for an extended period of time. Then, frequent assessment of the patient's physical health is necessary. This includes an on-going evaluation of hydration, nutrition and elimination. These patients will usually require assistance in personal hygiene and grooming, important not only for maintaining physical health of skin, mouth, and hair, but also in maintaining self-esteem. Helping a patient in the Quiet Room with activities of daily living conveys our message of caring for him and his integrity as a person. If the patient is receiving psychotrophic medications and is very agitated or depressed, he may not be able to relate possible side effects he may be experiencing from these medications. Nursing care involves an on-going assessment of possible side effects such as orthostatic hypotension, urinary retention, and parkinsonian symptoms.

Each time you visit the patient, evaluate his ability to handle all items; if any are misused, do not return them to the room too soon again. If a meal is not eaten but is thrown, smeared or dumped instead, another full food tray should not be offered a short while later but, rather, a sandwich or other finger food. It is difficult for nursing staff to withhold food because it is associated with nurturing and deprivation, but it is important for all staff members to make appropriate decisions in this area. The patient's ability to handle a sandwich, his medication, and contact with other people should be evaluated carefully and often to determine the amount of internal control and capacity for appropriate behavior that is present. Your goal is to return the patient to his social environment as soon as possible.

Effect on the Rest of the Patient Group

When one patient on a unit becomes upset and loses control, the episode has a significant effect on all the other patients on that unit. Initially, they may be in danger, so the staff should remove them from the vicinity of the activity, out of the path to be used in escorting the patient, and preferably to the other end of the unit.

At first, all staff members may be needed to assist in subduing the patient. Once the situation is under control, however, at least one person should remain with the patient group to answer questions and offer reassurance. Due to the anxiety these patients feel about what is occurring, they may make small requests of the staff or stand near the door to the Quiet Room in an effort to gain attention. This frequently results in curt and irritable rejection by busy staff members involved in drawing up medication, making phone calls, or other activities. This response serves to increase the anxiety of the group and creates more problems, but can be avoided if someone offers the support and immediate attention needed by the other patients.

The questions usually asked by patients include, "What's going on?", What's wrong with him (patient)?" "Why is he in the Quiet Room?" and "What are you (staff) doing about this?" The group is frightened of what is happening, fearful not only for their safety but of their own potential for anger and loss of control. They frequently identify with the assaultive patient and wonder what would happen to them if they were involved in a similar situation.

It is best to answer the questions in a manner which increases the group's sense of security and reassures them most effectively. That is, by giving a *positive* response which emphasizes what the staff is doing to exert external controls and help the patient. For example, "We are helping him (patient) to control himself", "It is necessary for him (patient) to be in the Quiet Room now" or "He (patient) is upset and we (staff) are offering assistance" are possible responses. Patients need reassurance about their own control and an opportunity to express their feelings about what is going on in their community. Community meetings or small groups are appropriate forums where the use of the Quiet/Seclusion Room can be discussed by staff and patients.

Patients who lash out in physical rage at staff or their environment are asking for help—for therapeutic limits and controls on their behavior. They are unable to express their need verbally and so they act it out in an urgent and violent plea for assistance. As professionals in a hospital setting, we all have a responsibility to respond quickly, appropriately, and firmly.

Not to do so is to tell the patient that he is not safe in our institution and cannot trust us to help him regain the internal controls and insights into his behavior necessary to his mental health and successful functioning.

"TERMINATION" IN THE STUDENT-PATIENT RELATIONSHIP

Barbara Stankiewicz Sene, M. S., R. N.

THE WORD "TERMINATION" SEEMS INADEQUATE TO DESCRIBE THE process of ending an interpersonal relationship which, if truly meaningful, results in learnings that will survive, mature, and bear additional fruit. This opportunity for learning is available to both the nursing personnel whose work or study involves the development of a therapeutic relationship with a psychiatric patient and to the patients involved in such a relationship. Yet, although the discipline of psychiatry has described conceptual viewpoints about the termination phase of psychotherapy and has proposed techniques to be employed in it, nursing literature does not yield a parallel repertoire of content.

This deficiency is particularly serious in view of the widespread use of the one-to-one student-patient relationship in the teaching of psychiatric nursing. It therefore seems timely to present information which will assist both the instructor and the student of nursing with respect to the termination phase of the student's one-to-one relationship with a schizophrenic patient. The limitations of such a discussion are obvious: because of educational, economic, and social factors this termination is usually an arbitrary matter rather than an outgrowth of treatment, and for this reason reference to criteria for determining when a patient is ready to end a particular treatment relationship has been excluded.

From *Perspectives in Psychiatric Care*, Vol. VII, No. 1, 1969, pp. 39–45. Reprinted, with permission, from Nursing Publications, Inc., 194-B Kinderkamack Rd., Park Ridge, N. J. 07656.

Past Experiences and Current Attitudes

The approach to the termination of a relationship with a patient is, of course, influenced by the student's personal attributes and attitudes. Frequently, students come from a cultural background which de-emphasizes the sad and frustrating components of separation. To illustrate, consider the festive mood which is cultivated at such occasions as graduation banquets, farewell parties, and wedding receptions. Feelings of sadness may be recognized and mentioned, but people usually do not examine these feelings in depth or assist each other to place them in perspective. Denial, suppression, and repression are encouraged, with the result that few students learn to talk about separation. The cogency of their affective involvement and personal impressions, be they success, failure, confusion, or growth, colors the screen through which they examine termination phenomena.

It has been consistently noted that patients often experience a surge of anxiety when treatment ends. Students have the same reaction, and for both, the rise in anxiety is accompanied by the need to master the unpleasant circumstances generating distress. It follows that students and patients are especially receptive to learning at this time. Despite the limitations of previous communication habits and attitudinal positions, both are charged with the task of capitalizing upon the emergent tensions by extending and cementing the learnings achieved in the course of the relationship. No matter what circumstance necessitated the separation, it is the responsibility of instructor and student to convey toward personnel a vivid picture of their commitment to maximizing learning at this point in the relationship so as to minimize the possibility of having the patient abruptly discharged without opportunity for a final meeting or meetings with his student.

Outstanding Psychodynamics of Termination

In nursing literature, Nehren and Gilliam[1] have discussed concepts of separation anxiety and object loss in conjunction with termination. Because therapist and patient are human, both are subject to a reactivation of earlier emotional experiences associated with the separation and loss of meaningful persons. A second potent influence rises from the fact that the patient has invested his energy so as to obtain important personal assistance from an external source. He is now expected to give up his dependence upon the unique individual who offers assistance and concentrated interest. Expectations that he will relinquish dependent behaviors practiced in relation to a specific person and that the helping figure will no longer fulfill his dependent needs mobilize feelings of anger and apprehension. Although levels of consciousness vary, both parties may experience some resentment at the demand that they give up satisfying behavior patterns and may anticipate some kind of a void in their forthcoming life satisfactions. Each needs to mourn his respective loss. [2, 3]

Experiential Meanings and Manifest Behaviors of Patients

When a one-to-one relationship is concluded, the patient who is schizophrenic may realize several experiences on a preconscious, unconscious, or conscious level or on two or all three of these levels. To him, separation represents deprivation and hence an injury to the self. His internal impression of rejection or abandonment may leave him with a sense of worthlessness or vulnerability—"If I were worthy I would not be deserted"; "I can be hurt"; "I can control the things which hurt me." He may fear future hurts or loneliness and wonder if he did something to cause the separation.

The patient needs to mourn, for he is losing a special atmosphere in which he has begun to measure and even to know the degree of freedom he has for sharing and exposing his most important self. Then too, he is losing a defined opportunity to learn and fears he may not learn enough in the future. He may feel guilty for not always having worked and for harboring negative feelings about his therapist. Sometimes he feels envious of the fantasized others who will replace him in receiving the attention of his special nurse.

Although a patient's attention may be divided between termination of the relationship and practical concerns associated with staying or leaving, certain behavioral manifestations of an emotional reaction to the concluding meetings appear with great regularity. If the patient is leaving, it is likely that these behaviors reflect concurrent feelings about separation from the hospital and other treatment personnel; however, all circumstances have similar dynamics and elicit the same responses. It often happens that the student has the most time available for being with the patient and helping him. The first, and probably most frequent, behavioral manifestation to be seen is usually regression. Typically, the patient's anxiety level rises; earlier maladaptive actions recur; he acts out his conflict by missing meetings entirely or in part; he may reiterate doubts previously voiced regarding the value of having a one-to-one relationship.

A second group of behaviors can be organized under the rubric "withdrawal from the relationship." A patient may adopt the method of quick closure, overtly rejecting his student by demanding cancellation of all meetings. Absence from sessions is another form of quick closure. An equally effective method is for the patient to attend meetings in a body but to participate on an insultingly superficial level. He may indicate that the student is no longer needed, saying "My plans are complete," or, "Dr. X will talk with me." Another patient will bombard the student therapist with angry behavior and even obscenity, causing her to retreat from their interactions.

For the student, a more bearable form of withdrawal is the gradual ending. Here, the patient presents some clues that he is ready to begin the process of separation. He may talk symbolically about separation, perhaps relating a story about the time the family dog died. Less covertly, he may discuss past separations he has survived. An alert student will begin to notice less affect accompanying the patient's expressed thoughts. He gives diminished attention to genuine concerns, shifts from one problem area to another, or asserts independent abilities—for example, "I've got my budget all worked out this week," "When I get the next letter from my mother I'll be able to answer it on my own this time."

Lastly, a patient may signify his inability to terminate by maneuvering to intensify and prolong the relationship. He may show helplessness through asking questions, exposing major problems previously untouched, and manipulating the student to make decisions for him. Sometimes his giving of a gift represents an attempt to incur a sense of obligation. It may also mask a feeling of anger toward a student who will not acknowledge his wish that the relationship continue.

Experiential Meanings and Manifest Behaviors Common to Student Therapists

The feelings of the student therapist who is ending a nurse-patient relationship are similar to those of the patient. Once discovered, this fact may be alarming to the student. Frequently she finds it difficult to acknowledge, label, and share her own reactions. Her ability to do so is influenced by her past experiences with separation and by the extent to which the learning atmosphere hinders or facilitates such disclosures.

Typically, the student devalues her contributions and is pessimistic about the patient's condition and prognosis. Occasionally, a student will admit to a sense of satisfaction at her own or the patient's achievement. More frequently, however, the student's accomplishments are buried in a heap of frustrated goals. A sense of guilt at the shortcomings of her own performance and investment may be activated. She may also feel guilty over her relief that supervisory sessions and meetings with the patient will be discontinued. She laments her unachieved goals and the continuation of the patient's symptoms. She, like the patient, experiences loss, for she will no longer obtain satisfaction from meeting the patient's dependency needs or watching his growth. Too, she is losing an opportunity to learn more. Oftentimes the feeling of loss is reflected in an angry attitude toward the institution or situation which demands termination of her relationship with the patient. The anger may be focused on the instructor who represents the authority allowing the change to occur.

Since in our American culture little encouragement is given to examination of the harsher realities of separation, it is usually the influence of instructors or treatment personnel that assists the student to engage in this process. Infrequently a student will spontaneously voice her feelings or will find in the literature data which lead her to open a discussion of termination phenomena. Most often, the instructor identifies behavioral data that indicate it is time to help the student.

The student most in need of such help is the one who completely avoids the subject of leaving both with her instructor and with her patient. Another who needs assistance is the student who begins to extend the length or frequency of her meetings with the patient, or who clearly demonstrates her reluctance to terminate by requesting formal continuation of the experience. Some students become more generous in giving to their patients; for example, they may increase their supportive comments, make optimistic remarks regarding the patient's abilities or his future, or present concrete gifts—coffee and doughnuts, a picture, a farewell party. Finally, there is the angry student who displaces her anger concerning termination and vigorously complains about the institution's treatment program, specific treatment, personnel, or the learning program itself.

The first step toward a constructive termination of the nurse-patient relationship is to recognize the intense emotional components of the process. Once these have been identified in student and in patient, they usually become manageable, and the student can proceed to consider alternative measures to employ with patients.

Guidelines for Therapeutic Alternatives

The following listing of guidelines for therapeutic interventions has been compiled with the hope that each therapist will select the approaches best suited to her relationship with a given patient. The list is not all-inclusive, but the suggested measures have been tested and proved useful.

The single intervention which is essential to all terminations of therapeutic relationships with schizophrenic patients is to establish with the patient the realistic fact of the impending separation and the separation date. This announcement is made to preclude, or at least lessen, the possibility that the patient will perceive the separation as a casting away of his self. A more dispensable but potentially reinforcing maneuver is to clarify the circumstances which make separation necessary. The student may reiterate the terms of the initial student-patient contract (for example, regular meeting over a given period of weeks), or she may state that the patient's discharge or transfer to another ward requires that their sessions be concluded for administrative reasons. This clarification serves to minimize the possibility that the patient will distort the reason for the termination of encounters.

In the final phase of therapy, nursing action is needed to decrease the patient's dependency on the student and her involvement in this particular relationship. The actions which the student may take are multiple. She may decrease the frequency or the length of her meetings with the patient. If this method is used, it should be discussed with the patient, so that he may view it as part of the separation process and not as rejection. The student may change the setting for meetings to one less amenable to discussion of highly charged personal conflicts or emotions. Again, it is preferable that the reason for changing settings is made clear to the patient; otherwise the student runs the risk of having the patient ascribe social attributes to the entire relationship. Once the student discloses her rationale, the way is paved for her to move into another constructive maneuver. She may proceed to encourage the patient to transfer his loyalties from her to other persons. For the schizophrenic patient, who tends to avoid involvement in any kind of relationship, establishment of interpersonal relationships at any level can be considered an accomplishment. The student who motivates her patient to play cards with other patients, to pursue a project in occupational therapy, or to enter into a therapeutic relationship with another staff member has been instrumental in furthering patient growth.

These therapist-initiated or therapist-cultivated methods to decrease patient dependency become unwieldy when the patient maneuvers to intensify the relationship and brings new problem areas to the student's attention. When this happens, the student's responsibility is to recognize the significance of the problem openly. Then, either she may redirect the patient toward attacking the problem with the help of another person, or she may support mental mechanisms which allow the patient to cope with his present situation.

As has been stated, the tension associated with termination can be used to extend and cement the learnings the student has achieved during the series of meetings with the patient. A touching and satisfying way to further such learning is for student and the patient to exchange verbally their memories of their shared experiences and feelings. I have found that a student generally expects her schizophrenic patient to spontaneously pour forth a description of the feelings he has had in his course of therapy and, if such a disclosure is not forthcoming, will attempt to elicit one with the over-used approach, "How do you feel about . . .?" This question may lead to an exchange of feelings, but unfortunately, the schizophrenic patient's notorious difficulty in recognizing and labeling his personal experience usually inhibits such a process. Instead, the student receives either no clear response or a gush of positive assertions which reflect the patient's view of what he should say in order to fulfill the expectations of the therapist student or the hospital system.

Another potentially useful approach is for the student to begin the exchange of affect and memories, thus serving as a model for thoughtful and genuine introspection. Prior to such action, it is again necessary that the student discuss her plan, feelings, and purpose with her instructor. If she does not utilize preceptory assistance at this point, she runs the risk of magnifying some of her own distortions and meeting her personal needs, excluding needs of her patient. Further, it is probable that objective discussion with an experienced person helps the student to develop a sound plan for approaching her patient.

The matter of exchanging memories deserves elaboration. One purpose of this action is to help the patient to remember the relationship as it actually was, including both the difficult and the satisfying aspects. Another purpose is to consolidate patient progress. In response to cues from the patient which indicate that he is ready to profit from a discussion of memories, the student may foster a review of how she and the patient spend time together, including a discussion of the gross areas they talked about in sessions and ways in which the patient has changed. Most patients, it might be hoped, emerge from such a review with a positive evaluation of therapy.

The student can encourage a favorable attitude by giving attention to the positive aspects and continuities in her treatment. In doing so she should not negate or disregard the patient's criticisms or complaints, for this behavior on her part would convey a serious lack of understanding. The more sensible policy is for her to acknowledge existing dissatisfactions and emphasize realistic gains. When a patient seemingly recognizes his improved grasp of troublesome areas, the student should help him to appreciate his own accomplishment. In so doing, she strengthens the patient's self-image as a person with potential for correction.

Another task of the therapist is to help the client to anticipate post-separation time. Typically, a schizophrenic patient has difficulty conceptualizing change in his daily time schedule. It appears that he either represses ideas pertaining to termination or thinks about termination in an abbreviated fashion. If no one attempts to influence his thoughts toward entertaining a clear picture of his future reality, he frequently experiences high levels of post-termination anxiety, as can be documented by numerous instances of patients who eloped, became assaultive, or had violent outbursts of anger, hallucinations, or delusions immediately following a student's departure. The student is responsible for helping her patient to anticipate differences in his life situation so as to lessen the possibility of massive regression.

Prior to giving this help to the patient, a student therapist must seriously examine the rationale for her policies regarding phone calls, letters, and future meetings. The traditional position is that there will be no meetings between student and client following their formal separation. This position is, of course, unrealistic if student and patient are likely to have chance encounters in the community. In such instances the student may acknowledge that such a possibility exists and explain that any interchange would be social in nature. Female students who are terminating relationships with male patients may be asked to date. They generally answer negatively and shunt responsibility for the decision to another authority—"My instructor doesn't think it's a good idea," "It's against hospital rules." If a student uses such an evasion, she blocks discussion of questions with potentially greater import for the patient. He may really be asking, "Would you or other women see me as a desirable escort?" or, "I want to date. Help me learn social limits." He may also be testing a nurse's professional integrity. In any case, preceptory assistance is needed if the student is to avoid rejecting her patient and to deal successfully with his genuine concerns.

In anticipating post-separation time, the student can guide the patient into planning for the future use of the time that has been given to the one-to-one meeting. Such planning protects the patient from feeling a sudden void when the usually scheduled hour is empty. When the patient is the one who is leaving the student, discussion may be centered on his goals for future treatment or on other sources of help. In the case of discharge, a review of the signs of approaching illness may help a patient to seek treatment quickly if he finds himself relapsing.

In conclusion, several points deserve to be underlined. First, not every student or every patient can become equally involved in working through separation phenomena; the quality of participating varies according to both parties' readiness and capacity for closeness. Second, special circumstances may arise (a death on the ward, a tragedy in the patient's family) which require that the student give attention to the new area and only touch upon the conclusion of the one-to-one relationship. Finally, it seems reasonable to expect that new approaches to psychotherapy will give rise to additional methods of teaching psychiatric nursing. In particular, the current trends toward telescoping the entire therapeutic process demand disciplined study of termination phenomena and preceptory relationships.

References

1. Nehren, Jeanette, and Naomi R. Gilliam, "Separation Anxiety," *American Journal of Nursing* 65: 109–112, Jan., 1965.
2. Schultz, Frances K., "The Mourning Phase of Relationships," *Journal of Psychiatric Nursing* 2:1 37–42, Jan., 1964.
3. Thaler, Otto F., "Grief and Depression," *Nursing Forum* 5:2: 8-22, 1966.

Bibliography

Bowlby, John, "Separation Anxiety: A Critical Review of the Literature," *Journal of Child Psychology and Psychiatry* 1:351–269, 1961.

Castelnuovo-Tedesco, Pietro, "The Twenty Minute Hour; An Experiment in Medical Education," *New England Journal of Medicine,* 266:6: 383–89, Feb. 8, 1962.

Chrzanowski, Gerard, "Termination in Psychoanalysis," (Goals and Technical Principles Evolving from Sullivanian Conceptions) *American Journal of Psychotherapy* 14: 48–62, 1962.

Hale, Shirley L. and Julia H. Richardson, "Terminating The Nurse-Patient Relationship," *American Journal of Nursing* 63: 116–119, Sept. 1963.

Hiatt, Harold, "The Problems of Termination of Psychotherapy," *American Journal of Psychotheray* 19, 4: 6–7–615, October, 1965.

Keith, Charles, "Multiple Transfers of Psychotherapy," *Archives of General Psychiatry* 14: 2: 185–19, Feb., 1966.

Pumpian Mindlin, E., "Comments on the Techniques of Transfer and Termination in a Clinical Setting," *American Journal of Psychotherapy* 12: 455–464, July, 1958.

Schiff, Sheldon K., "Termination of Therapy," *Archives of General Psychiatry* 6: 77–82, 1962.

CRISIS INTERVENTION

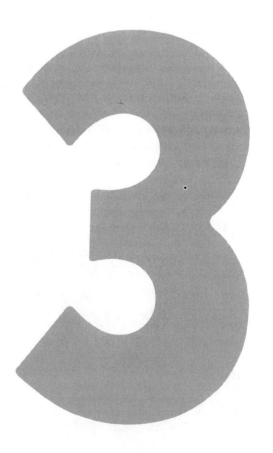

Introduction

The area of crisis intervention presents many challenges to nursing. Because, as Caplan has noted, crisis involves a turning point in one's life with a consequent reorganization of many aspects of an individual's psychologic structure, crisis situations represent both danger and opportunity. It is during the disorganization precipitated by crisis events that the basis for either positive or negative change is lain. Through an understanding of crisis theory, it is possible both to predict the outcome and to intervene in order to insure that the outcome for the individual and/or family will be positive. Appropriate and well-timed intervention in a crisis can be the critical determinant in the outcome. Ideally, intervention occurs on the level of primary prevention, before the crisis situation is fully formed, by identifying and working with potentially negative forces before they develop further. (See Unit I: "Assessment of a Family's Potential for Child Abuse.") For this to occur, however, the nurse must be aware of areas of high risk or vulnerability for her clients. This also requires that the nurse be able to identify the factors involved in a stress becoming a crisis, as well as understanding the components of normal and highly probable crisis situations. For example, the nurse who is working with a pregnant woman would fully assess the family situation and history of dealing with stress and change, anticipating that childbirth is a maturational crisis which varies in its impact depending on the individual and her support system. While this level of intervention is optimum, all too frequently intervention occurs at the secondary or tertiary levels of prevention. This level, however, is not too late to intervene humanistically and with a full understanding of the issues and course involved.

The unit focuses on the application of crisis intervention theory to a variety of case situations in equally diverse settings. Frederick takes crisis to the extreme in his discussion of specific modes of intervention in working with suicidal patients. His paper is invaluable for its check-list of suicidal precautions and its presentation of the components of primary intervention. An application of these factors to intervention can be seen in Fallon's description of her work with a suicidal woman. She makes the critical point that can be expanded to refer to all clients: we must be willing and able to listen fully and to help them understand that we are truly concerned with their well-being.

The next two articles in this unit present the emergency room as the setting for intervention. Burgess and Holmstrom describe the importance of recognition of the emotional crisis of rape victims, and the necessity of immediate intervention in order to prevent lasting psychological damage. They emphasize, as did Fallon, the critical element of a humanistic approach. Yowell and Brose describe another type of victim, one who is often treated as if he deserves to suffer: the drug abuse patient who is brought into the emergency room. As the authors indicate, such an attitude is counter-productive and potentially fatal. They discuss the four major types of drug abuse patients and the means by which psychological intervention can be initiated once the physiological needs have been met.

Last, crisis intervention is discussed in terms of a more long range, less critical incident focus. Miles and Hayes describe the development, process and resolution of a support group of widows whom they co-led. By utilizing such a framework, they enabled the members to work through their grief and redevelop new empathetic support systems. In this way secondary level intervention was successful in diminishing the impact of the crisis and in allowing normal griefwork to occur.

Similarly, Bayer presents an excellent example of a mix of tertiary prevention and primary level intervention with a primary care focus. She discusses a means by which nurses are frequently the most appropriate health practitioners for such intervention and can prevent physical health problems from being diagnosed as psychiatric crises.

Through these six papers, this unit provides a basis for crisis intervention in different settings and in a wide range of presenting problems. In each situation, it is clear that appropriate and early intervention can lead to prompt resolution of the crisis state or, at the very least, minimize the extent of the disorganization and circumvent the necessity for developing negative coping mechanisms. Here, the potential for nursing practice is unlimited.

18 THE ROLE OF THE NURSE IN CRISIS INTERVENTION AND SUICIDE PREVENTION

Calvin J. Frederick, M.D.

LIFE CRISES MAY BE PLACED ON A CONTINUUM of severity with a potential end point of the emotional dimension being suicide or homicide. The cessation of life is an ultimate termination of any crisis. The majority of us experience crises in various forms most of our lives. They can evolve from a number of causes: personal identity, school problems, difficulties with a job, marital problems, medical disorders, and financial trouble. Emotional crises usually have a common element: namely, difficulty with significant people in our lives along with an insecure view of ourselves. What makes suicide different from other behavioral disturbances? The disarmingly direct answer is simply despair and insufferable anguish as corollaries of the suicide trio: loneliness, helplessness, and hopelessness or other emotional disturbance includes all of these components simultaneously. A psychoneurotic may experience severe anguish or a schizophrenic may feel very lonely, but, unless suicidal ideation is present as well, all of these factors will not appear.

An encouraging aspect of a self-destructive crisis is that it frequently yields quite readily to intervention. Of interest to the nurse is the fact that the diagnostic acumen necessary for effective screening can be easily learned and applied by persons other than psychologists or psychiatrists.

Reprinted, with permission, from *Journal of Psychiatric Nursing and Mental Health Services,* January-February 1973.

Emotional crises are widespread demographically and represent all races and socioeconomic levels.

Frederick and Resnik[1] comment that crisis intervention in suicidal cases differs from traditional diagnostic and psychotherapy techniques in several ways: (1) It covers an entire spectrum of personalities and psychodiagnostic categories and thereby cannot be a unitary concept. In fact, there is no suicidal personality. Self destruction does not belong to any particular psychodiagnostic category. (2) The unique life and death component inherent in such behavior is not found in other mental health problems. (3) Stable and sensitive volunteers as indigenous workers are more important than in most other mental endeavors. (4) Innovation therapy approaches are especially needed since time worn procedures have not sufficed. (5) The thrust of crisis intervention is multi-disciplinary and multi-dimensional, involving psychological variables, public health, medical treatment, the law and cultural and social attitudes.

Mental health programs in this country have been too narrowly focused.[2,3] The most common procedure has been individual psychotherapy applied over a projected period of time in suburbia. The middle class housewife, living in affluent urban or suburban areas has represented the prototype of the ideal patient. Classical, intensive psychotherapy in an individual framework has been the mode of treatment, with the belief that those well-endowed verbally, intellectually, and financially, comprise the bulk of the patient clientele who are capable of utilizing psychotherapy effectively. This unfortunate parochial position has been self-serving and self-limiting. Other treatment procedures with a different frame of reference have not been characteristic of the helping modus operandi. The problems which most people experience are of a crisis type and require practical every day solutions and actions. Prolonged and intensive analytically oriented treatment is rarely necessary, although most of us would not deny the right to it for those who experience the need of it and can afford its temporal and financial demands.

The need for such crisis intervention is unmistakable. Although there were only three suicide prevention centers in the United States in 1958, currently our best estimate is that there are over 300 centers meeting basic criteria of a 24-hour telephone service, along with professional consultation and back-up. Where possible, an emergency mental health program should be developed as a part of a Community Mental Health Center so as to provide a complete range of services.

Knowledge of high risk groups is important for nurses as well as other persons in the mental health field. High risk means that, other things being equal, those individuals are more likely to constitute crisis problems in mental health and even take their lives more frequently than other persons in the general populations.

Some of the highest risk groups are the following: Persons over the age of 65, many professionals (such as some medical specialties, attorneys, and dentists), college age persons, and certain minority groups. Dentists for example have been shown to exceed the suicide rate in the general population by six or seven times. Paffenbarger et al[4] studied the records of former students at Harvard and Pennsylvania State University and showed, in addition to the high rates, the importance of a solid father figure in the home. Until recently suicide was regarded as a white middle class problem, but a number of minority groups such as American Indians, blacks, and young Spanish speaking persons have shown marked increases. Taboos in attitudes are still pervasive even among professionals as shown by Frederick.[5] There is a tendency to use intellectual defenses in order to handle the problem among professional groups.

Equivalent Forms of Self-Destruction

Menninger[6] and Shneidman[7] have commented about self-destructive behavior which is not obvious and unmistakable, but which has the same result. Menninger terms such behavior chronic suicide, while Shneidman speaks of sub-intentioned death with the decedent playing some partial, covert, or unconscious role in bringing forth his own death. A variety of behavior patterns can be viewed in this context as indicated by these examples.

A. DRUG ADDICTION AND ABUSE.   The proliferation of this drug abuse within the last few years has been so rapid that little definitive research exists to date: O'Donnell,[8] Dolkart, et al,[9] and Frederick[10] have all alluded to the possible connection between drug addiction and abuse and self-destructive behavior. After studying drug addicts released from the Public Health Service Hospital in Lexington, O'Donnell's work showed that the mortality rate exceeds the average on the order of 2.5 to 1 for men, and 3 to 1 for women. Among men about three times the expected percentage died from non-natural causes; that is, accidents, suicide, homicide and overdoses or withdrawal from drugs and alcohol. Dolkart et al[9] observe in studying suicidal preoccupation in young affluent American drug users that there are significant relationships between suicidal preoccupation and two chief aspects of yippie life styles, drug use and political protest activities. They found a direct relationship between frequency and variety of drug use and suicidal preoccupation. Suicidal preoccupation in a yippie subject does not seem to be an isolated phenomenon but rather part of a larger matrix of psychological disturbances including depression, anxiety, unresolved dependency feelings, and in older subjects, aggression. Suicidal preoccupation was shown to be related to extensive multi-drug use, social and personal isolation, and socio-political inactivity or indifference. Frederick et al[11] found a clear relationship between suicidal attempts and addiction as well as a much greater incidence of depression than in control subjects of comparable ages.

B. ALCOHOLISM.   It is probable that many alcoholics drink themselves to death literally and figuratively. Alcoholic addiction persists despite repeated warnings by doctors about the dangers of driving while under the influence of alcohol together with the physical debilitation which results. At least one suicide victim in five is alcoholic. The nine million alcoholics in this country bring about losses to society and families running into billions of dollars annually.

C. ACCIDENTAL DEATH.   Some one-car, one-driver auto accidents may be good illustrations of sub-intentioned death. Industrial accidents and those in our homes seem to be self-destructive more often than is generally believed. The term "accident proneness" is used too loosely, yet indications of previous self-destructive behavior appear at autopsy. Accidental deaths rank as the fourth leading cause of death in the United States while suicide has ranked around tenth for the last two decades. Preliminary evidence suggests that most near-fatal, one-car auto accidents are precipitated by personal stress upon the driver at the time of the event. This is frequently coupled with a personality type characterized by feelings of frustration and aggression, Mechanical failure of the automobile or poor road conditions do not play the important role which many believe. While few auto accidents are recorded as suicidal many of them may be just that.

D. EXCESSIVE SMOKING.   Despite all of the information from the Surgeon General's office regarding the deleterious effects of smoking upon health, many persons continue to smoke heavily. Whenever an individual has a serious respiratory ailment such as emphysema, a vascular disorder or any other medical problem evoking strong warnings against smoking by his doctor, does it not seem suicidal to continue smoking? The answer must be in the affirmative. If a person states that it relaxes him to smoke and that he needs to smoke, because he is nervous without it, then he probably should seek psychological help.

E. MISCELLANEOUS FORMS OF SELF–DESTRUCTION.   Other forms of risk-taking behavior such as auto and motorcycle racing suggest the possiblity of some self-destructive intent which may be operating at an uncon-scious level within the person. Such behavior may be rationalized by the view that the potential financial gain would be worth the risk, but the self-destruction intent may be present all the same. Indeed, one could ad-vance the notion that our entire society is more self-destructive than we might care to imagine when we consider pollution of the environment and our careless approach to handling such problems. Polluted lakes, rivers and air are dangerous to all of us and to our progeny and yet we continue to add to our own self-destruction.

Symptoms of Self-Destructive Behavior

A list of behavioral clues can prove helpful in pinpointing cases which are often missed by doctors and nurses alike. The author[12] has alluded to symptomatic clues for use for the school guidance counselor. There are others which ought to be helpful for the nurse.

1. Classical signs of depression always herald the possiblity of suicidal behavior. These are insomnia, anorexia or voracious eating, worry, mood change, and loss of sex drive. The observer should be cautioned, how-ever, against the belief that every suicidal individual will show clear depressive symptoms or that he is unlikely to take his life unless such clinical depressive signs appear. Many persons who are depressed do not commit suicide; while on the other hand, some do so who do not appear to have traditional depressive symptoms. Nevertheless, depression should always alert the nurse to the possibility of self-destructive be-havior.

2. The individual is apt to become more isolated, and morose than usual. This symptom may be discovered from speaking to a relative or close associate as well as the person himself.

3. Any change in behavior should be cause for alarm. Although these changes may appear in various emotional disturbances, it is likely to be an especially important clue with other tendencies toward self-destruction. If an individual suddenly goes for walks in the middle of the night, begins to eat at odd hours and displays other unusual forms of behavior, it could signal an impending act of suicide.

4. Arranging and ordering one's personal affairs such as insurance policies, or bank accounts, can be a corollary of self-destructive intent. Young persons are not apt to communicate with authority figures because they often lack faith and trust in them. Thus, if the young person says that he cannot talk to his parents or teachers, the nurse should be alerted to the nuances of such behavior.

5. Subtle attempts to communicate suicidal intent may occur such as giving away some valued possession, with comment that he or she may not be needing it any longer.

6. Previous suicidal intent or self-destructive acts should be noted. Threats as well as actual past acts are frequently precursors of future suicidal behaviors. The best predictors, other things being equal, of how an individual is going to perform in the future is the way he has performed in the past. Children may continue to poison themselves "accidentally" and require lavage only to continue this behavior until another pattern is developed or they expire.

7. Previous suicide within the family is consistent with potential suicide for all persons, especially if the event occurred before the individual became pubescent and if the relationship with suicide victim was close.

8. A drop in general efficiency occurs, along with a disturbance in interpersonal relationships. If the person has a regular job, such information usually reveals itself in reports of undesirable job performance.

9. The typical male profile discloses an inadequate relationship with the father or loss of the father prior to the time the son has reached the age of 16. Among lower socio-economic groups the father will have abandoned the home situation and evoke censure and bitterness from the mother. This will reflect itself upon the young man's concept of himself. Among higher socio-economic levels young males are apt to have a successful father who died while the son was young, left the home, or committed suicide himself.

10. The profile of young girls who attempt suicide is likely to reveal difficulty with the mother, especially if there is an ineffectual father figure in the home. The young girl often turns to a boy friend for support after having been rejected by her narcissistic mother. He then lets her down simply because he is not capable of satisfying her psychological demands, at least in her eyes. Often such a girl may believe she is pregnant whether she is or not, which supplies further impetus for a suicidal attempt.

Ward Behavior for the Nurse in
Charge of Self-Destructive Patients

Other than fellow patients, nobody is likely to observe hospital patients more than the nurse. Nurses can play a unique and significant role in diagnosing and reshaping suicidal and depressive behavior. The nurse is currently in a period of transition wherein the classical role of subserviency to the physician is being re-examined and questioned. The author[2] has perceived that the nurse probably constitutes a greater threat to the old medical model than any of the helping professions. They are apt to press the need for more independence as time goes on. Bell[13] has commented upon various nursing models in relation to suicide prevention which enlarge upon and expand current training procedures.

Known risks may bring about legal suit if the patient suicides. Precautions should be taken to assure the patient's welfare, as well as protecting the nurse and other professionals from suit. Considering the patient's interests first is a good way to accomplish both. Suicide is still a crime in some states, and persons can be liable for attempted suicide, even though such laws are not usually pressed. Special procedures should be routine for high risk patients. Suicidal precautions are not the universal rule in hospitals or clinics as much as one might imagine. The following precautions should be basic to patient care:

1. Remove dangerous objects such as razor blades, nail files, cords, belts, poisonous materials, drugs, and glass objects.

2. Maintain continuous periods of observation, especially during acute crisis.

3. If at all possible put the patient on a lower floor to prevent injury from jumping.

4. Do not place the patient in isolation. This may frighten an individual who is already afraid of his own impulses, add to feelings of despair and loneliness, and provide an implicit challenge or sanction to carry out the suicidal act. Arrange for other patients to be near and ask their cooperation with your handling of the person in crisis. They will probably know the essence of the problem in any way.

5. Observe the circumstances under which depressive reactions and/or suicidal behaviors occur. Discuss them with the therapist and change the contingencies for such behavior. Lack of socialization, expression of personal fears, and agitated depressive responses are signs of impending danger. Difficulty with sleeping, pacing, wringing of hands, and obsessive thoughts are all aspects of serious agitation. Take special note of medications which do not seem to be effective.

6. See the patient yourself and encourage talking as frequently as possible. It is not necessary for these periods to be lengthy, but they should permit the person an opportunity for ventilation. Tell the patient in a sincere manner to contact you if he really feels the need. Do not merely suggest, but instruct the patient emphatically and warmly that he *must* call you during suicidal stress. Inform him of the necessity to *always delay any self-destructive impulse* and call for help.

7. Provide alternative avenues of expression. Discuss what the person might have done instead of the suicidal act. Help him to engage in group activities in order to prevent isolation and withdrawal.

8. Commend the patient for any positive action, i.e. any non-suicidal, non-depressive response. It is important to reinforce positive responses to stress rather than negative ones. This will help to establish self-control over suicidal impulses. For example, give the person a ward task which he can accomplish successfully.

9. Never interpret behavior or confront an acute suicidal patient with what you think his behavior represents. You may be wrong and heighten the problem, thereby making the patient feel much worse and thus precipitate a suicidal response.

10. In cooperation with the primary therapist, solicit the assistance of relatives or surrogates in an active follow-up program before the patient leaves the hospital.

Some of these crises concepts may be reviewed in more specific terms in Frederick and Farberow[14] and Frederick and Resnik.[15]

Primary Intervention

This kind of first line intervention has been termed "psychological first aid." Ordinarily it occurs before hospitalization is required. What to do in an emergency situation is something that all allied mental health personnel ought to know, particularly with suicidal persons. One need not be a physician to render first aid medically or psychologically. How should the nurse act when confronted with persons whom she believes might be suicidal? The follow-up period after hospitalization assisting in a professional treatment plan should also be the nurse's responsibility. Emergency treatment, per se, can be given by a variety of individuals. What should one do in such an emergency?

1. BE AVAILABLE.   Be there and be willing to listen. Many individuals in this dilemma have never encountered anyone who really wanted to hear them and understand what they really feel. Be willing to respond rather than simply reflecting feelings in a nondirective manner. That can be extremely frustrating to a person in the throes of a suicidal act. While not often psychotic the stress and lack of rationality in the patient at such times do not lend themselves to dealing with the lack of support which reflection is apt to create.

2. PROVIDE A LIFELINE.   Be a psychological lifebuoy. Try to establish some situation or resource for the individual to grasp psychologically. This may involve catering to some infantile and demanding needs. For the time being that should be done simply because we are interested in saving a life. Many depressed and self-destructive individuals are extremely dependent and demanding and have thereby frustrated other persons around them who do not how to handle this problem. Such a personality flaw can be dealt with later in treatment. One need not interpret

it in the beginning. One may call significant others or anyone else who may be helpful in saving the person's life.

3. SUPPLY DIRECT SUPPORT.   Be reassuring. Do not always attempt to handle everything yourself. Be ready to ask for consultation and assistance. Call a Suicide Prevention Center, crisis center, priest, professional person you might know, ambulance, police, or anyone else you feel would be necessary to help solve the situation.

4. EVALUATE

A. Evaluate the suicidal reality.

B. Evaluate the depth of feelings or intensity or severity of the emotional disturbance. The likelihood that a person will take his life does not always bear a direct relationship to the intensity of his feelings. A person can be extremely upset and not at all suicidal; on the other hand, he can be quite calm and very lethal once he has made the decision to take his life, all of which can be misleading. However, agitated depression is always a dangerous symptom.

C. Evaluate the resources available to the person; both his personal inner resources in terms of past behavior, and possible ego strength, and the outer resources existing in his life situation. If there are other family members who can be contacted and included as adjunctive resources, they can be used to provide additional support. If family members are detrimental to the effort, this fact should be quickly appraised. If the individual has no outside resources, then he is apt to be a more serious suicidal risk.

5. ACT DEFINITIVELY AND FOLLOW–UP.   Reach out to the patient and render aid. If the patient has difficulty verbalizing his thoughts and feelings, then help him do so. Ask if your appraisal agrees with his own thoughts, e.g. "I wonder if you have been thinking of taking your life for some time." "I want you to go to Clinic Y or Hospital Z." "I'm going to call the hospital for you." or "contact Dr. A for you"; then follow the procedure through to completion. The patient may not be able to execute all the plans without some assistance. In the long run the patient will probably appreciate your stability and firm, decision-filled action.

In clinics and hospitals if the doctor has given no instructions or suicidal precautions, especially if there are no printed hospital rules regarding such patients, the nurse should call the matter to the attention of those in charge. The nurse may be culpable for negligence in contributing to errors of omission in suicidal cases. In some instances the nurse may be sued along with doctor. The old idea that the doctor alone is responsible for the care and treatment of the patient is patently false in some jurisdictions, and the nurse would be well advised not to depend upon it for protection. The nurse's first duty is to the patient to provide reasonable or appropriate care. Reasonable care is that which would be given by another person with equal training in a similar situation . In this instance, it is better to be overly cautious than not cautious enough.

The nurse is universally viewed as a helping person. They should capitalize upon the role and use it to advantage. They should give the impression of self-confidence, personal strength and warm but authoritative resolution. Many lives can be saved while simultaneously developing an expanded and realistic role in diagnosis, treatment and training for tomorrow's nurses.

References

1. Frederick CJ: Resnik III.P: Interventions with suicidal patients. J Contemp Psychotherapy 2:103-109, 1970.
2. Frederick CJ: Future training in psychotherapy. Int Psychiat Clin 6:379-401, 1969.
3. Frederick CJ: Psychotherapy, Quo Vadis? Psychotherapy Bulletin 3:13-15, 1970b.
4. Paffenbarger RS, King SH, Wing AD, Chronic disease in former college students. IX Characteristics in youth that predispose to suicide and accidental death in later life. Amer J Public Health 59:900-908, 1969.
5. Frederick CJ: The present suicide taboo in the United States. Ment Hyg 55:178-183, 1971.
6. Menninger K: Man Against Himself. New York, Harcourt, Brace and World, 1938.
7. Shneidman ES: Some current developments in suicide prevention. Bulletin of Suicidology 2:31-34, 1967.
8. O'Donnell JA: Narcotic Addicts in Kentucky. Public Health Service Publication No. 1881 U.S. Govt. Printing Office, Washington, D.C. 1969.
9. Dolkart MD, Hughes P, Jaffee J, Zaks M: Suicide preoccupation in young affluent American drug users: A study of yippies at the Democratic convention. Bulletin of Suicidology 8:70-73, 1971.
10. Frederick CJ: Drug therapy and self-destructive behavior. Drug Therapy 2:49-68, 1972.
11. Frederick CJ, Resnik HLP, Wittlin B: Self-destructive aspects of hard core addiction. Paper presented to American Association of Suicidology District, March 31, 1972.
12. Frederick CJ: The school guidance counselor as a preventive agent to self-destructive behavior. NY State Personnel and Guidance J 5:1-5, 1970a.

13. Bell KK: The nurse's role in suicide prevention: Some aspects. Bulletin of Suicidology 8:70-73, 1971.
14. Frederick CJ, Farberow NL: Group psychotherapy with suicidal persons: A comparison with standard group methods. Int J Soc Psychiat 16:103-111, 1970.
15. Frederick CJ, Resnik HLP: How suicidal behaviors are learned. Amer j Psychother 25:37-55, 1971.

19 "AND CERTAIN THOUGHTS GO THROUGH MY HEAD . . . ."

Barbara Fallon, M.S., R.N.

IN THE UNITED STATES TODAY ONE PERSON DIES by his own hand every 24 minutes. This tragic loss of life may be even greater than the known statistics. Because self-destruction is surrounded by cultural taboos, it is suspected that many deaths by suicide are assigned different causal factors. In addition, authorities suspect that many so-called "accidental deaths," deaths from alcoholism and drug abuse, are, indeed, "hidden suicides," not included in the statistics. However, the reported suicidal death rate of 105 per 100,000, in itself, is appalling and is the cause of much concern among mental health workers (1).

For nurses everywhere, and especially for a psychiatric nurse working in the community, the specter of patient suicide is ever present. When a patient communicates suicidal ideas or threatens to take his life, how can the nurse intervene effectively to dissuade him? What can she do for the patient in this crisis situation?

Shneidman believes that in nearly every case of suicide there are hints of the act to come. He believes nurses are in a special position to pick up these hints and perhaps prevent the act because they are trained to observe certain aspects of human behavior. He says:

Every rescue operation is a dialogue: Someone cries for help and someone else must be willing to hear him and be capable of responding to him. Otherwise the victim may die because of the potential rescuer's unresponsiveness. (2)

It is this willingness to hear the patient and respond to him that is exemplified in the following account of a patient in suicidal crisis with whom I worked in a community mental health agency. The conclusions I have drawn from this experience are, I believe, the heart and substance of successful intervention in such a crisis situation.

A Patient In Crisis

Mrs. D., a housewife and mother of four children, was referred to the community mental health agency by a social worker at the school her oldest son, G., a boy of 15, attended. She was referred for support and help in coping with the behavioral problems of this son. Although I requested to see the father, too, he refused to come. Mrs. D. was discouraged about this because she thought that unless her husband was willing to participate, her involvement with counseling would be useless. In spite of Mr. D.'s refusal to be involved, I continued to see Mrs. D. on a one-to-one basis. The son, meanwhile, was referred by the school to another agency for evaluation and treatment.

Mrs. D. revealed a history of severe marital problems and described her husband as a "drinker," who was extremely harsh and punitive to the boy. She said her husband did not offer her any support in dealing with the problems of either the household or the children. Rather, his threats and acts of violence placed her in the position of "covering up" for her children so that they would not become the victims of her husband's rage.

The patient also felt responsible for her aged parents who lived in the same house. She tried to act as go-between and peace-maker among the different generations, with apparently dismal results. She expressed anxiety and guilt over this unhappy situation. She reported that in the course of arguments with her husband he had threatened to "get rid" of her parents. This caused her to become "upset" since she could see no alternative to the present living arrangements.

Mrs. D. had suffered from repeated peptic ulcer attacks for seven years and was taking medications, including chlordiazepoxide HCL (Librium), for this problem. She appeared quite angry at times when discussing her difficulties at home.

She also revealed a need for personal recognition and notice by ascribing responsibility to herself for situations not under her control. This caused her interactions with family members to be rather manipulative at times.

Due to the constant bickering and disharmony at home which resulted in an impoverished family life, underlying resentment and anger in Mrs. D., and increasing difficulties with the son. Mrs. D. was beginning to feel overwhelmed. One day during a counseling session. I noticed her manner become increasingly anxious. She was chain smoking, her face was flushed, and her hand visibly shook.

PATIENT *Sometimes certain thoughts go through my head.*

THERAPIST *What kind of thoughts?*

PATIENT *Sometimes I feel I'd like to shoot the children. I read these stories in the newspapers where a mother killed her kids and I understand just how she felt. That's what I'd like to do.*

THERAPIST *Do you have a gun?*

PATIENT *No. But I don't see any solution. It's just getting worse so sometimes I feel like shooting them.*

Further questioning did not elicit much more. I sought supervision from the director of the agency and our consulting psychiatrist immediately. That same evening I called Mrs. D. at home to assess her emotional state. She seemed in control, but I set up an emergency session with her and gave her my home telephone number so that she could call me "just in case those thoughts come back or you feel the need to talk to me." Two days later, I met with the patient again. The following is taken from that emergency interview.

THERAPIST *Have you had those thoughts about shooting the children again?*

PATIENT *Yes, I think about it sometimes.*

THERAPIST *How are you planning on doing it?*

PATIENT *Well, you need a gun to shoot someone.*

THERAPIST *You said you didn't have one. Do you have one now?*

PATIENT *No. I don't have one. I don't own one. I wouldn't have one in the house. I don't really want to shoot the children.*

THERAPIST *What do you really want to do?*

PATIENT *I would much rather kill myself and get it over with.*

THERAPIST *How would you do that?*

PATIENT *With pills.*

THERAPIST *Do you have pills in the house?*

PATIENT *Oh, sure. I've got lots of stuff . . . pills . . . in the house . . . sleeping pills, too. But then I think, "if I die, what will become of the children." I would have to kill them too. Of course, if I'm dead I wouldn't know what the kids will do. Probably they'd be all right but I don't know.*

THERAPIST *Have you given much thought as to how you'd go about killing them and yourself—at the same time or what?*

PATIENT *No, but mostly I thought about taking sleeping pills and finishing it for me.*

THERAPIST *Have you thought about doing this before now?*

PATIENT *Yes, a couple of months ago.*

THERAPIST *Did you tell anyone?*

PATIENT *No.*

THERAPIST *How about now? Did you tell your husband or anyone else besides me?*

PATIENT *Yes. I told my husband the other night after I saw you and told you.*

THERAPIST *What did you tell him? What did you actually say?*

PATIENT *I told him I felt like killing the kids or myself.*

THERAPIST *What did he say?*

PATIENT *He called me a coward and said I was taking a coward's way out and that I was just talking anyway. I told him I didn't care what he thought, I was going to kill myself.*

I discussed with Mrs. D. the apparently overwhelming aspects of her problems. I reassured her that even though she could not at the moment see them, there were alternatives and I would help her find them. I reassured her that I would not let her down, that I wanted to help her find solutions other than killing herself. I also pointed out that if she killed herself she would not be around to know if anyone cried over her or even felt sorry. I emphasized that all that would happen would be that she'd be very dead and could not undo it or come back. I then said that I thought a psychiatric consultation was necessary. She agreed to see a psychiatrist and an appointment was made right then for her to be seen that same afternoon.

After Mrs. D. had seen the doctor, I consulted with him. He concurred with my assessment of the situation. He said he believed Mrs. D. could be dealt with as an outpatient and approved of my counseling technique. Arrangements were made to continue consulting with him at frequent intervals and, if, necessary, on an emergency basis. That evening, I telephoned the patient and spoke with her for about 20 minutes. We discussed her visit with the doctor. She told me her family was aware of the situation and knew she had seen a psychiatrist.

The next day, I called her to reassure her that I was still interested in her. I offered, once again, to help her find workable solutions to her problems and I attempted to foster a more hopeful attitude within her. Mrs. D.'s voice sounded a little more relieved during this conversation and I affirmed our appointment for the following day.

When the patient came in for our session, she appeared less anxious than before. We discussed the situation at home and Mrs. D. said she had acted on my suggestion to talk with the children about not hiding things from their father. She said she also had inititated a talk with her husband, had told him of her discussion with the children, and, together, they had decided on a plan of action for disciplining the children. I supported Mrs. D. in this, but warned her not to become discouraged if her husband or children reverted to old behavior patterns. I reassured her that this was not unusual, but suggested that the set-back would be temporary if she could only keep on discussing her problems with her husband. We discussed this for a few minutes. Then I asked her if she still felt like killing herself.

PATIENT *No, I feel much more relieved. Like maybe things can work out. Maybe not great right away, but a little better. But I realize I upset you because you sent me to a doctor and called me at home so many times. I feel badly about that . . . to make you so concerned about me.*

THERAPIST *Well, you're right about my being concerned about you. You told me you felt like killing yourself. I became concerned because I care very much what happens to you. But, you don't have to feel badly about it. I didn't break up into pieces. I'm pretty strong and I can take it. So, if you feel that way again, you can call me anytime of the day or night. We'll work it out together.*

Suddenly, the patient began to cry. After a few minutes she regained her composure.

PATIENT *You did believe me, didn't you?*

THERAPIST *Yes, I believed you, I thought you were seriously thinking about it.*

PATIENT *Do you know why I am here today?*

THERAPIST *No, tell me why.*

PATIENT *(Starts to cry again . . . then composes herself) Because I did mean it the other day . . . and you knew that . . . you didn't think I was just saying it like he did.*

THERAPIST *Like who?*

PATIENT *My husband. You knew, all right. You kept calling me, I guess you did that because you believed me and you were worried about me . . . that's why I'm here.*

People are reduced to suicidal gestures because "of feelings of helplessness, a hopeless sense of inability to cope with their problems, and the unhappy conclusion that others do not care or are no longer listening"(3).

The person who entertains suicide is a person who is desperate, who sees no solutions to his problems, and whose plight is seemingly ignored by those around him. The person who destroys himself is the one whose S.O.S. went unheeded. Either through ignorance or indifference, those who might have helped turned a deaf ear to his plea.

To listen to our patients, to believe them, to care about them, and to be willing to help them conveys our real concern for their well being and our appreciation of them as valuable persons. It is this underlying concern and regard which may very well be the determinants necessary to turn the patient toward life.

References

1. Yolles, Stanley. Suicide: a public health problem, In *Suicidal Behavior*, edited by H, L. P. Resnik. Boston, Little, Brown and Co., 1968, pp. 49–50.
2. Shneidman, E. S. Preventing suicide. In *Suicide*, edited by J. P. Gibbs. New York, Harper and Row Publishers, 1968, pp. 255–266.
3. Farhi Row, Norman, Crisis, disaster, and suicide: theory and therapy. In *Essays in Self-Destruction*, edited by Edwin S. Shneidman. New York, Science House, 1967, pp. 384–385.

Bibliography

Bellak, Leopold, and Small, Leonard. *Emergency Psychotherapy and Brief Psychotherapy.* New York, Grune and Stratton, 1965.

Heilig, S. M., and Klugman, D. J. Social worker in a suicide prevention center. In *Crisis Intervention,* edited by Howard J. Parad. New York, Family Service Association of America. 1965, pp. 274–285.

Shneidman, E. S., and Farberow, N. L. Eds. *Clues to Suicide.* New York, McGraw-Hill Book Co., 1957.

20

WIDOWHOOD

Helen S. Miles, B.S., R.N.
Dorothea R. Hays, M.S., R.N.

THE CONCEPT OF THE WIDOW AS A WEAK and defenseless person in need of protection is accepted in our society. Yet, the American widow usually discovers to her surprise that society reacts with indifference and even hostility to her sudden transition from wife to a person plagued by complex problems for which there can never be any adequate preparation. Little is done to help her. Relationships change and economic, financial, legal, and other problems often confront and overwhelm her.

We surveyed the services for widows in our community and found that social activities and therapeutic counseling were available. But we could find no services for recently bereaved widows aimed specifically at crisis intervention by group leaders with professional preparation. As experienced psychiatric nurses who understand the behavioral aspects of grief and crisis, we believed that bringing widows together to discuss their experiences, to learn from each other, and to gain mutual support might prove valuable. The Nassau County (Long Island) Chapter of the American Red Cross agreed to support our plan since the personal disaster of bereavement could be considered a part of its mandate to alleviate human suffering and improve the quality of life. In accordance with Red Cross policy, we charged no fees.

Our goals were to reduce pain, to try to prevent psychosomatic illness, and to help the women move toward new personal growth.

We would be supportive and encourage the women to discuss their experiences and feelings in relation to the loss of their husbands. We were prepared to discuss current concepts of grief and crisis informally and to make available reading lists on bereavement and the general problems of widows. We contacted various social and recreational organizations for information to pass on as needed. We arranged for resource persons who would talk on such special topics as social security, vocational guidance, and estate law, if group members wished.

Anticipating that some widows might have deeper psychological problems and might benefit from counseling and therapy, we checked on resources for referrals. We planned for weekly two-hour sessions in a comfortable room with plenty of coffee and cookies.

We publicized our program through newspaper and radio announcements and by distributing a leaflet, "The First Step," through local organizations and the social security office.

Twenty-eight women whose ages ranged from the early thirties to the late fifties attended the first session. They were given name tags which also showed their hometowns. They differed in levels of education and economic status, yet all had in common their widowhood.

To reach the women and to uncover their most pressing problems quickly, we asked each of them to write down responses to two questions: "What bothered you most when you lost your husband?" and "What are your biggest problems now?" We also asked how long each had been widowed.

Many women wrote that loneliness, abandonment, fear of being alone, hurt, pain, and inability to function bothered them most. They mentioned anger, resentment at their change in status, and regrets about not being with the husband when he died or not having talked with him enough. Some were upset about others' tactless comments and some were concerned that they would not be able to care for their children alone.

The women talked readily about their feelings of loneliness, isolation, anger, and guilt in response to our brief review of the phases of mourning and of the lack of understanding and support for widows in our society.

Loneliness was the major current problem for these women. Some women expressed guilt feelings about their needs for tenderness and love. Those most recently bereaved had problems in dealing with finances and plans for the children. The women who had been widowed 10 months or longer mentioned problems in becoming more self-confident and independent, making new friends, finding jobs, and planning for the future.

Talk came easily during the first meeting. The need to be heard was so strong that often several women spoke at the same time, turning to neighbors when they could not get the attention of the whole group. At the end of the two hours, the women said that it felt good to talk with people who listened, cared, and understood. They no longer felt so different and alone.

In the following weeks, requests from working widows for evening sessions led to the formation of a second group. Additional daytime requests required a third group. We also received calls and letters from widowers and from divorced women whom we could not accommodate.

Since the beginning of the program in January 1973, a total of 12 groups have been formed. Each of the groups met once a week for two hours during a three-month period. Of the 220 women involved, approximately two thirds continued regularly in each group.

The topics that these women select to discuss can be divided into three areas: intrapersonal, interpersonal, and material problems.

INTRAPERSONAL PROBLEMS   The widows' feelings of being wounded, less of a woman, and quite inferior and incapable formed the core of these discussions. They expressed a sense of aimlessness, as if life had lost all meaning and direction. Guilt feelings were often connected with depression and wishes for, as well as fear of, death. Some said their duties to their children were all that kept them going. They wished they had done more for their husbands, for example, being more strict about diet. They wished they had talked more about their problems. Some even felt guilty about being alive. Others experienced the physical symptoms of their husbands' illnesses. One woman feared that her own ill health hastened her husband's death.

But the overwhelming experience they expressed was loneliness. In contacts with other people, the often gauche, insensitive, and uncaring treatment of others coupled with their own hypersensitivity and anger often resulted in anguish for these women. They were acutely aware of not being called or invited or of being snubbed on the street. Yet it hurt to have to explain the husband's death to everyone and to listen to advice, such as get a job, go out more, be cheerful, and stop crying. It hurt, too, to be invited out and then feel like a "fifth wheel" as they listened to couples happily planning a future for their still intact families. They were particularly sensitive to women who complained about their husbands or fussed about trifles.

Their heightened sensitivity and low self-esteem often prompted many fears—being alone in the house, leaving the house, driving, and joining a group. Some feared burglars and obscene telephone calls, being talked about by neighbors, being treated as sexual prey, or being taken advantage of financially.

Most of the women seemed to have a strong desire to solve their problems. To counteract fears and anxiety, they bolstered each other's courage and offered real advice and help. They wanted to be treated as persons, not as "widows." They wanted respect, not pity. As they discussed their anger, they realized that their friends' distancing might stem from fear of death, both for themselves and for their spouses.

IINTERPERSONAL PROBLEMS   Dating and sexual needs were a problem, particularly for the younger women. At first, the women found that not having any sexual feelings was comfortable. When these feelings returned, there was guilt and then a time of looking for a person exactly like the dead spouse. For other women, learning dating behavior again was difficult. Holidays, mother's and father's days, and anniversaries, especially of the husband's death, increased depression.

Children were a special area of interpersonal problems. The pre-school child has difficulty understanding the finality of death. He has a concrete picture of his father being in heaven and waits for him to come back. The concept of burial was hard for these mothers to explain or even to mention. An elementary school-age child talks about his dead parent in the present tense and tries to take over some of his work. A teen-ager often is having such a difficult time with his own adolescence and grieving that he cannot tolerate seeing his mother act weak. Therefore he may not mention his dead parent and does not permit the living parent to mourn openly. A young adult man often refuses to help with the chores his father used to do, as if he were afraid he'd have to fill the father's role at home and be tied down at an age when he needs to become free and independent of parents. An older adult child generally is helpful. At times, especially in some Italian and Jewish families, he is too protective of his mother.

MATERIAL PROBLEMS   These problems involve the concrete difficulties that occur with houses, furnaces, broken-down cars, burned-out fuses, wills, social security, lower income, lost credit ratings, and preparation for and securing new jobs. Group members found sharing hard-earned experiences particularly valuable.

Summing Up

We found that the groups went through two phases that kept recurring alternately. In the first, one or more women talk freely about their feelings and difficulties and occasionally cry a little. The rest of the group responds with validation and support as well as some advice. In the next phase, which may be the beginning of the next meeting, stories of courage and success and how members cope by taking a course in auto mechanics or by planning a first trip away from home are recounted. This is greeted with applause and admiration from the group.

The process is influenced by the frequent coming and going of members. We found it necessary to retrace our steps repeatedly. But we also noticed that as core members got to know each other better, they began to exchange telephone numbers and plan mutual visits and outings together. This usually occurred about the fourth or fifth meeting. They also began to contribute food and coffee and to help clean up.

We expected some anger directed at us for having husbands. Only once did we suspect that a joking remark carried a message of anger, but we made no attempt at validation. We felt included as caring people and perceived as warm and giving. The group effect on us was that of sensitizing us toward our own marital relationships—at first fearing the possibility of loss and then becoming more appreciative of our husbands.

Because of other professional commitments, we were able to lead jointly only two of the original four groups. We did conclude, however, that co-leadership is more effective with groups as large as the ones we experienced, especially when members are involved in highly emotional topics. All succeeding groups have had two nurse leaders.

Although we have concluded our work with 12 groups, many members formed groups in their own homes, with more social activities. We are willing to provide counsel if requested, but our involvement does decrease in response to the gradual emerging leadership among the participants themselves.

Because of our experiences with our first groups, we have been limiting new groups to 16 or 20 persons. We encourage members to remain for all 12 sessions, during which the experiences of loss and grief are explored together. We also suggest that members might be interested in forming their own groups with no time or membership limits and with a minimum of professional leadership at the end of the three-month group meetings. The purpose would be to receive and give continuous support and to explore social and recreational opportunities.

We are also hoping to organize groups for widowers with a male discussion leader. We do not believe mixed groups are feasible because, although the grieving process is the same, the problems are different.

Professional involvement in the problems of widowhood is new and there is much to be learned and done to help these persons adjust successfully. While this is happening, the attitude of society as a whole toward widowhood must also be examined and changed.

21 THE RAPE VICTIM IN THE ER

Ann Wolbert Burgess,

D.N. Sc., R.N.

Lynda Lytle Holmstrom, Ph.D.

FORCIBLE RAPE IS ONE OF THE FOUR MAJOR violent crimes in the United States, and it affects the lives of thousands of women each year. FBI *Uniform Crime Reporting* indicates an 11 percent increase in the number of reported rapes in 1972. Although there has been a significant rise in the past three years in reports of forcible rape, little exists in the way of support services for rape victims. One service, a Victim Counseling Program, was begun July 20, 1972, as a voluntary collaboration between Boston College School of Nursing and the Boston City Hospital Emergency Department. The program provides 24-hour-a-day crisis intervention service for rape victims. To the best of our knowledge, it was the first such program in the Boston area and one of the first in the United States.

A psychiatric nurse and a sociologist, the co-authors of this article, staff the program. Originally, services were for adult victims. However, in December 1972, the Pediatric Walk-In Department of the Boston City Hospital requested the staff's services and, thus, the program began to include child victims of rape, attempted rape, sexual assault, or molesting. The police, the district attorney's office in Boston, and one private hospital also began to make referrals.

The counseling program is a nurse-to-nurse referral service functioning in the following way. The rape victim comes to the Emergency Department of the Boston City Hospital and is seen by the triage nurse, who calls the gynecologist and then both counselors, who come immediately to the hospital regardless of the time.

The counselors talk with the victim, family, friends who accompanied the victim, and the police to gather as much data as possible for assessing the crisis.

The nurse-counselor makes a follow-up telephone call within 24 to 48 hours to further assess for psychological and physical state of the victim. Weekly telephone calls continue until the crisis state stabilizes. When cases become ready for court, often the crisis is reactivated and longer follow-ups are required. An evaluation and termination telephone call is made at the appropriate point, or home visits are made in selected cases where a telephone is not available.

In our early work with over 80 victims, we saw certain patterns which have major implications for nursing management.

The act of reporting a rape sets into motion a complicated process. The victim is often swept along by the day-to-day workings of the police system, the hospital system, and the legal system. She is caught up in a process which is routine to the authorities, but new to her and most often not completely understood by her. More may be done for her or to her than she expected.

Most of the rape cases we have seen at Boston City Hospital were referred by the police. The police either advised the victim to go or brought the victim to the hospital. This is important for nursing management, since it means that the woman has had to deal not only with the sexual assault, but also with the police. Even though many women are grateful for their help, talking with them is one more stressful situation for the victim.

Furthermore, in most of the cases, someone other than the victim was involved in reporting the rape to the police. Someone other than the victim made the decision to call, acted as intermediary at the request of the victim, or persuaded the victim herself to call. During the confusion which follows rape, it often is hard to determine exactly who made the decision to notify the police. It was clear, however, that in a considerable number of cases with which we were concerned, other people took it upon themselves to make the decision for the victim. In our sample, such persons included mother, father, brother, sister, grandmother, roommate, friend, fireman, and stranger. Part of the counseling process involves talking with these persons also.

Medical Process

Once at the emergency ward, the attention the rape victim receives depends on the protocol of the particular hospital. At Boston City Hospital, the victim is generally seen for medical and counseling services within an hour. The priority of treatment is first, medical. This includes obtaining a brief history, diagnosing general trauma, performing a gynecological examination and laboratory tests, and providing treatment for such health concerns as prevention of pregnancy and venereal disease. Second is psychological treatment, assessment and counseling. Referral—gynecological, medical, and psychological follow-up—is third.

The gynecologist examines the victim and writes the medical and gynecological report. He generally records in the patient's words a brief history of the time, place, and circumstances of the sexual assault. Statements on the patient's general appearance, physical and emotional condition, bruises, lacerations, and torn or bloody clothing are recorded.

In our sample, the general physical examination of rape victims for signs of trauma indicated a significant proportion of victims suffered trauma, bruises, and lacerations, as the chart below shows.

Close to half the women are threatened with an actual weapon. Bruises to the body were from the weapon or the assailant's hands or fists. Struggles on the ground often resulted in abrasions of the legs, arms, and back.

Symptoms of trauma were reported more frequently than were found on examination. For example, many women reported that assailants put their hands around their throats and threatened to kill them if they did

SIGNS OF TRAUMA IN 80 VICTIMS

	HEAD	FACE	THROAT	CHEST	ABDOMEN	BACK	ARMS	LEGS
Trauma	19	23	13	9	7	15	20	17
Lacerations	3	11	3	1	—	—	2	4

While 147 marks were visible on physical examination, not all violence left visible signs.

GYNECOLOGICAL PHYSICAL FINDINGS

	PERINEUM	HYMEN	VULVA	VAGINA	CERVIX	ANUS
Bruises	7	2	9	4	10	5
Lacerations	3	5	3	4	2	3

In addition to the 147 visible signs of violence found in the general physical examination, 57 more were found by the gynecologist.

not do as the assailants demanded. Most of the women, fearing death, complied. Often there were no visible signs of trauma with these reports. In our sample, 21 victims reported being physically held by the assailants and 12 had verbal threats of danger without the presence of an actual weapon.

Twelve of the 80 victims required medical, surgical, or orthopedic consultation in addition to X-ray services to confirm a diagnosis secondary to the rape diagnosis.

During the gynecological examination, a water-moistened speculum is used to preserve all evidence. The examination for trauma includes observation of the external genitalia, perineum, cervix and vaginal wall for trauma and lacerations. Specimens are obtained from the urethral orifice for bacteriological testing for venereal disease, from the cervix for cytology and Papanicolaou staining, and from the vagina and cervix for chemistry and sperm testing. The physical findings are shown in the chart below.

Eight of the 80 victims did not receive speculum pelvic examinations. Copious vaginal bleeding required immediate vaginal packing and hospitalization of one victim. The hymen ring was intact and thus just a swab of the vaginal wall was taken from four patients. Two victims were not examined because of their pain and anxiety and one patient refused a pelvic speculum examination.

Women were usually concerned about the possibility of pregnancy resulting from the rape but none in our sample became pregnant. To guard against pregnancy, the gynecologist prescribes diethylstilbestrol. Women have sometimes heard of the medication as the "morning after pill" or it is explained as a "chemical D and C." This medication should be started as soon as possible and certainly within 24 to 36 hours to prevent implantation of a fertilized egg.

A variety of factors influence the physician's decision to prescribe medication of this type. Current birth control practice of the woman is one factor. Seventeen of the 80 victims were either on oral contraceptive pills (11 women), had an intrauterine device (4 women), or had had a tubal ligation (2 women).

Phase of the menstrual cycle is another factor. For women who were raped midway in their menstrual cycle, the concern about pregnancy was greatest. Even those women close to their menstrual periods were given prescriptions if they wished. Ten of the 80 victims were raped during their menstrual periods. These women had extra trauma from the tampon being pushed into the posterior cul-de-sac. The gynecologist removed the tampon on speculum examination.

Fear of exposure to venereal disease was a major concern of almost all women in our sample. Routine medical treatment was to administer procaine penicillin intramuscularly. Oral antibiotics were prescribed for those victims allergic to penicillin.

While venereal disease is a major concern at the time of the rape, a number of women will develop acute vaginal infections which may become chronic. Women need to be seen for follow-up six weeks later, and we recommend they be seen again six months after that, to be sure they have not contracted a venereal disease, especially syphilis.

Psychological Process

For most women in the sample, the rape represented a crisis with either psychological or social consequences. This was made overwhelmingly clear both from data collected from the interview at the hospital and during the follow-up telephone counseling.

The counselors were regarded by the victims as part of the emergency ward treatment team. Access to the women at this point in the crisis facilitated the therapeutic aspects of the counseling relationship. Most women responded favorably to the presence of the counselors and responded equally well on follow-up telephone calls. One victim said:

It is easy to talk with you, a stranger. It is good the hospital has something like this. So many people might tend to blame the woman. It's good to talk to someone who doesn't.

The ease or difficulty a woman has in talking about the rape experience may be viewed as her verbal style. The hospital system places demands on the victim to answer questions and describe the details of the rape. Victims respond to this in different ways. Some victims, because of their natural talking style or their youth, find this pressure to talk difficult and have a defensive reaction. Other victims respond to the pressure to talk with relief. It gives them a chance to ventilate some of their feelings. The verbal styles of the victims in our sample ranged from quiet to guarded to verbal to talkative. Often there were shifts from one style to another within an interview.

According to our data, one-half of the women in our sample were verbal and talkative and half were on the quiet and guarded end of the spectrum. Both styles are normal and it is important that nurses be aware of this variance.

The emotional style of the victim refers to the style that is normal for her in expressing her feelings. One's emotional style tends to become exaggerated under stress and having to talk about the rape experience to a variety of persons is one such stress for the victim.

In our sample, two styles were observed: In the *expressed* style, feelings of fear, anger, or anxiety were expressed verbally or shown through such behavior as crying, shaking, smiling, restlessness, and tenseness. In the *controlled* style, feelings were masked or hidden and a calm, composed, or subdued affect was seen.

Patients' responses ranged from fear, restlessness, tears, and anger to smiling, calmness, and composure. Some women had several of these responses during the course of one interview.

The primary reaction of almost all women to the rape was fear, that is, fear for their lives. To them the behavior of the assailants represented an act of violence.

A 35-year-old woman, who was grabbed by an assailant at four-thirty in the afternoon as she left her apartment to visit a friend, said:

I felt terror. I was so scared I could think of nothing else but fear. There was no other feeling present. I don't know what I am going to do now (tears). I cannot even walk on the street. This is the worst experience of my 35 years. Nothing so terrible has happened before.

In another situation, a 20-year-old, married student was waiting for a bus when a car stopped and three men pulled her into the car. This young woman said:

I spent the whole time while I was riding in the car [blindfolded] thinking of the girl [in a recent newspaper story] locked in the closet who was murdered.

A 23-year-old hospital employee walking home after the 3:00 to 11:00 P.M. shift was pulled into some bushes off the main sidewalk. She said:

I tried yelling but he put his hand around my throat. I have never been strangled, but he tightened his hand so hard that it hurt so bad. I couldn't do anything. I was frightened of dying—the thought of being killed when the rape was over.

A significant number of women show their feelings by tears and crying as well as other signs of being visibly upset such as shaking. They find it difficult to talk about the incident and cry when describing the very painful parts. Women have said things like, "I will never be normal again," and, "I wish he'd killed me."

The expressed emotion of anger may have a variety of targets: the assailant, the act of rape, the police interrogation, the hospital system, the counseling service, the court process. All are appropriate foci for the victim's feelings.

When they expressed anger toward a procedure in the emergency ward, they generally spoke of the pelvic examination. One statement captures the distress of the woman:

The pelvic was quite depressing at the time. To have to get undressed again and get up on that table and go through almost the same thing again of something being stuck into you was awful.

Another victim directed her anger at the assailant. She said with bitterness:

It is not fair that he should be running around having a good time while I have to go through this—to have to take medicine that will make me sick. Why should I have to go through this?

This victim had been raped before. Thus she knew already one of the side effects of the medicine and talked about it at the hospital. For most women, the nausea and abdominal pains from medication to prevent pregnancy will be a new experience.

Still another women expressing her anger at the assailant said:

I was angry. I could have torn him apart if he had not had the knife. I was outraged that he would do such a thing, that he would have the gall.

A certain number of women expressed feelings by smiling. Sometimes

when feelings are unbearable, the victim defends psychologically or sub-
stitutes another feeling such as avoidance: As one woman who smiled occasionally during the interview said, "Laughing is better than crying." As
another example, a 20-year-old woman returned to her apartment after
work and was raped six times by a man wearing a ski mask and rubber
gloves, who had broken into the apartment and was waiting for her. During the interview, she would cry occasionally when describing the upsetting parts. She also laughed several times. The laugh was used as a way of
avoiding feelings. She would say, "Really, nothing is wrong with me," and
laughed as she said it. She substituted a laugh for the painful memory of
the attack.

Women who seemed calm and composed said they were controlling or
hiding their feelings. They would say, "I will probably be depressed later
when this really hits me." Also, many women were seen in the
emergency ward in the middle of the night (between 1:00 A.M. and 5:00
A.M. was the most frequent time) and these women were often exhausted;
they had not slept since the previous night. This calm exterior might have
been a sign of sheer exhaustion.

A 20-year-old woman was assaulted in the hallway of her apartment
building by an assailant who had followed her and her roommate home
from a local college night place. The roommate was able to telephone the
police, who arrived in time to apprehend the man in the act of rape. At
4:00 A.M. during the hospital interview, the victim said, "I feel so tired. I
know I seem calm. The reaction may hit me later." It did.

Other victims who also presented a controlled, calm outward appearance found it important to present a "strong" appearance and to have
people think everything was fine and that there would be no problems.
The woman would say, "I'll be fine; you don't have to worry." Or the
woman would talk about the rape in a controlled, emotionless way. This
was her style of coping.

Many women said they were "in a state of shock" and "feeling numb."
They would say, "It doesn't seem real; I can't believe this happened," or
"I just want to forget it; I don't want to remember."

Discussing the rape, the women often associated it with related issues.
The woman's sexuality was one such issue. Some discussed previous
sexual activity, forced sexual acts and/or rape, and the loss of virginity
from the rape. One women said, "I remember my first sexual experience;
the guy just jumped on top of me." A 24-year-old woman said, "I have always hated men. I don't like sex. This is the last straw. I am puritanical
about sex." The possibility of pregnancy was also a concern. One woman
said, "I don't believe in abortion; but I wouldn't want the baby."

Losses, especially past relationships with men, are another theme in the concerns women have after being raped. Former engagements and other breakups in male-female relationships are often discussed. One woman talked of the death of her husband seven years previously. Another woman talked of her divorce three years previously. Still another talked of her suicide attempt as a response to her loneliness after her divorce.

Concern over future relationships, especially how to cope with men, was another theme. For example, a 21-year-old woman said:

My fiance will be enraged [at what happened to me]. I feel so bad. He didn't want me to come to school here. Now he won't want me to stay and I have one semester left.

A newly married, 20-year-old, college student said:

It's like being unfaithful, but I couldn't help it. I'm afraid my husband will have the feeling I let him down. I had a religious upbringing; my family will overplay the idea that sex with anyone outside of marriage is worse than death. I could never tell my family that this happened to me.

Nursing Implications

Three assumptions underlie the theoretical framework for counseling the rape victim: (a) the rape represents a situational crisis for the victim which is disruptive of her life-style; (b) the victim is viewed as a consumer of emergency health services—medical and psychological; and (c) crisis management of the rape victim is actually the practice of primary prevention of psychiatric disorders.

The nurse in the emergency ward is in an optimal position to have major therapeutic impact on the experience of the rape victim in the hospital system. There are ways to make the woman's hospital experience less traumatic.

Periodic interdisciplinary staff conferences should be held by the emergency ward team. Staff feelings and attitudes about rape victims as well as current research findings on rape would be important for staff education.

Time is an important factor in working with the rape victim. The police may be waiting for further questioning, and laboratory tests and treatment need to be instituted as quickly as possible for maximum effect. Delays should be avoided. The triage nurse should view the victim as high priority.

The woman should not be left alone, if at all possible. If a nurse is not available and there is to be a delay for the physician, encourage family or friends to stay with the victim for emotional support. This is a good time for the nurse to make a psychological assessment of the rape victim.

A separate examining room is preferred to allow the woman privacy to fully describe the circumstances of the incident. The woman should not be rushed in her talk, as she may interpret this as being forced through the system. Force in any form may symbolize the rape experience.

The prevailing attitudes in society are not on the side of the victim. Many myths exist, leading people to interpret rape solely in sexual terms rather than in violence terms. Staff members may show their bias and ambivalence about rape victims through such statements as, "The woman is just faking," or, "This isn't a real rape case," or, "I don't believe half the stories I hear."

Any attitude which blames the victim will serve only to abort any therapeutic relationship before it has a chance to develop. Listen carefully to the victim as she relates her experience and leave moral and legal judgments to others. The nurse should be nonjudgmental.

The humanistic skills of the nurse will make a major difference in how the victim feels she has been treated at the hospital. The victim should be encouraged to talk. She has many feelings and thoughts about the rape and she often wants to talk if she feels someone will listen. Talking helps people to feel better and this, in turn, gives understanding of their reactions to the incident.

If the nurse also listens carefully she can understand the distress of the woman. When a person is understood, she is no longer alone and is more in control of her situation. Listening and understanding are important skills in counseling.

A special dimension of listening and understanding is to help the victim bear the feelings she is trying to express. Sharing the pain is an emotionally strengthening experience for the victim of rape.

The technical skills of the nurse are an important part of the overall nursing management of the rape victim. An important part of preparing the victim for the physical and gynecological examination is to find out if she has ever been examined.

For some women and especially child victims, this will be the first pelvic examination. The woman needs to know what is expected of her and what the physician will be doing and why. Often the gynecologist explains this, but reinforcement by the nurse will help the woman feel involved rather than being the object of things that are being done to her. She has just been through an experience where consent was not part of the procedure, and so cooperation with her in the hospital treatment is essential for therapeutic care.

The nurse can arrange for the physical comfort of the woman in the hospital. Victims in our sample have needed such items as safety pins, needle and thread to mend torn clothing, drinks of water to relieve their thirst, cigarettes to decrease their anxiety, and tissues to dry their tears.

Many women complain of feeling dirty and request a place to wash. Many have been raped outdoors. Some have been urinated on. Water and a basin would be important equipment to have available after the medical examination is complete. Mouthwash is also a helpful item to provide for those women (of whom there are many) who have been forced to have oral sex.

Health education is another service. The nurse is the appropriate person to further emphasize and elaborate on the prescribed medical treatment for the woman. She should ask if the woman understood what the physician advised for treatment, ask if the woman has other questions, be sure the woman understands the side effects of the penicillin (discomfort at the site of the injection) and the diethylstilbestrol (nausea, vomiting, vaginal spotting), and advise the woman to come back to the gynecological clinic or see her own gynecologist for follow-up examination and culture for venereal disease and infection.

Discharge planning is needed, too. Rape victims often do not have transportation home. Their money may have been stolen, and they often leave the hospital at night. When the woman is ready for discharge from the emergency ward, the nurse should be sure the woman has transportation home or wherever she is going. Abandoning the victim is not therapeutic. The hospital might work out arrangements with appropriate community resources (such as police) for those situations where family or friends are not available to take the victim home.

Crisis Center

As rape crisis centers are developing, emergency departments might have the referral telephone number available for the woman. Ask the woman for permission to give her number to the crisis center with the understanding that the follow-up person from the center will take the initiative in contacting the victim. All women should have access to a follow-up service, if at all possible.

The therapeutic nursing management of the rape victim sets into motion a series of administrative, humanistic, and technical skills of the helper. To be a "genuine" victim in our society means that one must have people available who can accept and acknowledge that something extremely disruptive has occurred in one's life. In other words, the victim's claim to having been victimized needs to receive confirmation from others. If, however, the staff's attitude appears to be that "nothing has happened" to the woman, or if the attitude that "she asked for it" clouds the issue of physical and psychological trauma, the humanistic approach will be lost.

It does not take a psychiatric nurse or nursing clinician to talk with a rape victim. It is vital that all nurses have such counseling skills.

22 WORKING WITH DRUG ABUSE PATIENTS IN THE ER

Sharon Yowell, M.S., R.N.

Carolyn Brose, M.S., R.N.

YOU JUST FINISHED LAVAGING THE BARBITURATE OVERDOSE PATIENT. He's withdrawn. Whenever you try to do anything for him, he shouts, "Don't bug me!" How can you approach this patient? How can you help him to start looking for a better way to cope with his problem? He probably won't accept follow-up care unless you can help him in recognizing his need. What about the paranoid amphetamine abuser? You don't want to sedate him because, when he crashes, sedation may exaggerate his depression.

These are some of the problems that an emergency room nurse faces in working with the patient who abuses drugs. These patients are often disruptive and the ER atmosphere can intensify their reactions. Treatment of the physiological effects of a drug overdose is, of course, the first priority. But because the ER often is the person's first contact with professionals, helping him recognize he needs additional assistance is the second priority.

Attempts to understand why some people abuse drugs have included research into the personality structure of drug abusers and research to determine why they use chemicals to cope with their daily problems. Early research showed that drug abusers' personality characteristics are related to the basic need for personal control—a desire to control their level and experience of stimulation, to control metabolic processes, to modify social role or status, and to modify experiences of time and distance, particularly in relation to other people (1).

Chemicals can do all of these things. By selecting the appropriate drug, one can speed up, slow down, feel pleasure, be awakened or anesthetized to pain, alienation, or almost any other experience. Time and space can be modified so that one is isolated from or in touch with everything in the surroundings.

At first, analysis of these characteristics appeared to be a key to understanding the drug abuser and thus to controlling drug abuse. However the need for personal control is common to all people, not just drug abusers (2). We all control how much television we watch, what and how much we eat or drink, how much we smoke, and the activities we take part in. Most of us try to choose the people we spend our time with and regulate how closely we become involved with them.

Therefore, knowledge of personality characteristics alone does not provide sufficient information to aid in reducing drug abuse. A more constructive approach to the problem might be to focus on the person's *need* to adjust his situation by using chemicals, rather than to concentrate on "what's wrong" with his personality structure (3). A two-year study of 600 drug abusers, sponsored by the Johnson County Council on Drug Abuse (Kansas), indicated that similar environmental and personal coping patterns are displayed by people who abuse each of the major classes of drugs. Those studied were 14 to 25 years old, and came from middle class suburban communities. The majority were voluntary participants in an outpatient drug treatment program (4,5,6). This study's findings dispel the notion that there is a typical drug user, and discourage attempts to find out why people take drugs (7).

A more critical problem is to determine how drug abusers can learn the skills necessary to create alternatives to drug abuse in dealing with the stress in their lives. There is a fine line between use and abuse of drugs, alcohol, food, or anything else. But, chemicals have a different potential for abuse, depending on their pharmacologic action.

The risks in using drugs vary, depending on the interaction of five factors:

- the individual's personality
- the desired or anticipated effects of the drug
- mood when the drug is taken
- the specific chemical used
- the interplay of these factors and the person's social situation.

Reactions to the same drug taken by the same person at different times or in different situations may vary considerably.

Our recommended therapeutic approaches to drug abusers in the emergency room are based on the environmental and coping patterns observed among drug abuse patients in the Johnson County Drug Abuse Council study. We have related this information to the reactions commonly seen with each group of chemcials.

Barbiturate Abuse

The barbiturate abuser has, or believes that he has, little control over his life. He perceives that he is under too much pressure, derives too little satisfaction, and has too little power and too few skills to deal with the people and stimulation surrounding him. He reduces these pressures by numbing his mind and body.

Long-term barbiturate abuse perpetuates passivity, lack of involvement, and isolation. The person avoids change, conflict, and new experiences, and becomes increasingly resistive and pseudo aggressive.

In the ER, the barbiturate abuser may appear intoxicated. Behavior will be extremely labile,—he is whining or crying at one moment, loud and abusive the next. The typical response may be resistive, "Let me alone. I can do what I want to." Actually, relief from the pressure of having to relate to others and from the frustration of not knowing how to relate is perhaps the only satisfaction and pleasure this person experiences.

Similar behavior is exhibited by people who use alcohol or prescribed sedatives to unwind after a very stimulating or frustrating day. These substances depress the body, and supply temporary relief. The fine line between drug use and abuse is illustrated by society's acceptance of these actions to tune oneself down.

Drug abusers come to the ER voluntarily or they are brought in by police, family, or friends. When a barbiturate user appears by his own choice, he usually has been frightened by the potential effects of mixed or unknown drugs.

Treatment of central nervous system, respiratory, or cardiovascular depression from barbiturate overdose is the first priority. Treatment often consists of gastric lavage, stabilization of vital signs, and dismissal. After lavage, the patient is kept physically active and stimulated while the absorbed barbiturate is metabolized.

This patient should not be dismissed to care for himself. If his release cannot be prevented, the ER staff must insist that he be accompanied by his friends, even when he appears fully conscious and in stable condition. If the person is addicted to barbiturates, especially to extremely high doses, withdrawal symptoms can begin after release, with severe cramping, nausea, and delirium; and may progress to convulsions and death.

For these reasons, the barbiturate addict is usually admitted for gradual detoxification.

Any environment, but especially an emergency room, may be very stimulating to the barbiturate abuser. Contact with other people often is perceived as intrusive, as bugging or hassling. Typically, this patient believes that others are incapable of providing positive input into his life. Many barbiturate abusers come from homes with nagging parents or spouses, and from situations where accusation and blame are constant.

For some people, the crisis period in the ER may be the only time any real therapeutic intervention is possible. Defenses are down; the patient may be reachable. However, firmness and patience are necessary to overcome resistance to suggestions. Resistance stiffens when the barbiturate abuser feels he is being forced to do something against his will.

The best approach at this time is to be firm but not confront. You may have to be somewhat intrusive to penetrate the patient's defensive shields, but don't encroach on his power to make decisions, or you will be shut out just as quickly and firmly as everyone else.

In the ER, the barbiturate abuser needs acknowledgment that life has been miserable. Let the patient know you are aware that he is the only one who can make any real change in his life. He needs to hear that the option he chose has not worked well but that there are other options. At this time, objective, nonjudgmental feedback helps most. Avoid asking why or how or telling the person "you should." Any probing or advice may be taken negatively. Assure the patient of your interest—"I'm not going to leave you alone. I would like to talk with you more."

If the person does begin to listen, he may develop sufficient trust to make a short-term contract that he won't use drugs until a specified time when he can consider his alternatives without the barbiturate's influence.

Roosa's model for reaching a decision, SOCS, may be helpful (8). SOCS stands for situation, option, consequences, and simulation. This is a problem-solving approach that defines the situation in the person's life, and the choices open to him, and relates these to potential consequences. In practice, SOCS may be used as follows:

I think the Situation is_____.
What do you think?
I think an Option is_____.
What do you think?
I think the Consequences of that option are _____.
What do you think?

Staff can simulate situations and practice this technique on each other until they feel comfortable using it.

Follow-up of the emergency treatment is vital. Just giving the person a phone number is not follow-up.

Opiate Abuse

Like the barbiturate abuser, the person who takes opiates tends to withdraw from pressure, and to feel little satisfaction with his life or control over it. The depressive effects of opiates on the central nervous system effectively block out the problems of dealing with frustrations. The euphoria is superb. There are no problems.

Generally, the opiate-addicted person has more succesful interpersonal relations and tends to be more aggressive than the barbiturate abuser. The barbiturate abuser is apt to be sensitive, sorry for himself, and introverted. The opiate abuser is more extroverted.

Once addicted, skillful manipulation and active involvement in the drug culture environment are necessary if he is to avoid the intense physical pain which occurs when he cannot obtain the opiate. The costs of these drugs are high, and habits very quickly become very expensive. Many opiate addicts may turn to theft or prostitution to support their habit. Physical dependence, and high tolerance are all commonly present.

For these reasons, and because of the life-style associated with long-term opiate abuse, this person is rarely seen in an ER except in deep coma or death. Rather than seek medical assistance, and risk legal complications, the opiate abuser who has taken an overdose often counteracts the depressive effects by injecting stimulants. When this person is brought for help, nalorphine (Nalline), a narcotic antagonist, rapidly reverses the depressant effects. It may also precipitate withdrawal symptoms in physically dependent persons.

As with the barbiturate user, such a crisis period may be the only time effective intervention can be started, because the person's defenses are down. An approach similar to that used with the barbiturate abuser is best for the person who takes opiates.

Amphetamine Abuse

Amphetamines probably have the highest potential for abuse because tolerance develops quickly and necessitates higher and higher dosages. Oral administration is often replaced by injection to obtain sufficient stimulation or highs. Subjecting the body to high doses of amphetamines over a prolonged time is extremely destructive, physically and psychologically.

People who take stimulants often have very high expectations of themselves and believe they are failures if they do not achieve these goals. The person who opts to take stimulants is usually one whose environment is too demanding. They are people who feel they want to, or must, accomplish more than they have time to do.

The person becomes more active to cope with external pressures and demands. When higher doses of amphetamines are necessary to reach and maintain the desired high, oral ingestion frequently is replaced by injection.

Amphetamine abusers fall into a vicious cycle. Following injection, the person feels intense stimulation and excitement—the rush. Hours later, depending on the dose taken, the stimulation vanishes and depression occurs. Commonly known as the crash, this mental and physical depression is often accompanied by suicidal ideas.

Amphetamine abusers can take a potentially lethal dose (1,000–5,000 mg./day) with no apparent adverse physical effect (9). They may speed up for three or four days, then crash awakening with a ferocious appetite and depression. To alleviate the pain, they begin the cycle again, with the same results. The body cannot tolerate constant, intense extremes of stimulation and depression. In time, marked psychological and personality changes occur.

During the high, perception becomes distorted because every stimulus is experienced acutely. The person can very easily become erratic, aggressive, violent, hyperactive, and extremely suspicious. Marked impairment in judgment is evident. He may shut himself in a room without windows, furniture, or light, and still have all the stimulation he can manage.

For a patient exhibiting these behaviors, the ER is perhaps the worst place to be. The lights, noise, rapid movements, and strange people and voices can cause or increase panic.

The first step in this patient's care is to manipulate the environment. Do not approach him too closely—he may perceive your motion as threatening. Take him to a room where there is minimal activity. Dim the lights and explain calmly everything that you are doing, to the smallest detail. Speak slowly. Slight movements—scratching your nose, folding your arms—can be perceived as potential attack. Don't whisper to others. Suspiciousness and paranoia are usual in these patients, and they often misinterpret innocent gestures or comments.

It is not wise to push or intrude in any way when dealing with the amphetamine abuser. Tomorrow means nothing. Even 10 minutes is too far in the future for any planning. By keeping your distance, allowing friends or family to remain nearby, and explaining everything you are doing, before you do it, you may prevent aggressive behavior. Be especially careful not to do something inadvertently that you promised you would not do. Also, don't say "I won't hurt you" and then give a painful injection.

Avoid talking about feelings. Keep all communication simple: "I'm not going to touch you," "What do you want me to do for you?" "I'll tell you everything that I am going to do before I do it." If possible, determine what he wants. If it is a cigarette or a place to stay until the effects of the drug wear off, grant these requests as soon as possible. Ideally, depressants are not given to this patient because the depressive phase will only be deepened when the effects of the amphetamine wear off. If the panic becomes extreme, depressants will be necessary.

Hallucinogen Abuse

The person most likely to abuse hallucinogenic drugs, usually has not found much stimulation in life, his environment seems dull and uninteresting, or confusing. None of society's values seem to make sense. Meaning, imagination, and differences seem to be painfully lacking.

D-lysergic acid (LSD) and certain other hallucinogens can produce acute sensitivity to visual, auditory, and tactile stimuli, and extremes of happiness and sadness, peace and anxiety. At times, the user experiences deep personal insight or religious union with others. These feelings may be very pleasurable. For others, the experience is a stressing, frightening escape from a dull existence to a horrifying one.

Anxiety and panic are usually a result of the novice's reaction to the hallucinating experience, rather than a direct consequence of the drug. A person can forget that what he is experiencing is caused by the drug and he may fear that he is going crazy.

As with the amphetamine abuser, manipulation of the environment is helpful. Permit friends to remain in the ER and reduce external stimuli as much as possible. Reassure the patient that what he is experiencing are effects of the drug, that they will end, and that someone will stay with him until he can manage by himself. Lavage is not advisable for this patient; he may see the tube as a snake being forced down his throat.

"Talking down" from a panic reaction is the most effective help. The talk down is a gradual redefining of the bad experience into something less frightening or even pleasurable. Begin to elicit information from the patient. Ask what he is experiencing and what he sees or hears. When the person describes something frightening, focus on its more positive aspect. If the person claims he is being attacked by green and purple men, you might respond. "Green and purple! That's a color clash." Because of the patient's suggestibility, he can easily focus on the colors rather than the 'attackers.' Pick up the cues and follow through with what the person is describing. This process may take several hours, so let the patient's friends take over or call for additional assistance.

The emergency department is not an after-hours psychiatric clinic. However, just as emotional support of the critically injured patient is a necessary part of emergency care, so psychological support of the drug abuse patient is an ER responsibility. Patient workloads and staffing determine how much time and support are given to any patient. In the best situations, the crisis may be the beginning of rehabilitation for drug abusers. At the very least, they deserve emotional support while they are in the ER and referral to other agencies for follow-up care.

References

1. O'Connor, W A *Four Criteria for Chemical Abuse.* Paper presented at Missouri Social Work Conference. Drugs and Alcohol, held at Kansas City, Mo., April 1971.
2. *Social Implications of Drug Abuse.* Paper presented at Annual Conference Kansas Psychiatric Association, held Sept. 1971.
3. *Echosystems Theory and Clinical Mental Health.* (To be published)
4. *Drug Intervention Group Handbook.* Washington, D.C., U.S. Dept. of Justice. 1971 (Mimeographed).
5. And Others, *Who, What, Why of Drugs.* Paper presented at Industrial Drug Seminar. Greater Kansas City Association of Industrial Nurses held at Kansas City in June 1972.
6. Crosbil, Q I *The Environment of a Community Drug Program for Youth: Resources, Use, and Benefits.* Lawrence. University of Kansas, 1974. (Unpublished doctoral dissertation).
7. Barker, R G *Ecological Psychology,* Stanford. Calif., Stanford University Press, 1968.
8. Roosa, J B *SOCS Situation, Options, Consequences, Simulation: A Technique for Teaching Social Interaction.* Paper presented at American Psychological Association Annual Meeting, held in Montreal, Aug. 1973.
9. Smith, David The trip. *Emergency Medicine,* Dec. 1969, p. 32.

23 EASING MENTAL PATIENTS' RETURN TO THEIR COMMUNITIES

Mary Bayer, B.S., R.N.

"SHE WIPES HER NOSE ON THE CURTAINS."
"HE does weird things like urinating on the front lawn."
"She sits and rocks and talks to herself all day."
These were laments from boarding home staff members about boarders who were, until recently, back-ward patients in the state mental hospital.

If the staff members were shocked, so were the patients. At least, in the mental hospital, their odd behavior was more or less accepted. Already shocked by change from the familiar to a strange "home," they now had to endure the disapproval of their caretakers.

Most of these staff members had neither the experience nor education to understand these patients who had been in back wards anywhere from 15 to 40 years. The need of both groups for follow-up service was so great that such a program became my first priority when I was employed by our rural mental health center, the Tri County Mental Health Services, Rumford, Maine.

At that time, the state mental hospital, the Augusta Mental Health Institute, was releasing many of these patients, some to their own families, many to boarding homes. The hospital had been making some referrals to our branch of a tri county mental health center which served Oxford County, but, for the most part, the referral slips remained in a drawer. The center did not have the staff nor the time to follow through.

Today, four years later, a thriving continued-care program has changed many of the hospital's discharge procedures. For the patients, the program has cut rehospitalization rates and, when patients are readmitted, has reduced the time they stay. Boarding home personnel understand them better, and so does the community. Local people are beginning to regard the state mental hospital as a rehabilitation center for people with emotional difficulties, not a dumping ground for deviants.

The community in which these changes have taken place is a rural county with a population of 43,000, mostly working class people. A mountain range divides Oxford County in half, and we have an office on each side.

When I was hired as the sole nurse in the mental health center, I was expected to assume a case load immediately. I had adequate time, however, to assess and plan my role in the clinic. Attending meetings with our staff and others, I learned more about the discharge patients and the boarding homes.

Many of the patients were elderly and had various chronic physical problems. Their discharge papers poorly documented their physical problems, and the hospital was not referring them to local physicians. When discharged patients became physically ill, boarding home proprietors wanted to return them to the state hospital. The hospital, however, refused to readmit the physically ill unless they were also psychotic, and most were not.

Frequently, if a patient "didn't work out" at one boarding home, a health and welfare worker transferred her or him to another home, or custodians exchanged patients without informing anyone else.

The state division of hospital services, which licenses nursing homes, had begun to inspect the larger boarding homes. The small (three-to-six-bed) boarding homes, though, and the one-to-two-bed foster homes seemed accountable to no one at that time, and abuse of patients was suspected in many cases.

I began visiting the tri county unit of the state hospital on a weekly basis, getting to know staff and Oxford County patients. (In keeping with current trends, the hospital had recently regrouped patients by place of geographic origin rather than by diagnosis or degree of violence.) I conferred with the unit chief and the team leaders about mutual concerns.

Within a few weeks, Nan Brizindine, a staff nurse at the hospital, was freed from most of her former responsibilities to work with me in defining a liaison-nursing position. She and I began to plan what we termed a "sustaining care" program. As we planned, Nan spent two days a week out in the county and three in the hospital.

We hoped to replace the word "aftercare," with its connotation of second-class citizens and care, with a new concept, "sustaining care." To us, this implied *caring* and *advocacy*.

Our first tasks were to win organizational support and to identify the needs of patients who were soon to be discharged from the hospital. At a joint meeting with our agency supervisors, Nan and I explained that we planned to use the nursing process to execute the project. We carefully outlined for them the steps of assessing, planning, implementing, and evaluating. We agreed to keep our supervisors updated in writing every two weeks, and they gave us free hand.

Together, we designed an assessment tool to evaluate patients' physical, emotional, and social status. Using the assessment data to draw a baseline of health, we would be able to measure subsequent changes.

Shortly after, we found that we needed to assess the homes that accepted patients. In the past, patients had been placed anywhere there was a vacancy, with little attention to the specific needs of either patient or placement facility. We designed an assessment tool, which we could use uniformly with all of the small boarding and foster homes. We planned to correlate the data with each patient's assessed needs and, by careful planning, decrease the movement of patients from home to home and from home to hospital.

Using the tool, we systematically surveyed the foster and small boarding homes in Oxford County and filed copies of the completed forms at the hospital and at the mental health center's clinic. These made a ready reference describing the patient's environment and, when a vacancy occurred in a home, gave the hospital an objective profile of the home available.

Within a month, Nan and I had established the following priorities:

- To systematize discharge planning
- To coordinate referrals from hospital to community agencies
- To provide inservice education for caretakers (foster and boarding home proprietors and staff, family members)
- To increase patient advocacy
- To better use community resources for these patients
- To design and justify a liaison nursing position which eventually one person could fill.

Our top priority was to systematize the existing discharge procedure. To do this, we divided the procedures into three phases: *predischarge*, *convalescent status*, and *discharge*.

During the *predischarge* phase, hospital personnel would identify patients for discharge. Using the assessment tool, the liaison nurse would assess the patient. The staff would begin resocialization, make referrals, identify the placement home, and make an appointment for the patient's evaluation at the mental health center.

We designated the *convalescent* phase as a 30-day trial period in which the patient would live in the community. While she was adjusting to her new environment (75 percent of our patients were women), the patient would return to the hospital without going through the admission procedure again.

During this 30-day phase, the liaison nurse would visit the patient in the home and would present her case to the therapist assigned by the mental health clinic. She and the patient together would be seen at the clinic and she would report back to the hospital staff.

The *discharge* phase was to begin after completion of the discharge papers. At the time of her discharge, the patient was to receive a one-month supply of medication and a clinic appointment for evaluation and medication review. The liaison nurse would send a summary of her hospitalization to the clinic.

In the ensuing months, the liaison nurse would visit the patient in the home bimonthly for at least three months or until the clinic staff and caretakers could supply the support. She would also make monthly visits to all the boarding homes and foster homes in the county to provide continuing education for the staffs.

As soon as we had explained the new plan to the hospital staff and incorporated their suggestions into it, we began the new discharge procedure. Everyone seemed enthusiastic and cooperative, probably because all staff had been involved from the beginning and it was theirs, too.

Then came an obstacle. Nan moved out of the state. The position of liaison nurse could not be filled for several months, but the hospital staff overextended themselves to keep the project alive until Bernie Mickeriz, a nurse who had worked for many years in the local community hospital, volunteered.

Bernie is accountable only to the clinic administrator in the mental health center and to the hospital unit chief. Her salary is paid by the hospital but her major base of operation is in the community.

On her days at the hospital, she attends morning intershift meetings and conferences where the staff discuss only Oxford County patients with her. The patients know the days to expect her visit and approach eagerly saying, "Oh, I'm so glad to see you!" or they might say, "Good, now you can tell me how my mother is."

Bernie is always consulted before a discharge. Often, the staff seem to have as many questions about the "outside" as the patients do, because they frequently ask, "How's Betty (or Bob) doing these days?"

At the mental health center, she serves as advocate for former state hospital patients, insisting that they be given the same staff time and consideration as the center's short-term patients. At each staff center meeting she presents cases and the staff frequently ask for news about the patients they have had to hospitalize.

She visits the largest (35-bed) boarding home weekly to provide staff support and informal inservice education. Once a month, she and the clinic psychiatrist visit this home to review boarders' medications. Three years ago, no one was reviewing medications, and the staff knew nothing about caring for psychiatric patients. Then, they would refer to the boarders as "those people," as if the former patients were creatures from another planet.

During monthly visits to smaller homes, she has often intervened early, thus preventing severe physical problems or exacerbation of mental illness.

One afternoon a week, she attends the day treatment activity program held in a church basement for foster home residents. She observes individual progress and visits with the caretakers when they come to pick up their boarders. Several of them are so interested in the meetings that they attend the full two-hour session each week to learn new skills.

Bernie also acts as patient advocate with others in the community, meeting often with clergy, physicians, law enforcement officers, community health nurses, and various volunteers.

While this is a success story, there have been problems, too. Right at the beginning and for some time after, we had difficulty justifying to the hospital staff our reason for strongly emphasizing patients' physical status. We pointed out that medical care was substandard in the institution. I was able to cite specific patients who had been discharged while suffering serious chronic medical problems that had gone unnoticed in the hospital.

As we started the program, we also interviewed community physicians. We found them reluctant to get involved with expatients from the state hospital, because the hospital never furnished any referral information. Patients frequently had abdominal scars and the physicians would ask, "What's been removed?" or "What's left in there?" The patients did not know. The physicians said they would be receptive to seeing these patients if the hospital would furnish decent referrals.

As awareness of the need for more comprehensive medical care grew, the hospital administration soon changed policies. Hospital physicians began giving thorough discharge physical examinations to each patient and making findings available to the discharge planners. Within a few months, they initiated yearly checkups as well.

As the project gained visibility statewide, administrators began to question why this role should be filled by a nurse. Why not someone from another mental health discipline? they asked. However, we believed then as now that this must be a nursing position rather than a social work position.

By the time this question was raised seriously, we had documented cases where a nurse's knowledge of normal physical conditions and development and her ability to quickly detect deviations had been important in crisis intervention.

In one case, an elderly woman in a remote boarding home began acting strangely. The caretaker thought perhaps her medications should be changed. When we responded to the call, we thought that she had had a cerebrovascular accident. We sent her to the hospital, where our suspicions were confirmed.

In another case, a woman was thought to have a "bad chest cold." The nurse had to arrange hospitalization immediately because of pneumonia. Another woman was thought to be regressing into her former hebephrenic state. Her trouble was fecal impaction, which she was trying to evacuate.

These incidents may seem unconvincing evidence to city people, as health care services are readily available in cities. But the distances and the general lack of knowledge about health maintenance in rural areas make the problems different. Rural people tend to try home remedies, ignore the problem and hope it will go away, or wait until the health situation reaches a crisis.

We were amazed, too, that problems which, to us, were obviously related to physical illness caused most caretakers to assume that the patient was "going crazy again." Once a nurse, who was versed in physical, emotional, and social assessment, began visiting the homes on a regular basis, many problems were solved in the early stages. The caretakers also began to learn that mental patients are also human beings, vulnerable to the same physical ailments that can affect anyone.

WORKING WITH GROUPS
AND FAMILIES

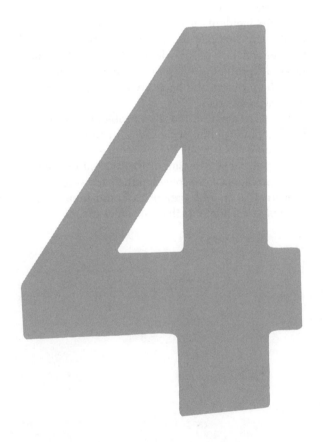

Introduction

In many settings, nurses are involved in formal and informal groups on a daily basis. Nurses can, with a basic knowledge of group dynamics, coupled with experience in analyzing group behaviors, make valuable contributions in both leader and membership roles. Diabetic and newborn care classes, ward and therapeutic community meetings, activity groups, floor staff conferences, and psychotherapy groups are only a few of the kinds of groups nurses organize and lead. The extent of nursing responsibility for specific groups is dependent upon the kind of group and on the nurse's preparation and experience. Professional nurses today are frequently expected to assume group leadership roles, but should, in return, expect to receive adequate support and supervision for their group work.

The advantages of working with groups are many. One of the most effective arguments for a group approach has always been that in the same amount of time a practitioner can provide attention to several clients instead of only one. The most important reason for working with groups, however, is not the timesaving effect, but the opportunity groups provide for using the positive forces of mutual support and the rich variety of insights and experiences which several individuals can bring to bear on the same concerns or problems. A skillful group leader or member is readily able to recognize and enhance the development of behaviors which contribute to meeting the group's goals. Skill is also necessary in order to recognize and manage successfully those problem situations that invariably arise whenever several people attempt to work together under even the most favorable circumstances.

Like group therapy, family therapy is a relatively new treatment modality in psychiatry and mental health. Nursing has always been concerned with treating the individual without isolating her/him from the family and community systems; it is therefore not surprising that a number of nurses are preparing for and functioning in the role of family therapist. Family therapy as described here is not treatment of an individual while including the family; it involves assessing and treating the family system itself as the client. Working with a family system requires specialized techniques and training to deal effectively with the complex communication patterns existing among people whose relationships extend into the past and continue beyond the relatively small amount of time spent with the therapist(s) in clinical sessions. For these reasons, undergraduate students and nurses without special preparation usually do not assume the role of family therapist or co-therapist. However, knowledge of the goals and methods of family therapy may facilitate referrals and support for family therapy by generalist nurse practitioners, and, at times, the kinds of family therapy techniques described in this chapter may be appropriately incorporated into generalist practice.

Swanson's (1969) article provides several checklists helpful to new and experienced group leaders. Specific suggestions are offered in response to questions about the value of group activities for psychiatric clients, goals for group work with this population, how the group members should be selected, and which leadership styles will be most effective. Answers to these questions are drawn from theory and research in the area of group process and group therapy and give the reader a brief summary of the final checklist for self-appraisal, a guide which can be used for evaluating group and leader functioning at various stages of group development.

Realistic goals and techniques for group work with a difficult client population—the psychotic elderly—is the subject of the paper by Yalom and Terrazas (1968). Among the topics discussed are how to select group members, meeting place and seating arrangements, how to begin the interaction once the group has been assembled, and how to manage such common group problems as monopolizing, silences, and bizarre behavior. Numerous examples from the authors' own experiences with these groups illustrate their suggestions and cautions, which are applicable to many kinds of groups, and give this article special value for new group leaders.

The article by Brandner (1974) is about a health-maintenance, growth-promoting type of group whose members were not diagnosed patients. The setting was a women's center, the leaders were nurse practitioners in private practice, and the group members were respondents to newspaper announcements. The program was designed to help each woman "discover her own potential for growth and self-reliance" by bolstering self-confidence and increasing problem-solving skills. Brandner describes how the groups were started, how the sessions were structured, the kinds of women who participated, and some of the answers individual participants found in the short-term groups in their search for self-definition and self-actualization.

Miller's article introduces the family systems approach with a brief history of family psychotherapy and a review of the theoretical concepts such as feedback, steady state and information processing that form the basis for this treatment modality. The family with a "sick" member is assessed and treated· as an open social system responding to stress; individual member behaviors are evaluated in terms of what they contribute to the function or dysfunction of the system as a whole. Miller discusses specific assessment and intervention techniques derived from the systems approach and gives examples from her own practice with a dysfunctional family.

A different approach to diagnosing and intervening in problematic family communications is the subject of Padberg's (1975) article on bargaining as a therapeutic maneuver. As described here, bargaining can be used both to reveal where communication breakdowns have occurred and expectations remained unmet as well as to clarify communications and expectations among family members. In this context, bargaining becomes, as the author relates, "not simply a matter of someone winning or losing" but a means toward the end of clear and direct family communications.

The final article in this unit, by Harris and Fregley (1971), concerns the role of the nurse working with a family in crisis in the setting of the home and community. Harris worked with a family consisting of two parents, thirteen children, and two grandchildren over a period of five months, during which time the family underwent four major crises. She describes here, in considerable detail, how she helped the family deal with each crisis and emerge strengthened by the experience.

24 A CHECK LIST FOR GROUP LEADERS

By Mary G. Swanson, M.N., R.N.

WORKING WITH GROUPS OF PATIENTS HAS BECOME
ONE of the most frequently used approaches in psychiatric nursing,
particularly in large federal and state mental hospitals. In some of these
hospitals the goal now seems to be to have every patient, every nurse,
and every psychiatric aide participate in some kind of patient group every
week or even every day. In many hospitals the more experienced and bet-
ter-prepared nurses serve as co-therapists or even group leaders in group
therapy, as leaders of remotivation groups, and as organizers or leaders of
special hobby or interest groups. They are also often expected to participate in the training and supervision of psychiatric aides who lead remotivation or hobby groups.

Many nurses who, when they accept emp loyment in large mental hospitals find that group work is included in th ir assignments, lack preparation for this responsibility. True, most graduate programs in psychiatric
nursing now provide training for work with groups of patients, especially
in formal therapy groups. In most basic nursing programs, however, little
or nothing is taught about group techniques; the psychiatric nursing
courses are focused almost entirely on teaching the students to function
effectively in a one-to-one relationship with patients. Thus, the area of
group work with psychiatric patients is one in which many graduate
nurses find they need some additional reading, observing, and training
after arriving in their job settings.

From Perspectives in Psychiatric Care, Vol. VII, No. 3, pp. 120-126, 1969. Reprinted with
permission, from Nursing Publications Inc. 194-B Kinderkamack Rd. Park Ridge, N.J.
07656.

Values of Group Work

Several reasons account for the increasing use of group work in psychiatric hospitals. At first glance the main reason might seem to be economy in the use of staff, which in large hospitals is almost never numerically adequate to provide a one-to-one relationship for every patient who could benefit from it. However, economy is not the only reason; there are therapeutic values for a patient in group interaction which supplement the benefits he can derive from even a very satisfactory one-to-one relationship. Some of these values are:

Socialization; increased self-confidence and enjoyment in interacting with groups of people.

Moving out of the dependent and self-centered role of patient and regaining the feeling of interacting with a group and becoming more aware of and responsive to the feelings and ideas of other people.

Increased sense of well-being. This goal is sometimes the only realistic one for group work with chronic patients with considerable organic brain damage or with fairly advanced senility. It is a legitimate goal: when a patient cannot be "cured" it is still worthwhile to make him as happy and comfortable as possible.

Practice in problem solving as a member of a group. Such activity helps the patient to recognize and take into account the opinions and suggestions of others and to develop an increased flexibility in sometimes working to influence other people and sometimes changing his own opinion in response to what he learns by listening to them.

Clearer realization of how one's personality and actions appear to others. For a patient to persist in denial when a group of his peers express an opinion about him and his problems is harder than for him to insist that his therapist does not like him or understand him.

The impact of group pressure in the direction of conformity rather than toward deviant or unhealthy behavior.

The development of psychological insight into one's unconscious feelings. The responses of group members to a patient's disclosures can facilitate the development of insight. Also, many patients gain some insights by realizing their similarities to some of the other patients who are describing their situations and feelings.

Diminution of the feeling that many psychiatric patients have of being alone and unique in their suffering from emotional problems.

Increased hope that one may improve, derived from the observation of other patients who are improving during therapy.

An opportunity to practice an alternative method of handling anxiety, anger, or despair for the patient whose usual response to such emotions has been to withdraw and regress rather than seek out other people to help him cope with these emotions more successfully.

A stimulus to the practice of clearer communication with others derived from the patient's realization that others cannot understand his present mode of communication or that he is not receiving communication from others adequately.

Formation of relationships with other patients which often result in more interaction among patients on the ward between group meetings and less sitting and staring into space during hours when activities are not scheduled.

Increased feeling of community with others and the consequent lessening of the anxiety and anger that accompany feelings of being shut out and ignored by other people.

This last-mentioned benefit is supported by some evidence that simply being required to function as a group member is therapeutic, even if the group does not discuss psychiatric problems. One study which seems to demonstrate this is the experiment by Anker and Walsh[1] in which matched groups of long-term schizophrenic patients were assigned either to group therapy or to produce plays for the entertainment of the hospital population. The plays were not psychodrama, but were selected by the patients from books of plays. The group therapy was in charge of a trained therapist, but the drama group had no staff help except for a recreation leader who was told to help the patients obtain materials for scenery, costumes, and so on but to furnish no other leadership. Observations and tests of the two groups over a one-year period indicated that the drama group had made the greater improvement.

One can only speculate about why the activity group members improved more than the patients in the therapy group. One possibility is that if destructive or deteriorating personality changes can take place without a patient's conscious knowledge of the process, reconstructive changes can also take place unconsciously when conditions encourage such change. Apparently cooperative interaction with peers in and of itself was enough to produce some constructive changes even without development of the insight which, in chronic schizophrenic patients, is so difficult to achieve without arousing the anxiety, despair, and opposition that may make them regress when talk is directed to their problems, failures, and traumatic experiences.

The following checklist contains a set of considerations about which a nurse or other staff member undertaking the leadership of a group of psychiatric patients would find it profitable to become self-conscious. Some of the items have been suggested by literature from psychology on group techniques; others reflect questions that have been asked or problems that have arisen with nursing personnel new to group work. The items fall into two categories: those which pertain to the decisions that should be made before a group is started and those which relate to the abilities needed by the leader.

Preliminary Decisions

In planning to initiate a patient group, the leader might well answer the following questions.

What do I most want to help the members of this group to achieve? Among the possible goals are:

Socialization.
Independence and initiative.
Increased sense of well-being.
Learning to cooperate in problem solving.
Productivity from work on a project of mutual benefit.
Insight.
Stimulation of energy and interest.

On what basis shall I choose my patients?
Mixture of personalities and diagnostic categories. Many experienced group therapists feel such a mixture is the most beneficial arrangement for the patients.

One special problem, such as drinking, epilepsy, blindness, orientation to the hospital, or preparation for discharge.

Similar diagnosis. This criterion would be a very difficult one to use with groups of withdrawn psychotic patients, but groups of neurotic patients sometimes work well together, as do groups of drug or alcoholic addicts.

Similar ability in verbal expression and abstract thought.
Emotional Level.
Sociometric similarity—that is, putting patients who like working

together in the same group. This can be done by getting patients to indicate preferences in individual interviews before the group is established.

The patient's choice that results from permitting each patient to choose one of several available interest groups.

How large will my group be? Why this size? How is the size I select related to group goals? If the group goal is to apply pressure outside the group, a large group is effective (as with a political party or a labor union). If the group goals include the full functioning of every member, a smaller group (five to fifteen) is better.

What type of leadership shall I try to maintain? Why?

Democratic. Such leadership results in more friendliness, group mindedness, motivation, and originality.

Authoritarian. More work is done, but more discontent, hostility, and dependency may develop. Nonetheless this type of leadership may be better in some kinds of group therapy, especially short-term therapy in which the aim is suppression of sensitive material and the patients' acceptance of practical arrangements for living, in contrast to long-term therapy aimed at the patients' development of insight into their unconscious feelings.

Laissez-faire. The quality and quantity of work may be less, but this approach may be best for some chronic patients who need to be placed in a position of setting up their own organization.[2,3]

Checklist for Self-Appraisal

How do I appraise myself as a leader according to the following criteria? In which areas would I like to improve?

Am I successful in reducing the patients' anxiety about participating in this group?

Do I let the patients become acquainted with me before the group begins?

Do I relate to patients with warmth, supportiveness, and nonthreatening humor during the orientation phase?

Do I arrange for comfortable surroundings & refreshments if appropriate.

Do I exhibit a matter-of-fact, businesslike attitude if the group includes many patients who tend to be suspicious of direct friendliness?

Do I reward participation or otherwise promote progress toward group goals? Do I use verbal conditioning, smiling, nodding, and so on, or more direct praise or statement of approval?

Have I established expectations among the patients that participation is the group norm? This is most easily done while the patients are new in the group. The most frequent error of new group leaders is to make a long preliminary speech at the first session.

Am I successful in drawing out persons so that all members participate? The leader achieves this goal by:

Accepting contributions.

Making reluctant individuals feel their ideas are wanted and needed.

Preventing talkative individuals from dominating without rejecting them.

Keeping discussion and activity moving forward.

Accepting the feelings and attitudes of all participants as valid points for consideration.

Protecting individuals whom other group members might attack verbally.

Accepting conflict or disagreement in the group as therapeutic if it is expressed with reasonable appropriateness.

Do I "wait out" pauses? Usually the group "takes over" more after the first few pauses.

Do I hear the ideas and feelings expressed and restate them accurately in shorter, more pointed, clearer form? In this way the leader shows he is paying attention, understands what is said, and accepts the views of the person who expresses them. This kind of acceptance does not always mean agreement, but in demonstrating it the leader shows that he respects the right of every member to contribute.

Am I sensitive to nonverbal communication from group members? For example, silence can connote concentration, hostility, or lack of interest, and it is important for the group leader to know which of these attitudes is being reflected. She also should be able to identify restlessness and other feelings reflected in nonverbal communication.

Do I ask questions which stimulate problem-solving behavior? Among such questions are those which clarify situations that have been unclearly described, those which inquire about the emotions surrounding a situation, and those which promote investigation of alternative solutions. The questions should be difficult enough to keep the patients interested. Good questions direct exploration along fruitful lines as well as prevent the persistence of thinking in areas where failure has repeatedly been experienced. Questions which the group members see as threatening rather than helpful should be avoided.

How much did I learn about each patient before the group started?

How well am I keeping up contact with the patients between group sessions and learning about them outside of the group? Knowing group members well enhances the leader's ability to ask questions of the appropriate member if the occasion arises. Also, if patients already know and trust the leader, they are more likely to feel secure in answering questions. Knowing the patients also enables the group leader to promote group cohesiveness by pointing out the similarities among some group members or to promote interaction by pointing out differences in viewpoint or in experiences among them.

Do I summarize as the need arises? This important skill can be used to:

Move the discussion along.

Indicate progress.

Restate the problem in new form in light of the discussion.

Point up the fact that differences exist in the group and that these differences are part of the problem.

Am I receiving genuine feedback on the verbal level? If not, why are patients not telling me what they think and how they feel?

Do I maintain standards that are high enough to keep the group interested and to prevent fake questions and the selection of tasks that are too easy or too difficult?

Do I keep the group moving toward new problems and activities as they tire of old ones and thus promote a sense of momentum?

Am I varying techniques and formats for meetings in order to keep interest up? Some possibilities are:

Pictures and equipment, relevant to topics being discussed. It is desirable for these materials to be collected with the help of a patient or a patient committee.

Role playing.

Goal-directed fantasy, a technique which involves helping the patients to talk about things they would like to do as part of the motivation program. [4]

Psychodrama.

Didactic sessions characterized by lectures which give patients information that is new to them followed by discussion.

Film followed by discussion.

Outings.

"Guest leaders"—that is, volunteers or other staff members expert in some topics of interest to the group.

Group tasks selected and approved by the group.

Group recreational activities selected by the group.

Do I display ingenuity in arranging for the group to do its own work? The leader should not perform any task, however small, that a patient or a committee of patients could do. Even such a small job as arranging the chairs in a circle for the meeting should be left to the group members if they can accomplish it. Is my attitude that of getting the group to learn to solve problems with me, or do I tell them what to do?

Am I alert to every opportunity to give the group as much real power to make choices as possible? Patient groups usually prove to be more conservative than staff when they are permitted to make choices and may often be trusted to make appropriate decisions about matters that affect them. Some psychiatric hospitals now permit patient groups to have considerable choice in setting schedules for their unit, making and enforcing many of their own rules, and setting up most of their own recreational programs. The effective group leader limits himself to supplying essential facts and clarifying the areas of choice without suggesting the decision. For example, if the group has decided to have a party, the leader might have to tell them what the amount of money and the times available are, but should let the group decide how to spend the time and money as long as the decisions are within permissible limits.

Do I turn activity and responsibility over to group as soon as possible and keep turning it back to them as needed? In many psychiatric patient groups the turning of responsibility back to the group has to be repeated frequently.

Am I using group deviants wisely? The quantity of interaction increases when a deviant is in the group, and recognition and discussion of differences of opinion make a group more active. However, in some cases the leader should intervene to prevent a deviant from being subjected to a harmful degree of scapegoating. Among psychiatric patients, scapegoating seems to occur most often when there is strong external pressure on the group or when an especially odd or deviant patient arouses fears in the other patients that they may resemble him. When strong pressure for scapegoating appears in a group, direct suppression is not always the most effective way of stopping it; the leader should also look for and deal with feelings of individual worthlessness among patients, fear of revelation of weakness, and fear of similarity to the scapegoat.

Am I contributing to group cohesiveness? Cohesiveness is highest when goals are strongly desired and agreed on and when the means for achieving them and the norms are agreed on. The leader can facilitate cohesiveness by encouraging the group to make its own choices, to talk out and resolve differences, and to review and alter goals as needed. The leader of a group of psychiatric patients can usually work best by helping the patients do the work of facilitating progress toward their own goals, but if there is an influential group member who tries to persuade the group to adopt unhealthy goals, the leader must sometimes exert her influence to help the group maintain goals that will be therapeutic for the members. This threat to therapeutic goals is most likely to occur in a group of adolescent patients or in one with several adult sociopaths.

What am I doing to develop leadership among the patients?

Rewarding it?

Encouraging the ability of some patients to draw out others?

Encouraging the patients to direct questions and remarks to each other rather than to me?

Sitting back quietly whenever possible?

Am I encouraging shared or circulating leadership among the patients instead of merely replacing a "staff leader" with a "patient leader"?

Am I bringing in new members or removing present members from time to time when therapeutic considerations indicate this?

Am I bringing new members into the group at the best time for them? Research has shown that many people seem much more attracted to interaction in groups when their anxiety is high because of changes in or uncertainty about their own situations. This finding would seem to indicate that the best time to move many patients into a group is when they have just been brought into the hospital or moved to a new setting within the hospital or when changes in staff or in hospital procedures have increased their anxiety.

Is the group actually moving toward goals? How can I facilitate this progress more? Most group progress occurs when the group has chosen goals and agreed on methods of reaching them. If it is not possible for the patients to choose all of their goals, maximum progress will occur if they see the goals as important to them and agree on ways to reach them. Progress is also facilitated if the group leader keeps the group aware of gains they are making, and keeps further goals visible to them.

Am I flexible enough to revise goals as patients progress or other circumstances change?

Probably no group leader will ever reach the point where she can honestly respond "Yes, I always succeed in doing this" to every question on this list. But the group leader who, as she periodically checks her performance against the list, finds that her answers are progressing from "sometimes" to "often" to "usually" will not only experience the rewards that come from observing improvement in patients, but also the satisfaction that occurs when one realizes one's own growth and one's increasing effectiveness in working with patients.

References

1. Anker, J. M., and Walsh, R. P., "Group Psychotherapy, A Special Activity Program and Group Structure in the Treatment of Chronic Schizophrenia," *Journal of Consulting Psychiatry*, 1961, 25:476–481.

2. White, R., and Lippitt, R.: "Leader Behavior and Member Reaction in Three 'Social Climates'." In D. Cartwright and A. Zander (eds.) *Group Dynamics*, Row Peterson, Evanston, Ill.: 1953, Ch. 40.
3. Mullan, H., and Rosenbaum, M.: *Group Psychotherapy*, New York: Free Press of Glencoe, 1968.
4. McClelland, D.C., "Toward a Theory of Motive Acquisition," *American Psychologist*, 1965, 20:321–333.

Bibliography

Armstrong, S. W. and **Rouslin, S.**: *Group Psychotherapy in Nursing Practice*, New York: Macmillan Co., 1963.

Goldstein, A. P., Heller, K., and **Sechrest, L. B.**: *Psychotherapy and the Psychology of Behavior Change*, New York: John Wiley and Sons, 1966.

Lewin, K., Lippitt, R., and **White, R.**: "Patterns of Aggressive Behavior in Experimentally Created 'Social Climates,'" *Journal of Social Psychology*, 1939, 10:271–299.

Maier, N.: *Psychology in Industry*, Boston, Houghton Mifflin Co., 1965.

25 GROUP THERAPY FOR PSYCHOTIC ELDERLY PATIENTS

Irvin D. Yalom, Ph.D.

Florence Terrazas, M.A., R.N.

PSYCHIATRIC PATIENTS OCCUPY OVER 50 PERCENT OF THE hospital beds in the United States. The majority of these are psychotic, elderly patients, hospitalized for many years and generally considered intractable to therapy. Several studies have demonstrated the efficacy of therapy in groups for this population, though many traditional group therapy techniques must be adapted to fit (1,2).

We have worked with groups of psychotic patients whose average age is 60 years and whose average hospital stay has been 15 years. We have found certain group therapy techniques to be particularly relevant to these patients.

To understand how to do therapy, we must first understand what we wish to accomplish. Confusion occurs when one attempts to describe the goals of group therapy. There are, in fact, many group therapies, and the goals of the therapist depend on which type of therapy he is practicing. It is possible to arrive at a rough classification of group therapies by ordering them along a continuum of goals of the therapist. We must keep in mind that the goals of the therapist are largely a function of his patient population.

At one end of the continuum are ambitious intrapersonal goals such as personality reconstruction, while at the other end are such goals as remotivation, resocialization, and the reestablishment of adaptive methods of dealing with everyday life problems. Some therapy techniques most appropriate to groups near the personality-reconstruction end of the continuum are intensive exploration of personal history and fantasy material, as well as interpersonal confrontation, while entirely different techniques are most useful for groups with different group therapy goals.

What are realistic goals for therapy groups composed of chronic "back ward" psychiatric patients? Nurses assigned to these wards often become pessimistic and discouraged about their work. Some patients are so dependent and regressed that the nurses' role often becomes an ungratifying, custodial one. We have found that group therapy for these patients has much to offer, provided that realistic, attainable goals are formulated.

The elaboration of these goals must start from the premise that the majority of the patients in such groups will remain permanently institutionalized in either a psychiatric hospital or a nursing home. Any other premise would have been unrealistic and inconsistent with the degree of pathology, chronicity, and unavailability of family or community resources of our patients.

Building on this premise then, the major goal of therapy for such patients is to rehumanize their lives. A characteristic feature of many chronic wards is the degree of estrangement that exists among the patients. Patients may sleep in adjoining beds for years and yet avoid all meaningful interaction. Friction may result from this lack. A major therapeutic assumption is that improvement of motivation for and skill in communication will enrich the ward lives of our patients, enable them to use the extra ward facilities and, by expanding their life space, prepare them for transfer to a more autonomous residential institution.

Other goals are part processes of this major goal. We wish to reduce the isolation of patients, to enable them to reexperience bonds with others, and to increase feelings of group morale or cohesiveness. The reduction of bizarre behavior, the strengthening of adaptive personality traits, and the resolution of specific ward problems are all appropriate therapeutic goals. Given these goals, what techniques are useful?

Beginning The Group

COMPOSITION OF THE GROUP   The first task of the therapist is to select members. Since we could find no reports of systematic evaluative studies of this type of group, our guidelines had to be generalizations from clinical observation. Many clinicians have found that group functioning markedly deteriorates if the number of active members falls below 4 or 5. The maximum number of patients for this therapy format is approximately 12. We have found the optimal range to be 8 to 10 members.

Mute patients can profit from group attendance. Nonverbal cues often indicate that these patients are actively involved in the group. A verbal group cannot absorb too many nonverbal members, however, and still maintain active interaction. The hostile paranoid patient presents the greatest challenge, and few groups can absorb more than one or two of these patients.

Patients who have such severe organic deterioration that they cannot comprehend the group conversation or who are incapable of consistently identifying others do not profit from group therapy. One must not, however, develop undue pessimism about organic brain disease. It is well known that there is not a one-to-one correlation between organic brain damage and organic-like symptomatology (3). Even severe memory loss and disorientation may diminish considerably when the psychologic condition of the patient is improved. In general, heterogeneity is desirable in regard to sex, diagnostic categories, and interpersonal behavioral styles. We recommend meetings of approximately 45 minutes duration twice weekly, for at least six months.

Initial anxiety is diminished if the therapist clearly states the purpose of the group. A simple statement such as, "We are meeting to get to know each other better," may suffice. One may elaborate further by commenting that many patients experience difficulty in meeting and communicating with others and that the group is designed to help the patients in this respect.

ESTABLISHING TRUST   It is well known that important group norms are established early in the course of a group and that, once rooted, they are difficult to change. It is highly advisable, therefore, that the therapist begin immediately to help the group establish a nonthreatening, trusting atmosphere. A useful guideline is the general strategy of ego enhancement.

When the therapist is presented with diverse material, he should attempt to focus on the ego enhancing apsects. For example, a paranoid patient attacked the therapist for asking her too many questions. She accused him of intrusiveness and of invading her private life. The therapist replied that he liked people who were honest enough to let him know just where he stood and that he admired her ability to speak her mind. The patient responded thenceforth far less defensively and assumed a responsible role in the group. We, of course, are not suggesting idle flattery. Unless the comments are based on real feelings within the therapist, they are without therapeutic value.

Angry, suspicious patients are often imprisoned within the vicious circle of an environment which responds to their hostility with hostility. It is important for the therapist to check his initial tendency to respond angrily to the patient's anger and, instead, to comment on the patient's feelings of loneliness or worthlessness underlying the anger. In general, one should attempt to discourage behavior that is socially self-defeating and reinforce socially adaptive behavior.

COMMON THEMES   Meetings assume heightened meaning and interest for patients when the groups focus on issues relevant to all or most of the members. The therapist should alert himself to the emergence of these themes and reinforce them whenever possible. These may range from shared experiences in the group or in the hospital, such as ward activities, diet, staff personnel, to more meaningful shared feelings such as loneliness, feelings of isolation from family, and discouragement about the future.

Groups generally progress from discussion of safer, more superficial issues to concern with more affect-laden themes, and therapists should not expect groups to deal prematurely with these latter issues. Individual members differ in ability to deal with emotionally important areas and should be encouraged to proceed at their own pace.

INCREASING INTERACTION   Since a major goal of therapy is to improve interpersonal communication, the therapist should continuously strive to increase the patients' awareness of each other and to encourage their interaction. A convenient beginning is to work on the names of the group members. Rarely, in our groups, do many patients know other group members' names. Often, it is useful for the therapist to ask the patients to find out the others' names, since this encourages them to address one another directly.

Comments by patients to therapists should whenever possible, be rechanneled to another patient. Thus, if a patient comments to the therapist about another patient, the therapist may ask that the patient speak directly to that other person. The transfer of responsibility to patients may increase their interaction. A verbally active patient can be complimented on his contribution to the group and his verbal facility and asked to help some of the silent members learn to speak in the group. It is highly likely that helping another patient builds the helper's self-esteem and is thus doubly therapeutic.

Therapists should help to point out similarities between group members. When a patient expresses a feeling or a concern, the therapist can ask whether others have experienced similar feelings. The patients are encouraged to describe these concerns directly to each other. Feelings of isolation and loneliness diminish when patients become aware that others are experiencing similar feelings.

Interpatient feedback should be encouraged. The therapist, for example, can ask each patient to comment about a particular patient's strengths or talents. Nonverbal patients can be included by asking each member to guess from facial expression or nonverbal cues how that patient is feeling today. Maladaptive interpersonal behavior can be constructively pointed out. For example, one patient was inattentive and continually interrupted others. The therapist asked one of the group members to talk about how she felt when she was interrupted. The therapist approached this in a constructive fashion by pointing out that this response was not desired by the interrupter, who, in fact, wished very much to please others. Often this type of intervention must be reinforced many times before effective learning occurs, and therapists must expect that many of their interventions will appear to fall flat.

GROUP COHESIVENESS   A cohesive group confers a sense of acceptance and belonging to its members. The therapist, accordingly, should continuously attempt to strengthen group cohesiveness. The less a group needs to depend on the therapist, the more cohesive it becomes. Leader-dominated groups (for example, many remotivation groups) rarely achieve any degree of autonomy and may tend to perpetuate dependent attitudes in patients. Techniques described already, such as increasing intermember focusing on member similarities and encouraging patients to assume group responsibility, enhance cohesiveness.

The composition of the group should be kept fairly stable, since frequent turnover retards the sense of group identity. Members should be encouraged to express their feelings of loss when patients miss meetings or stop attending. Periodic nonverbal group activities—canteen visits, walks, or other projects—can also increase group cohesion.

Therapists tend to create self-fulfilling prophecies. The enthusiasm or faith—or their lack—of the group therapist is highly contagious, and therapists who feel considerable pessimism about therapy should have an opportunity to discuss this with supervisors. Feelings that group therapy is senseless can result in behavior which insures therapeutic failure. If, on the other hand, the therapist demonstrates his respect for the group by consistent attendance, by placing high priority on therapy time, and by asking their permission to invite observers to group sessions, patients will soon come to share his positive evaluation of the group.

THERAPISTS' ROLE   We have found that groups of chronically ill patients do not fare well with detached, aloof therapists. The therapist who reports his immediate feelings to the group serves as a model to the patients in this regard. Some therapists relate some pertinent autobiographical material to the group. Questions directed toward the therapists should be answered directly and clearly. It is helpful for the patients to see the therapists as real persons who have feelings and unanswered questions themselves. If there are cotherapists present, they may at times disagree or express their feelings to each other in the group. This helps the patients to differentiate the therapists as separate persons rather than as impersonal figures in white uniforms.

PHYSICAL SETTING   The meeting place and seating arrangement of the group are important. A permanent meeting place free from distraction is desirable, as it provides stability and continuity from meeting to meeting. A rather small, close circle is more desirable than a large, open one, since physical proximity promotes intimacy and cohesiveness. If any member feels great anxiety because of the closeness, he should, of course, be encouraged to participate from the distance most comfortable for him at the time. Another advantage is that chronically ill, elderly patients often have impaired hearing and, as a result, fare better in a small circle.

From our clinical observations, we have found that group interaction is also increased when the co-leaders sit on opposite sides of the circle. Chronically ill patients frequently are more inclined to talk to a staff member than to another patient. With physical separation of the therapists, the focal points of the communication pattern are dispersed, thus increasing the probability of including more of the patients in the network.

Specific Problems

THE MONOPOLIST   The patient who monopolizes the group often creates a significant problem. The task of the therapist in this situation is complex. He must stop the monopolist from consuming all the group time. Otherwise, the other patients cannot profit from the group and will eventually grow to resent the monopolist. At the same time, the therapist must not so threaten the monopolist that other group members will be reluctant to speak, lest a similar attack be their lot also.

If the therapist considers the axiom that whenever a monopolist appears there is also present a group which allows or encourages the monopolization, a reasonable strategy suggests itself. The therapist may wonder aloud why that certain patient is shouldering the entire burden of the meeting or why others in the group are letting that patient do all the work or all their talking for them.

SILENCE   Many of our groups periodically lapse into silence, which often creates more anxiety for the therapists than for the patients. Some therapists, to avoid prolonged silences, try to force participation by asking patients overobvious or childlike questions. Although immediate tension may be reduced, this approach, in the long run, tends to infantilize patients.

One can best manage silence in groups by treating it as a focus for the discussion of feelings. Therapists may, for example, comment on their feelings of uneasiness and inquire how the group members feel about the silence. If silence persists, therapists may look for underlying feelings, such as an important theme left over from the previous meeting or some other source of tension or sadness in the group.

BIZARRENESS   Not infrequently, patients present bizarre delusional or hallucinatory material. For example, one patient opened the meeting by saying that she had been dead since 1937 and had been buried in a burlap bag. The therapist chose to ask everyone in the group whether she looked dead. The patient responded defensively and irrationally to every comment made, and her bizarreness was accentuated by this strategy.

Another patient told the group that she was going to leave the hospital by saving a dime a week to pay for her cross-country journey to a nonexistent state. The group also attempted to confront her with the folly of her plans, the result again being an accentuation of the bizarreness. Delusions, by definition, are fixed false beliefs and are impervious to rational confrontation. Groups which attempt to dislodge a delusion are inevitably frustrated and the delusional patient is made to appear even more strange.

In these instances, we would suggest that the therapist look for aspects of the patient's communication which are shared by others and which will include rather than exclude her from the group. With the first patient the therapist might have said he wondered if other patients had not at times felt dead or empty inside. In the second example, the therapist might have commented on how much the patient wanted to leave the hospital and rejoin her family.

Another method utilizes the interpersonal effects of the patient's bizarre behavior. One patient with chronic schizophrenia persistently disrupted his group by inappropriate laughter in response to auditory hallucinations. The therapist, at one point, said to the patient, "John, I want you to hear something that may be very important to you." The therapist then went around the group and asked every patient to guess why he thought John was laughing.

Each patient advanced a reason ranging from, "John thinks we're fools and he's laughing at us," to "He's trying to get attention," "He's silly," and, "He's crazy." John was then asked whether he knew that people could get so many different and conflicting ideas about him. Although John did not appear to be highly involved with the other members, he abruptly stopped the inappropriate laughter when he was in the group.

As a general rule, we would caution therapists against investigating pathology in the groups. Neophyte therapists often err by exploring pathology in order to uncover original causes. This search, a product of mass media glamorization of psychiatry, is fruitless and often harmful. The more an individual is perceived by others as different, strange, or crazy, the more others tend to exclude him. Exclusion and isolation will beget anxiety and despair, which further intensify the maladaptive behavior of the patient.

PATIENT UNINVOLVEMENT   In every chronically ill group there are patients who manifest apparent disinterest by lack of participation, distractability, autistic behavior, sleeping, or refusal to attend a meeting. Therapists are often frustrated and discouraged by the apparent intractable lack of involvement. Group development research shows, however, that intimacy is a stage that occurs late in a group's development. Chronically ill, hospitalized, psychiatric patients have profound problems in intimacy, and the therapist must employ a more sensitive yardstick to measure change in this area. Our patients do not lack the desire for closeness and involvement, but are enormously threatened by closeness.

This point should be clarified by the therapist, since group members accept and understand fear or distrust far more easily than boredom or disinterest. Patients must be allowed to proceed toward closeness at their own pace, but the therapist must provide constant opportunities. Patients who refuse to attend the group should be encouraged to sit in the room, even at some distance and be reassured they need only listen.

In summary, group therapy has much to offer the psychotic elderly patient. By setting realistic goals, by increasing patient interaction, by focusing on patient strengths and similarities, and by building group cohesiveness, the therapist can demonstrate that pessimism about therapy with this population is unwarranted.

References

1. Ross, Matthew. Review of some recent treatment methods for elderly psychiatric patients. *Arch. Gen. Psychiat.* 1:578–592, Dec. 1959.
2. Linden, M. E. Significance of dual leadership in gerontologic group psychotherapy; studies in gerontologic human relations. *Int. J. Group Psychother.* 4:262–273, 1954.
3. Rothschild, D. Neuropathological changes in arteriosclerotic psychoses and their psychiatric significance. *Arch. Neurol. Psychiat.* 48:417–436, Sept. 1942.

26 WOMEN IN GROUPS

Patty Brandner, M.S., R.N.

SOMEONE READS OUR ANNOUNCEMENT IN THE NEWSPAPER AND our phone rings. The person at the other end usually begins "I need something in my life—a job or college or—but I'm not sure I can handle it. I've never done much. . . ." The caller realizes I'm listening closely, and she says, "I've never told anyone this before" and rushes into the story of her situation, relieved. She often concludes with the questions asked in our publicity announcement. And then, "Do you have room for one more in your group?" I assure her she has a place and tell her where and when.

In my mind I add her story to the variations I've heard, all sounding the same theme: "I want recognition as a worthwhile human being." I understand because I've wanted it too. In fact, that's the reason why our mental health support groups for women were planned.

Early in 1973 the first publicity for our "Who Am I?" series appeared. Evelyn and I, the "two mental health nurse therapists" in an independent practice partnership, had signed a contract for facilities and sponsorship for publicity with a newly created organization in our community that was seeking—in the words of its own publicity—"to change society's expectations of women through research, education and communication" and providing "a forum to enable women to help themselves and each other." It seemed a logical partnership. We were interested in offering preventive and educational mental health support groups and needed clients and a place to practice, and the center—called the Women for Change Center—needed programs. We pay it a percentage of our fee.

Our plan for the series of four two-hour sessions is based on the concept of primary prevention which "aims toward further strengthening individuals who enter the process from a condition of health even though the joining a group is an indication of need."[1] We want to help women develop feelings of self worth and the ability to solve problems, to look at roles for themselves in the future, and to learn to channel their feelings for enhanced relationships. Our fee is low, and women can join the groups before they may need more extensive costly therapy. However, we're aware of the community resources if follow-up help is needed.

To supplement the group sessions and to give participants a view of other women's ideas and values, we have drawn up a booklist that we distribute to them (see page 273). As we read books we can recommend, we include them. WFC Center has begun a library for women so that Evelyn no longer lugs a suitcaseful from her own collection. We've compiled, and continuously bring up-to-date, a "Choices" list of activities and involvements for women that we believe provide enhanced opportunities for exercising their skills and talents. A questionnaire which we send to them one month after a series' end is designed to evaluate the experience for the women and for ourselves. And by the second session, each woman has a list of the names, addresses, and telephone numbers of the group members for use during and after the series.

Before we start a group, we make a return call to the women who have phoned in response to our publicity. The call gives us an opportunity for further exchange of information and helps the woman decide whether our series is really what she's looking for. At the same time we learn more about the potential make-up of each group. The caller chooses the morning or evening group, depending on whether she works in or outside her home. She may ask about babysitting facilities—like the mother whose children were recovering from chickenpox when the series started. (We quickly polled the center staff and group members about their families' immunity and told her to bring the children along.) Other problems, like a husband's resistance to his wife's involvement, aren't as easy to solve. However, when a woman decides to attend in spite of his resistance, we support her self-reliance. Sometimes a woman needs more extensive help than the group offers, and we suggest other resources.

We meet with our groups on the second floor of a 40-story, glasswalled skyscraper in downtown Dallas. With the help of comfortable cast-off chairs donated by WFC Center members, we've been able to offer a

---

[1] U.S. NATIONAL INSTITUTE OF MENTAL HEALTH. *Current Ethical Issues in Mental Health.* Based on workshop at 47th annual meeting of American Orthopsychiatric Association, held at San Francisco, Mar. 1970 (DHEW Publication No. (HSM) 73–9029) Washington, D.C., U.S. Government Printing Office, 1973, p. 10.

homey-looking room in spite of the floor-to-ceiling glass enclosing us. We arrange the chairs in a close circle near a table piled with books and the booklists we distribute. Coffee supplies and ashtrays stand ready. The idea is to create an atmosphere more like a social gathering than a therapy session. We've discovered, though, that once we're engrossed with each other, even wind and rain pounding the glass can't disturb us.

As the first meeting begins, Evelyn and I match faces with the voices we've heard on the phone and point out that each woman already knows one of us. We try to help move the women past conventional first-meeting stiffness into the warmth of new friendships by encouraging informal talk while all gather and settle into the circle.

Getting Started

The search begins. Our aim for this first session is to stimulate thinking about a woman's individual identity in today's society. To encourage increased awareness of women's roles, Evelyn and I tell about ourselves. We then review the series' goals and pass out the booklists. Next, as each group member tells about herself, common interests and concerns emerge. These surprise many who believed they were alone with their problems.

A 60-year-old woman hesitantly mentions she'd like to get a college degree, but is afraid her family will laugh. "I went back and got a degree after being out of school 22 years," says a middle-aged group member, and the first woman sits up straighter, eyes sparkling.

A very young mother cuddling her tiny baby, explains, "My husband and I are separated, and I didn't have anyone to leave the baby with tonight." Then she says, "I'd like to continue college on my scholarship, in case my marriage ends. But the baby's so young, and I don't know anyone to keep her while I'm in class." An older mother who has told us her children are teenagers leaving home, looks wistfully at the baby and asks, "Can't your mother keep her?"

During further discussion it becomes obvious that the older woman fears the end of her mothering role and yearns for a grandchild to relieve her anxiety. But the young mother firmly answers, "I'll raise my own child. My mother has raised hers." Another group member says, "That would be the easy way out, to be the eternal mother. But if you've done a good job mothering your kids, they'll want to leave and raise their own families." We all silently think of the future for these two. Changes for both will require confidence, courage, and all the help we can offer.

This is our cue to lead the discussion into awareness of society's attitudes which limit women's choices for fulfillment. Humor and laughter explode as we all review the ridiculous situations both men and women encounter in our culture. Seriousness returns with discussion of how to retain a sense of personal worth in a world which continues to build barriers against women and dehumanizes us all.

Anger at the inequalities rises. I take this opportunity to point out that aroused feelings can lead to actions aimed at changing the situation. Finally, it's obvious that each individual will have to discover her own potential for growth and self-reliance as a step toward changing society. To push the process Evelyn asks the women to make a list of "self-likes" to read at the next session. This activity reminds the group member all week of the previous meeting's interactions and stimulates awareness of herself.

Self-Likes

The second session begins with the reading of the self-likes lists. At first the women protest, "My list is short because I could only think of the things I *disliked* about myself." I tell them, "It may not be acceptable to brag in society, but it's encouraged in our groups. What's more, we want you to take the lists home for re-reading and additions."

Many self-likes are qualified with a "but." We gently admonish that we want to hear only positive statements with no buts. Group members make suggestions: "List 'honesty.' You told us last week you had never liked women." With a blush, the lister writes down another quality she can value.

It amazes us that "intelligence" is so seldom listed. We believe that women who come to a preventive mental health program are intelligent, and this leads to discussion of the reasons why a woman might consider it a liability to be "smart," believing that "showing my brains" will lead to being called "aggressive and unfeminine."

Most women don't include "being a woman" as a self-like, although they might list "I like my ability to mother, but. . . ." The alerted members quickly pounce on the qualifier and encourage the sheepish lister to cross it off. Yet the disclaimers continue to come even as the next one reads her list.

Belonging

As mutual acceptance and support become apparent, the women dare to be more open about themselves and their feelings. One woman, active for years as a community volunteer, exclaims, "This is the first time I've ever been at meetings where the focus is on *me* and not on doing something for someone else. I really feel I can discover who I am!" For many women it's a revelation to think about themselves and their own emotional needs, exciting to consider themselves first without guilt and put husband, children, church, and community temporarily aside.

But time is short and there are more questions to consider. Evelyn asks whether it might not become a problem to use their newly discovered potential. "Where will you go from here?" A woman who has happily told us she now feels ready to go out and find a job, softly says, "But I've never even had an interview. I don't know if I dare." Depressing thoughts threaten the group. I remind the women that we have two more meetings and, at the next one, "we'll work on successful problem solving as a step up to maintain your strengths." In preparation we suggest that, during the week, they think over ways they cope with their problems, the patterns or techniques they use to make decisions.

Problem Solving

By the third session some of the women have already put their reinforced self-confidence to work. "My husband and I had a long talk and decided to try our marriage again. He's keeping the baby tonight," the young mother proudly tells us. The group is as pleased as if she were a sister or daughter. She goes on: "Talking with him wasn't easy. We fought a lot. I couldn't have stood up to him as I did, for me and the baby, if you all hadn't made me feel more sure of myself." And though we're going to miss having the baby there, we know it's a sign of progress.

We all realize that this marriage will present future difficulties that require decisions, and Evelyn and I are ready with our ideas. I point out that, for successful solutions, the problem has to be defined clearly, the choices and consequences considered, and then a decision made. Sometimes the process is stopped at the first step, as a woman says, "I want to finish college, but," then overwhelms us with an avalanche of reasons why she can't. When the other women's suggestions for solutions run out, there's the realization that "finishing college" isn't the problem. What she's really looking for is something to keep her mind active while she stays home with her children. Then, with the problem redefined, the group can help her with more appropriate choices.

Where Am I Going?

Evelyn and I encourage the women to formulate goals for themselves, a process made easier by their self-examinations in previous sessions. But some women refuse to set goals; they fear "success" can lead to more responsibility—and greater risk of failure. We examine this cycle of fear in the context of our sexuality.

In this group (as in others) we hear various women tell of their talents and ambitions, as yet underdeveloped or unpursued over past years. Now we hear a group member tell us she didn't take the law school entrance exam she'd been studying so hard for. We're stunned. Her efforts toward her goal had become our success symbol. I ask, "But why didn't you take it?"

"Because, as I told you, my husband is a lawyer. Oh sure, he said I'd pass the exam easily as you all did. But as the date came closer, I began wondering what would happen with the two of us practicing law. I'd be doing what I always wanted, but maybe at the expense of my marriage. I just don't think my husband could stand the competition if we were both in the same business. I'm not ready to take that risk. My son needs a father; I love my husband."

We nod with understanding as we deplore her dilemma. Then we rally to help her find other less threatening goals, hoping that with success and self-confidence, she can reach again for the bigger objective. Discussion of the success-failure cycle continues until I ask the women to prepare for the last session by bringing at least one future goal for the group's consideration.

How Do I Get There?

We meet for the last time, and the women come early and linger late. Evelyn and I have the next series to look forward to, but this group is feeling a sense of loss. Optimism is encouraged with a discussion of future plans aided by our "Choices" list of community resources (see next page).

As the end comes closer, we ask each woman to write a brief unsigned evaluation of what the group has meant to her. Finally, reluctantly, our new friends leave, and Evelyn and I remain to read the evaluations—a cold word to describe the warmth of the writing.

Evelyn and I sit and talk over the lives we've encountered in this group and we fantasize about their futures. We know some of the women will stay in touch with us, sometimes continuing as clients in our therapy groups or in individual or marital counseling. Others will call to talk over plans or to tell us of new steps upward. We've learned from these women—of their intelligence and talents, their strengths and capacities, their warmth and womanliness. They have become a part of our experience, a spur to greater efforts in offering supports for our "sisters."

WHO AM I?   HOW DO I GET THERE?
                        WHERE AM I GOING?
. . . Some CHOICES that may apply in your individual situation . . .

1. Continue with leaderless group.
2. EXPLORE: 8-week course, $25; children, $10.
3. Other Women for Change courses: Membership $10 per year. Newsletter subscription ($2) keeps you posted. Newly-Single Woman, Transactional Analysis Vocational Counseling.
4. Private Therapy with Evelyn or Patty, sliding fee.
5. Support-therapy group, Evelyn and Patty, on-going, 1 weekly 2-hour session, limited to 6-8, time/place to be announced.
6. Specific Agency Therapy: child guidance, family guidance, pastoral counseling, Jewish family service, community mental health centers. These agencies have sliding fee scales.
7. Churches: special courses, discussion groups, programs, workshops, seminars, special-interest groups.
8. YWCA: courses, interests, physical conditioning, parent-child.
9. Voluntary Action Center.
10. Park Department: swimming, tennis, art, dance.
11. Body Relaxation: yoga, belly dance, aerobics, gymnastics. (Caution: Check out any health spa for unethical practices.)
12. Health Needs: dental; immunizations, information on communicable diseases; well-baby, prenatal and geriatric clinics in neighborhoods; Dallas Association for Parent Education for OB/GYN referrals, classes, parent education programs; women's health; family planning and maternal health clinics, contraceptive and abortion counseling; Women for Change counseling/health task force.
13 Reading: Dallas Public Library, Great Books and American Institute for Discussion study courses. Available at libraries are films, records, newspapers, art, journals, magazines.
14. Re-entry in Job Market: changing careers, vocational testing, individual or group counseling, resume writing, interviewing, etc.
15. Women for Change: volunteer; task force member, office worker.
16. Reentry to Educational System: credit courses for degree or non-credit community college courses. Catalogs available at colleges.
17. Women's Groups: WEAL, NOW, League of Women Voters, Women's Political Caucus, Republican/Democrat Women's groups, United Church Women, American Association of University Women, Women's Coalition.
18. Physical Conditioning: modern dance, ballet, movement.

19. Maple Lawn Service Center: AAUW Day Care Center.
20. Volunteer Service: may give you emotional rewards and prepare you to re-enter salaried employment with more confidence, knowledge, and experience. A way of developing your talents and discovering new potentials.
21. Time Off for Yourself: planned for regular intervals.
22. Trip with Women Friends: to conferences or conventions, or sight-seeing.
23. Outdoor Exploration: camping, hiking, canoeing, skiing, boating, swimming, picnicking with congenial companions. (Children are often delightful companions!)
24. Hobbies: needlework, crafts, woodworking, etc. Sometimes these activities lead to job ideas, talents, awards. (See displays of women's talents at the state fair.)
25. Writing: talented *women* writers are needed for many different types of publications.
26. And, finally, a word for involvement in politics: at least *vote*. Women make up one half our population as well as being half the citizenry with a stake in political decisions. Contact with our elected representatives is desperately needed if women are to have a voice in the way our country is run. Women who have been elected to represent you in government, need your support; they do not have an easy job in a traditionally male endeavor. Let Eddie Berenice Johnson, a Dallas representative to our state legislature, hear your views about the concerns of women and children.

Prepared by Evelyn Wormser, R.N., M.S., and Patty Brandner, R.N., M.S. The list actually used gives such specifics as persons to call and telephone numbers. Copyright on that list is held by the two nurses.

Readings for Group Participants

Bettelheim, Bruno. *Informed Heart.* Rye, N.Y., Avon Books, 1971, $1.50.

Boston Women's Health Book Collective. *Our Bodies, Ourselves.* Boston, The Collective, 1973. $2.95.

Button, A. D. *The Authentic Child.* New York, Random House, 1969. $5.95.

Friedenberg, E. Z. *The Vanishing Adolescent.* New York, Beacon Press, 1959. $3.95.

Goble, Frank. *Third Force: a Psychology of Abraham Maslow.* New York, Grossman Publishers, 1970. $7.95.

Gornick, Vivian, and Moran, B. K. *Women in Sexist Society.* New York, New American Library, 1972. $1.95.

James, Muriel, and Jongeward, Dorothy. *Born to Win.* Reading, Mass., Addison-Wesley, 1971. $4.95.

Keyes, Ralph. *We, the Lonely People: Searching for Community.* New York, Harper and Row, 1973. $6.95.

Luthman, S. G. *Intimacy: The Essence of Male and Female.* Freeport, N.Y., Nash Publishing Corp., 1972. $7.95.

Madow, Leo. *Anger; How to Recognize and Cope with It.* New York, Charles Scribner's Sons, 1972. $7.95.

Martin, Del, and Lyon, Phyllis. *Lesbian-Woman.* New York, Bantam Books, 1972. $1.50.

Moustakas, Clark. *Creativity and Conformity.* New York, Van Nostrand Reinhold Co., 1967. $2.95.

Nin, Anais. *Under a Glass Bell.* Chicago, Swallow Press, n.d. $1.50.

O'Neill, Nena, and O'Neill, George. *Open Marriage.* Rye, N.Y., Avon Books, 1973. $1.95.

Overstreet, B.W. *Understanding Fear in Ourselves and Others.* New York, Harper and Row, 1971. $.95.

Previn, Dory. *On My Way to Where.* New York, Bantam Books, 1972. $1.25. (also a record.)

Rogers, Carl. *On Becoming a Person.* New York, Houghton-Mifflin Co., 1970. $3.25.

Roszak, Betty, and Roszak, Theodore. *Masculine/Feminine.* New York, Harper and Row, 1970. $2.45.

Rubin, T. I. *Angry Book.* New York, Macmillan Co., 1970. $1.25.

Seaman, Barbara. *Free and Female.* New York, Fawcett World Library, 1973. $1.50.

Sheresky, N., and Mannes, M. *Uncoupling: the Art of Coming Apart; A Guide to Sane Divorce.* New York, Viking Press, 1972. $7.92.

Ms Magazine. $9 a year.

The Liberator. (1404 Grant Avenue, Ft. Worth, Tex. 76106) $3 a year.

Membership in Women for Change. $10 a year.

Human Behavior Magazine. (Subscription Dept., P.O. Box 2810, Boulder, Colo. 80302) $14 a year.

27 SYSTEMS THEORY AND FAMILY PSYCHOTHERAPY

By Jeanne C. Miller, M.S.

A Brief History of Family Psychotherapy

THE INVESTIGATION AND TREATMENT OF EMO-
TIONAL DYSFUNCTION have long been the concern of nurses, physicians,
and other clinical practitioners. For some time, individual psychotherapy
has been considered the treatment of choice for emotional illness.
However, the increasing numbers of patients identified as suffering from
emotional dysfunction have necessitated the advent of methods that more
realistically meet the needs of persons seeking professional assistance.

Family psychotherapy as an approach to emotional dysfunction was
born in the early 1950's. Prior to that time, theorists and clinicians briefly
acknowledged some concern for the patient's relationship with his family.
In the 1950's, however, Bowen, Jackson, Wynne, Bell, Ackerman and
others began extensive investigation of family processes and the relationships between these processes and emotional disturbance. These men
were the first to consider the family unit as the central focus of therapy
rather than an adjunct to individual therapy with the identified patient.
These researchers then began defining their discoveries about family relationship systems.

Because classic analytic psychiatry does not adequately describe the
relationships observed in families, new concepts and to some extent new
terminology have been developed. During the two decades since those
early discoveries, the search for theoretical explanations of the re-

Reprinted, with permission, from *Nursing Clinics of North America*, Vol. 6, No. 3, September 1971.

lationships between family systems and emotional dysfunction has produced a variety of interpretations. Presently there are many family investigations in progress. There still are no adequate explanations for emotional dysfunction. However, systems theory as applied to the family unit provides useful guidelines for continued research into the problem.

The Family as a System

The family may be described as a system. Von Bertalanffy, the originator of general systems theory, defines a system as a set of units with relationships between them.[4]

Systems are of two types: open or closed. Closed systems are those sets of units with relationships between them whose output depends solely on the system and not at all on external input. In contrast, open systems receive input from the environment and depend on interaction with the environment for change.

For this discussion the family is considered an open social system. As an open system, the family exhibits characteristics of self-regulation. Other self-regulating systems have been described fruitfully in terms of feedback control. A system in which output becomes a part of or modifies input exhibits feedback. Input from the external environment may be thought of as a stimulus to the production of some given output. A system showing negative feedback has the capacity to compare input expectations with output and to minimize any differences. A system showing positive feedback, on the other hand, tends to maximize such differences.[7]

For example, an input expectation from society to a family is that individuals should not steal cars. If Johnny, the son of the family, in fact steals cars, then Johnny's parents, as part of the feedback loop, may exert pressure on their son. If this pressure results in a decrease in Johnny's stealing, then the feedback may be described as negative. If, however, the parental pressure leads to an increase in Johnny's delinquent activities, the difference between input expectation and output has increased. The feedback may then be described as positive.

Feedback as a concept is helpful in clarifying certain observed characteristics of families, one being the tendency of families to maintain a steady state. In this discussion, steady state refers to unvarying output from a system over time. This does not imply that a system may not maintain different steady states at different times. However, in one period of time, the output remains relatively constant.

For instance, within the ghetto, there is an input expectation from the ghetto community to the families that children will learn behavior that helps them to survive in the ghetto. If a family has an adolescent member in a college preparation program, the family is likely to be subject to pressure from the school. The pressure may take the form of requests for family support for the daughter as she learns behavior that will prepare her for college. This behavior, which the school expects, may not be useful to the adolescent in her struggles for survival within the ghetto. For this and many other reasons, the family may resist pressure from the school by preventing the daughter from attending class or by encouraging her participation in antisocial activities that are necessary for survival in the ghetto. These family processes may serve to maintain an unvarying output from the system: namely, members who can survive in the ghetto but who are not prepared to leave the ghetto.

If, however, the daughter persists in her college preparation and does leave the ghetto, a new steady state may be attained by the family: namely, all children may go to college. This exemplifies the idea that families cannot be adequately described as simple feedback systems. In the case of all children of the family going to college, the system matched output to input apparently by selecting a new input expectation: that of the school. This example also illustrates the growth-producing potential of positive feedback. The changed output, daughter goes to college and leaves ghetto, reinforces the input expectation for other children to go to school.

In this example, primarily one input expectation was considered: namely, that the children should learn to survive in the ghetto community. There are multiple factors affecting a system, including numerous other inputs that were not mentioned in the above illustration. This points out a deficiency in the conceptualization of the family as a simple feedback system.

Furthermore, inputs into families may be stored over time by memory. An open social system, such as a family, has the capacity to compare output with stored input. Because memory of a system may distort input over time, this also contributes to the family functioning and makes it something more than a simple feedback system. [8]

Finally, an open social system, in contrast with a simple feedback system, appears to be capable of producing output that is not explainable in terms of observable input. This suggests that multiple factors interacting with one another can so affect the system that a variety of results or outputs may be produced in spite of the fact that the same initial conditions existed in the system in all cases of varied output. This phenomenon has been labeled equifinality. [7]

Another systems concept that is useful in studying families is that of a basic program or template that serves as a guide for family functioning. [7]

This basic program is part of the initial information gathered by the system through input and internal feedback. It becomes stored information and is referred to by all family members over time. The program contains parental ideas on behavior of a good mother, good father, and good child, and rules by which each of these persons should live. Modification of this basic program is possible through new inputs. The capacity for modification is obvious in parental expectations of themselves with their first child and their usually relaxed ideas about the same issues with the third or fourth child.

Stress and the Family System

Stress as a concept seems to be closely associated with theories of emotional dysfunction. Therefore, the relationship between stress and family functioning will be considered here.

James Miller identified certain recurring patterns of open systems in coping with stress.[8] He suggests that as stress increases, the functioning of systems at first improves and then gradually worsens. This has been observed in families coping with a crisis. Initially, families function more efficiently, but as the stress continues, the family system may gradually disintegrate.

As stress increases, first one and then another of the sub-systems usually will be involved in coping with the stress, until all components are involved. For instance, parents experiencing marital conflict may attempt to keep the stress within their own sub-system. However, as their disagreements mount, more and more of the children may become involved in resolving the difficulty.

Varying levels of stress may be tolerated by different parts of the system.[8] For example, what constitutes intolerable stress for one member of a family may be moderate stress for the rest of the system. A mother may be grieved by the loss of a dear friend. She may collapse and be unable to function. The other family members may share her grief, but continue to function at a satisfactory level.

The "Le Chatelier principle" may also be applied to families. This suggests that a stable system under stress will move in the direction that tends to minimize the stress.[7] This includes such situations as a family's maintaining that they are really a well-adjusted family in spite of the fact that a member is hospitalized for a psychiatric disorder. Frequently, the family justifies this perception by pointing out the difficult pregnancy experienced by the mother prior to the patient's birth, or the drugs that the patient received as a newborn. In this case, the stress is the possibility of the family seeing themselves as something other than a well-adjusted family. The movement is in the direction of rejecting the "sick member" as a means of maintaining the status quo and minimizing the stress.

Information Processing in the Family System

Communication, as an aspect of information processing, is an important determinant of family functioning. Characteristically, more information is transmitted with less effort within the system than is transmitted over the system's boundaries.[8] This concept is obvious when a family is seen in therapy. The family possesses much more knowledge about itself than does any other system in the family's environment. Therapists may see families for years without acquiring a fraction of the knowledge about the family that the family members possess. Some family secrets never cross the family boundaries.

Information transfer is affected by stress. As stress increases, information is interpreted in a fashion to relieve stress.[8] Also, in periods of increased stress to the system, stress-reducing messages are given priority over neutral or stress-producing messages. A mother may distort a doctor's inquiry about pregnancy with a disturbed child as an indication of the doctor's belief that there indeed was something wrong with the child long before she had any interpersonal contact with him. This relieves stress for her, as it allows her to assume that she is, therefore, not responsible for the behavior of the child.

As the system matures, information processing becomes more efficient. Messages are transmitted with relative ease over noisy channels and more efficient codes are used.[8] The ability of some husbands and wives to transmit messages more and more efficiently after thirty years of marriage illustrates this principle.

Systems or sub-systems may transmit information through other systems or sub-systems. The success of such a transmission depends on the extent to which the external system is under the control of the system using it for transmission.[7] An example of this principle may be seen in a pathological process that develops when a child becomes the shunt for parental or marital transmissions between parents. It is possible that this principle helps to explain to some extent what happens in the "family projection process" described by Bowen.[2] Usually, in this process, the needs of one or both persons in a two-party system are not being met. A child becomes the focus of the problem between the parents and the two-person system is stabilized because of the control it possesses over the child sub-system. However, if there is interference from the controlled system, it is possible that the original two-person system will become dysfuntional. Symptoms may represent interference from the child sub-system.

Systems program and store information which may be substituted for a currently transmitted message.[9] This stored information allows a wife to assume that her husband will be angry when he discovers that she bought a new dress, in spite of the fact that she has not yet informed him of her purchase.

Dependence-Interdependence in Family Systems

Sub-systems or components and their relationships with each other must be explored in the study of family systems. One particularly interesting concept is the state of dependence among sub-systems. Miller suggests that one system is independent of another if all variables in the first undergo alteration in ways uncorrelated to alterations in the second.[9] The amount of correlation is a measure of the degree of dependence among subsystems.

In all families there is some emotional interdependence among subsystems. However, as Bowen has pointed out, in dysfunctional relationships there is an inordinate degree of dependence.[2] The concept of differentiation as a characteristic of maturity has part of its origin in this principle. The degree to which one member is dependent on the emotional functioning of the system and other members in the system is the degree to which he is undifferentiated.

The final characteristic of a family as a system refers to the family's potential for growth. This characteristic is also related to the process of differentiation. As a family grows emotionally, it moves toward increased differentiation of its members, more obvious boundaries between its members, and more dispersed decision-making.[8]

Exploring The Family System
Through Family Psychotherapy

Family psychotherapy may be considered an open system with self-regulating capabilities. Some major inputs to the system are: (1) ideas of the therapist about family systems, (2) ideas and feelings of the family about the family, and (3) society expectations about the family.

When beginning consultation with a family, it is first necessary to get a general picture of the family as a whole.[2] At this time, the system development as well as the ongoing family process can be investigated. For example, Mr. and Mrs. Zylo sought assistance for their 13-year-old daughter after she spent a weekend away from home without permission. In the *first interview* with the Zylos the consultant inquired about the ages and sexes of the children in the family. Information was gathered about the health of the children and their adaptation to school and peer relationships. The parents' observations about differences between the children were noted. Mr. and Mrs. Zylo were asked when they first recognized that their daughter was having problems. Any outstanding changes that might have affected the family were recorded. The consultant also made observations of the Zylos' behavior during the initial interview. The following observations were recorded: Mrs. Z. cried frequently throughout the session; Mrs. Z. talked a lot while Mr. Z. spoke only rarely; Mr. Z. looked at the floor much of the time his wife was speaking; Mrs. Z. sat in the same position throughout the interview; Mr. Z. smoked half a pack of cigarettes during the two-hour session; and Mr. Z.'s hand shook noticeably throughout the session.

The second area of investigation is the parental sub-system.[2] Mr. and Mrs. Z. were asked about their courtship and their early days of marriage. Mrs. Zylo talked about her first marriage. Inquiries were made about the births of the three children, with particular attention paid to prenatal and postnatal thoughts of the mother about the children. Mrs. Z. was asked to identify changes that she thought the children had caused in her first marriage. The ages of the children at separation, divorce, and remarriage were noted, as well as any reactions of the children to these events. The occupational status of both Mr. and Mrs. Z. was recorded as well, as any changes in these since their marriage. Any changes in geographical location of the family were also noted. Mr. and Mrs. Z. were asked about any changes in their relationship since marriage which they considered important. Deaths of close friends, siblings, or parents of Mr. and Mrs. Z. were recorded. The consultant asked about the general health and illness patterns of the couple, and dates and duration of major illnesses or injuries were noted.

The third section of the family history is concerned with the extended families of both spouses.[2] In this part of the interview the consultant asked about parents and siblings of Mr. and Mrs. Z. Such information as ages, sexes, geographical location, general health and illness patterns, and intensity of relationship with extended family members was recorded. Inquiries were made about Mr. and Mrs. Z.'s grandparents and aunts and uncles. The same information was compiled about these members of the extended family.

These three major areas of discussion provided the consultant with a general picture of the family system over time.

Family psychotherapy is based on the hypothesis that the identified patient is only one symptom of the family's dysfunction. For this reason, it is helpful to see all members of the family together to evaluate the relationship system as a whole. The Z. family sought assistance for their daughter. The consultant first acquired a family history from the parents and then asked Mr. and Mrs. Z. to bring all the children to the second interview.

During the *second interview*, the consultant asked questions of all family members and made observations of all members' behavior. An attempt was made to determine the general degree of differentiation of each family member. As mentioned in a preceeding section of this paper, differentiation refers to the degree of independence from the family's emotional interdependence.

Emotional interdependence exists in all families.[2] However, the degree to which a member is dependent on the system for approval differs among families and individuals. The following observations were made in this second family session. Mrs. Z. reported getting knots in her stomach when she thought of the "patient." During the session the "patient" scowled each time her mother spoke. The same daughter did not show any external reaction when her stepfather spoke. Mrs. Z. cried each time the "sick" daughter spoke. The other daughter, age 15, did not respond verbally to anything said by her sister. The son, age 18, answered some questions which the identified patient directed toward her mother. Mr. Z. did not initiate any statements. However, when Mrs. Z. began to cry he handed her his handkerchief, without her request, and made a supportive statement to her. Mr. Z. did not directly address any of the three children. He reported that he had never disciplined the children, as he thought that Mrs. Z. and the children would see him as interfering. All family members except the "sick" daughter stated that they had seen their family as well adjusted and happy prior to the outburst of symptoms. Mrs. Z. frequently used "we" when replying to questions that asked for her reactions or thoughts. The 15-year-old daughter reported frequent minor illnesses throughout her life with an increase in fatigue and colds since her sister's misbehavior. Mr. and Mrs. Z. stated that they saw this daughter as physically weak. The son reported early knowledge of his sister's acting out. He stated that he had not discussed this with his parents because he was afraid that his mother would "become too upset." All family members reported that Mrs. Z. became upset easily and that they tried to avoid upsetting her. Many other such statements were made by the family during this session.

Following an evaluation session with all family members, the consultant must decide who will be seen regularly in therapy. There are many different techniques that can be utilized with a variety of configurations of family members. However, the approach being discussed is one in which the two most responsible members (the parents) of the family are seen.

The rationale for this approach is based on the following concepts. First, the relational system of families is believed to be composed of three persons in a triangle. The consultant, when meeting with the parents, can function as the phantom side of the traingle, with his major efforts being directed toward objective observation and keeping himself free of the demands of the emotional interdependence of the system.[2] In this way his input differs from that of any other family member who might function as the third side of the triangle. Therefore, he will stimulate change in the system by adding a new input expectation. Second, the parents are the originators of the basic program for family functioning, and they hold positions of great authority within the family system. If the parents can bring about a change in their sub-system, the rest of the family system may also change.

If a child is the presenting problem (as was true in the Z. family), the parents are asked to leave the child at home and concentrate on studying the system and defining problems that exist between the two of them.

The basic goal of family psychotherapy or consultation is to assist individual family members as they move toward increased differentiation of self.[2] For instance, Mrs. Z., after numerous sessions, cried less frequently and became less completely invested in the lives of her children. She began to paint seriously, although prior to the sessions she believed that she should "take care of the family" instead of paint. She became less reactive to the "sick" daughter's behavior and to the physical illnesses of her other daughter. These changes in Mrs. Z. stimulated changes in the rest of the family system. Thus Mrs. Z.'s output became new input expectation for the family system and thereby stimulated a change in output from the rest of the system.

Consultation time is spent assisting the spouses in their defining of their thinking and feeling reactions. Each parent explores his relationships with his extended family as well as relationships between other members of the extended families, in order to get a broader picture of himself. This also provides the couple with an opportunity to get a clearer picture of one another. Furthermore, parents are frequently able to make comparisons between their relationships with their parents and their relationships with each other and their children.

During the consultation sessions, it is necessary for the consultant to define his beliefs about emotional dysfunction and family or relationship systems for the spouses.[2] He must be able to reinforce his statements of beliefs through his ability to function as a differentiated individual. He must constantly reevaluate his position within the therapeutic system. Thus the consultant must be aware of the feedback mechanisms and the input expectations he is providing for the family.

The following are some specific techniques that can be utilized in family psychotherapy. First, asking for thoughts instead of feelings can help members distinguish between their thinking and feeling responses.[2] Instead of asking how Mrs. Z. felt when she was crying, the consultant asked for her thoughts about a particular relationship or situation. In this way Mrs. Z. was eventually able to gain some thinking awareness of her feeling reaction.

Second, it is important to avoid focusing on the "sick" member.[2] This is difficult to accomplish because persons who seek assistance expect the "therapist" to treat and cure the "sick" member. However, by defining beliefs about family systems and by continually focusing on systems processes rather than the patient's behavior, the consultant discourages the parent's concentration on the "sick" member. Frequently, when parents become uncomfortable with the topic being discussed they will refocus on their "sick" member. This reverting to a "safe" topic illustrates the tendency of a system to ignore stress-inducing messages and to focus on information that may be stress-reducing.

A third technique is that of note taking as a means of keeping oneself less reactive to the emotional interdependence of the system.[1]

It is important that the consultant avoid fulfilling requests for solutions as well as for individual relationships with family members.[1] When the Z. family asked for advice, the consultant would inquire about Mrs. Z's thoughts on the subject and then ask for Mr. Z's thoughts or reactions to Mrs. Z.'s statements. Requests for private sessions by one family member can be discouraged by stating that all information discussed in a private session will be reported to the general family session.

Finally, consultants should avoid making content interpretations.[1] Focusing on process and allowing family members to discover their own interpretations are generally more useful than standard interpretations offered by the consultant. For example, Mrs. Z. reported, after nine months of consultation, that a recurring dream had changed. The longstanding dream was one in which she was being attacked by thousands of small snakes just outside her grandfather's home where she had lived as a child. In the dream her grandfather would frantically beat the snakes with a club. She would always awaken while he was still beating them. Her dream had changed, however. Now the dream took place in her own home. There was only one snake, and her husband and son very quickly killed the snake with little effort. The consultant asked Mrs. Z. what her thoughts were about the change. Mrs. Z. stated that she had been doing a lot of thinking about her relationships with her grandparents, her parents, and her husband and children. She said she had come up with a new working hypothesis about herself and these relationships, and that she believed that this brought about the change in the dream.

Families with an identified patient are anxious. As suggested earlier, they are stressed, and they attempt to move in the direction of alleviating the stress. Families attempt to lessen their state of anxiety, but change does not take place without accompanying anxiety. Therefore, the therapist should be able to accept anxiety in the family and to convey the message that anxiety is inevitable.[1] Although stress is uncomfortable it is rarely fatal, and it does not continue at an intolerable level forever. When one member of a family begins to change, anxiety is aroused throughout the system. The consultant assists the changing member to accept the anxiety and resist the temptation to revert to old output patterns that are being pressured for by the other members. If the changing member can continue to change, the remainder of the system also will change.

The consultation sessions should be focused on learning about family systems.[2] If the consultant can see the family as a system, and help the family to see itself thus, the clients will be encouraged to make observations about how the system works. Thus they will begin to view the family sessions as learning experiences rather than treatment sessions.

Mr. and Mrs. Z. discussed their family system for nearly a year. They explored their relationships within their extended families and postulated comparisons between the two systems. While they still have many years' work before them, systems theory as it applies to families has provided a basis for their continued exploration and resulting development.

Although this approach is still not completely defined, there is already much literature available which provides guidelines for those nurses or other clinicians or clinical practitioners who choose to investigate and treat emotional dysfunction from a family systems point of view.

Summary

Family psychotherapy as an approach to emotional dysfunction began in the 1950's. Since that time numerous nurses, physicians, and other clinical practitioners and researchers have studied and treated families.

This paper relates systems theory concepts to family unit functioning and consultation with families.

The family is described as an open social system. The systems theory concepts of feedback control, steady state, equifinality, information processing, basic program, stress, interdependence, and growth are fundamental to an understanding of the family as a system. Such an understanding is important for nurses, physicians, and other clinical practitioners who study and care for families.

Although there is still no adequate explanation of emotional dysfunction, systems concepts provide tools for continued exploration of the relationship between family processes and this dysfunction.

References

1. Bowen, Murray: The family as the unit of study and treatment. Am. J. Orthopsychiat., 31:40–60. 1959.
2. Bowen, Murrary: The use of family theory in clinical practice. Compar. Psychiat., 7:345–374, 1966.
3. Boszormenyi, Ivan, and Framo, J. L.: Intensive Family Therapy. New York, Harper and Row, 1965.
4. Buckley, Walther: Modern Systems Research for the Behavioral Scientists. Chicago, Aldine Publishing Co., 1968.
5. Buckley, Walter: Sociology and Modern Systems Theory. Englewood Cliffs. N.J., Prentice Hall, 1967.
6. Grinker, R. R., Ed.: Toward a Unified Theory of Human Behavior. New York, Basic Books, 1956.
7. Miller, James: Living systems: basic concepts. Behav. Sc., 10:193–237, 1965.
8. Miller, James: Living systems: cross level hypothesis. Behav. Sc., 10:380–411, 1965.
9. Miller, James: Living systems: structure and process. Behav. Sc., 10:337–379, 1965.
10. The Field of Family Therapy: New York, Group for the Advancement of Psychiatry, Report #78, 1970.

28 "BARGAINING" TO IMPROVE COMMUN- ICATIONS IN CONJOINT FAMILY THERAPY

By Joan Padberg, R.N.

"TELL ME ABOUT YOURSELF" IS AN EARLY THEME in any couple's relationship, and as the sharing experience continues, as the two become better acquainted, the question of getting serious is entertained, evaluated, and resolved. After marriage, new problems occur and these, in turn, bring new demands on the couple's capacity to communicate; that is, to listen, to understand each other, and to express themselves clearly and accurately. The positive relationship between communication and good marital relationship is well documented in the psychiatric and marriage counseling literature.

Communication has been defined to include all the procedures by which one mind affects another. This, of course, involves not only written and oral speech, but all human behavior. (Ruesch, 1961, p. 452) Communication is also a process by which meanings are exchanged between individuals with a common system of symbols. (Webster) Clear communication between persons, then, is necessary for a meaningful, understanding, and positive relationship.

From *Perspectives in Psychiatric Care*, Vol. 13, No.2, 1975, pp. 68–72. Reprinted, with permission, from Nursing Publications, Inc., 194-B Kinderkamack Rd., Park Ridge, N.J. 07656.

Lederer and Jackson (1968) have suggested that there are two major ways in which communciations between individuals break down. The first is a physical one: The persons speak to each other, but neither hears what the other says. Sometimes this failure is the result of a lifetime of non-listening. The second is when the message sent is not the message received: A problem occurs when the message has two or more possible meanings. The meaning, therefore, is dependent upon the interpretation of the listener, which may be different from the interpretation given by the speaker.

Ruesch (1961, p. 460) introduced the notion of therapeutic communication which, he says, ". . . differs from ordinary communication in that the intention of one or more of the participants is clearly directed at bringing about a change in the system and manner of communications."

Therapeutic communication is particularly useful in conjoint family therapy. The goal of any form of psychotherapy is to promote more effective functioning along with a reduction of intrapsychic distress. This holds true for the family as well as for the individual. Conjoint family therapy is a form of group treatment of two or more members of a naturally occurring group who are, to some degree, interdependent on one another; have existed as a group prior to therapy; and may continue to exist as a group following therapy. (Arlan, 1966) The therapist steers or maneuvers communications to bring about situations and message exchanges that eventually will bring about more gratifying social relations.

The bargaining process is one such maneuver for teaching the use of therapeutic communication among couples and family members. It is through the working out of the bargaining process that each family member sees not only himself and his needs, but also widens his vision to include other members of the family and, in so doing, becomes aware of how interdependent they are on each other. To make the family a cohesive unit all must give and take, but not without thoughtful effort and some sacrifice.

Bargaining is an agreement between parties, settling what each gives or receives in a transaction between them or what course of action or policy each pursues in respect to the other. (Webster) Lederer and Jackson (p. 178) define bargaining as a kind of reciprocal behavior . . . a "quid pro quo" or "something for something," and in the marriage process this means "If you do so and so for me, I will do such and such for you." In "quid pro quo is implied shared or exchanged behavior often automatic and out of the realm of consciousness"; that is, not deliberate or "conscious." Sussman's term for this kind of interchange is "reciprocity." Persons in a dyadic relationship do things for one another for which there are commonly shared expectations. (We engage in reciprocal acts because we expect to be rewarded.) (Sussman, 1968) Homans (1961) has suggested that the more one is rewarded as a consequence of his action, the more likely he is to engage in the same or similar acts later on.

Establishing a Quid Pro Quo

For a couple to establish a quid pro quo according to Lederer and Jackson (p. 285), it is necessary for them to understand two fundamental principles. First, the behavior and attitude of one partner always stimulates some kind of reaction from the other. Each partner must become aware of his own behavior and attitudes and recognize how they stimulate reactions in the other. Second, spouses differ in behavior and interests; therefore, if each behaves naturally and spontaneously, that is, without forethought, there will be conflicts between them. In establishing a quid pro quo, spouses soon realize that to maintain a marriage, each must sacrifice some of his natural and spontaneous behavior in respect to his partner's wishes and desires.

Steps in the Bargaining Process

Lederer and Jackson have outlined three steps in the bargaining process.

¶The spouses must examine their relationship to see if their past bargainings have been open or underground. When spouses are trying to straighten out a discordant marriage, the bargaining must be brought above ground and accomplished deliberately, consciously, and with stated goals.

¶Each spouse must examine his own attitude to determine if he is placing his promise of repayment too far in the future. Of course, the setting of common goals such as owning a home, buying a car, and the like, is another matter. What is being discussed here are negotiations concerning things, attitudes, or behaviors over which there is a difference of opinion. Each spouse wants his own way and since that is impossible, the negotiation necessitates a compatible compromise.

¶The third step is an estimation by the couple of that for which they are able to bargain. However, their differing opinions may be so great and their capacity for change so small they are incapable of negotiating a compromise on a particular subject of disagreement. (p. 273)

Here we are exploring something very important, namely, that since bargaining in marriage is a constantly occurring affair, it is not simply a matter of someone winning or losing. When one spouse yields to the other, he does so primarily to be yielded to in return. Over the long run, it is not a matter of winning or losing, but of negotiation and understanding. When each partner knows what the other wants and consciously and deliberately gives something for something, both parties are the winners. (p. 275)

One common misunderstanding about bargaining is the implied assumption that exchanges between two persons must be equal. Most of the reciprocal relationships that exist are based on exchanges that are unequal and often involve a different order of exchange. For example, a person receiving financial reward as exchange may give in return deference, honor, prestige, and respect to the other. In other words, there is little expectation that marital partners will reciprocate in the same order or with an equal amount. An understanding on this point is extremely necessary in order that bargaining patterns not become destructive by each spouse vying to be superior and win the upper hand. Bargaining, then, must not become an end in itself, but rather a means to a clearer understanding of the other's needs, and an aid to open communications. Once quid pro quo patterns have been established and accepted each partner can live from day to day with a degree of security. Each knows what the other wants and what to expect from him in return.

Clinical Data

The following is a clinical example of the use of the concept of bargaining in conjoint family therapy.

The R family was received for family therapy on referral from the mental health clinic. It was scheduled for ten sessions, two a week, lasting approximately one and one-half hours with all five family members present. The problems identified by the family were: alcoholism by the father, who is now on Antebuse; the prolonged hospitalization of the second child, which has brought financial hardship and contention between parents and siblings; a lack of cohesiveness and a breakdown of communications as a result of the problems.

Mr. and Mrs. R are in their early and middle thirties. Mr. R is a blue collar worker in the lower income bracket. He has been attending a mental health clinic for "drinking too much" and "nervousness." He is a small, pleasant, and friendly man, but rather quiet. Mrs. R is large in stature and attractive in spite of a visible eye defect. She is neatly dressed, as are the three children, and she is an immaculate housekeeper. Barry, age 7, reportedly does poorly in school, has an eye and hearing defect, and was very shy in the early family therapy sessions. Lisa, age 4, has a congenital spine defect. She wears braces and walks with a walker. However, she is usually held by her father during the family sessions. She is very verbal, outgoing, aggressive, demanding, and poses a discipline problem to her parents, but is not unmanageable by the therapist. Blake is 3 years old. His growth and development appear normal for his age.

The therapist and cotherapist were received into the family with caution by Mrs. R but rather openly by Mr. R, who had, from current and past experience, become familiar with group process and therapy expectations. The concept of bargaining was introduced in the third session and the participants were asked to consider what they would like to bargain for and with whom. The oldest child, Barry, who had remained silent but attentive during the first two sessions, was encouraged to interact with his parents at the bargaining table. The following are excerpts of verbatim notes taken from the group session.

MR. R: Well, actually, I can't think of a solitary thing that I'd like for my wife to do that she doesn't do. I mean I can't think of a thing, but she says she has . . .

MRS. R: (laughs) Yes, but what I want costs money.

MR. R: Money isn't everything.

MRS. R: It is almost. All I can ever do is think about it. I never get it.

NURSE: Now is your chance to make your wants known. I've heard you mention several things that . . .

MRS. R: Trouble is, nothin' don't ever come of it.

MR. R: Well, tell me, I won't know till you tell me.

MRS. R: Oh, Junior, I've been telling you for six or seven years, there's one little thing that you have *never* done . . . that is bring me home a little wild flower or something, you know, or some little cheap present just to show you care.

MR. R: A wild flower?

MRS. R: You say it foolish . . . you say it's foolish.

MR. R: (unbelieving) Bring you home a wild flower!

MRS. R: Well sure, you'd be bringing it to me.

MR. R: (almost inaudibly) I guess that's an okay request.

MRS. R: But you don't ever do it! (laughs)

MR. R: (laughs) O.K., I got your message.

The nurse then reviewed the request Mrs. R had made and Mr. R agreed to it.

NURSE: All right Mr. R, now it's your chance to request something to bargain with or for.

MR. R: Well, I still can't think of a . . . well, yes, it would thrill the daylights out of me if once on Friday, you wouldn't ask me "Honey, what would you like to have for supper tonight?" or "What are we going to have?" Just surprise me! I hate to make decisions on what we are going to eat on Friday or any other night for that matter (Friday is the day for shopping).

MRS. R: Well, if I bought what I wanted to, you might not like it.

A dialogue followed concerning shopping, spending, budgeting, "stretching the dollar," and spending the income tax return for clothes. Obviously, the real issue here was money and how it was spent and Mrs. R's apparent difficulty in budgeting the limited family income. Mrs. R showed surprise at Mr. R's apparent allegation and entered into a lively controversy over money matters and defended her position. Mr. R finally conceded that his wife really did very well with the small and rather unstable income that he provided.

The above dialogue is a perfect example of the first breakdown in communications as suggested by Lederer and Jackson, in that the spouses talk to each other but neither hears what the other has said. Incorporated in the dialogue is the notion of the message sent not being the message received. By each party stating, in the presence of a third person, the wishes and omissions often hinted about and the expectations often requested but gone unheard, the spouses listen and respond in an appropriate and forthright manner.

The quid pro quo between father and son was, again, a source of great surprise to the father. Barry bargained for his father to play football with him in return for going to bed when requested to do so. Mr. R said he was sure Barry was going to ask for a toy of some kind.

In the fourth session the bargains were discussed. Mr. and Mrs. R had fulfilled their bargains and showed some pleasure at their accomplishments. However, Barry had not kept his bargain, therefore he had not played football with his father. Barry's failure to keep his end of the bargain made him feel "left out" of the session and he asked to bargain again. Lisa also asked to make a bargain with her parents. The requests made were simple and easy to accomplish, again revealing wishes and desires unknown to the other family members.

In the fifth session, the bargaining proved successful for both parents and children. The children are now becoming more manageable and are showing an interest in being a part of the family decisions. There is less discord about taking baths and going to bed when requested and they are receiving some of their own small wishes in return. The family members are more attuned to one another's needs and expectations, and "private" bargaining (without aid of the therapist) is being encouraged.

Conclusion

This is a warm, loving family whose members seem eager to assist one another with the problems of family living. The parents responded well to the concept of bargaining as a means to clearer communications and as aid in rewarding or disciplining their children. It is generally accepted that one of the principal aims of conjoint family therapy is to improve the clarity and directness of communications within the family so that all members are able to participate appropriately and with some equality. The nurse therapist and family agree that progress has been made in opening channels of communications. The children have assumed some responsibility for their behavior and are attempting to lessen the conflict and rivalry among themselves. Teaching to assist this family with communication problems is ongoing even after the formal sessions are ended.

References

Arlan, Monroe S., "Conjoint Therapy and the Corrective Emotional Experience," *Family Process*, March 1966, Vol. 5, No. 1, p. 92.

Homans, George, *Social Behavior: Its Elementary Forms*, New York: Harcourt, Brace and World, 1961, p. 53–59.

Lederer, William and Jackson, Don, *Mirages of Marriage*, New York: W. W. Norton and Co. 1968.

Ruesch, Jurgen, *Therapeutic Communication*, New York: W. W. Norton, 1961.

Sussman, Marvin B., "Adaptive, Directive and Integrative Behavior of Today's Family," *Family Process*, September 1968, Vol. 7, No. 2, p. 240.

Webster's Seventh Collegiate Dictionary, Springfield, Mass.: G. C. Merriam Company, 1963.

INTERVENTION AND INVESTMENT IN COMMUNITY MENTAL HEALTH
A Family in Crisis

By Faye Gary Harris, M.S.
and Marilyn S. Fregly, Ph.D.

WHILE STUDYING FOR A MASTER'S DEGREE IN PSY-
CHIATRIC nursing, I worked for five months with a family of seventeen
members who during this period underwent four major crises. My
method of therapy was based upon the preventive psychiatry model of
Gerald Caplan and the crisis theory of Erich Lindemann.

The Higgins Family

The Higgins family, consisting of the parents, thirteen children, and
two grandchildren, live on the west side of Chicago in a rapidly changing suburb. The drab, overcrowded buildings with broken windows,
rickety staircases, and dank odors symbolize the basic discouragement
the inhabitants feel toward their lives. The same incohesive structure
is found in the family unit, huddled in a thrown-together style, each
member "doing his own thing" wihtout much awareness of the consequences of his individual actions on the others.

Reprinted with permission, from *Nursing Clinics of North America*, Vol. 6, No. 4,
December, 1971.

My introduction to the family occurred when the principal of the grade school where I conducted group therapy with emotionally disturbed students referred Mrs. Higgins to me. She had come for help in dealing with her 10-year-old son who attended the school. Our first meetings were at the school, but because of baby-sitting problems we agreed to meet in her home. In the home we were surrounded and frequently interrupted by her many children. The conditions were not exactly ideal for a satisfactory interchange, so we often used the telephone in the evenings as a means of holding a one-to-one conversation.

Mrs. Higgins is a 35-year-old black mother of thirteen children and has two grandchildren. The children range in age from two months to 24 years. Though living under deplorable conditions, she keeps herself and her children clean. She also seeks self-improvement for them and herself. She related with some enthusiasm her experiences in the adult education program held at night at the community school, her parts in plays there, and how she tutors her younger children with their homework, as well as preparing them for school in the morning.

Her interest in her children showed on our first meeting in the principal's office, a familiar place for her but a relatively strange one to me. She knew the physical structure of the building and was pleased to show me around—to the ladies' lounge, to her children's classroom and to the rooms of teachers she knew. She assumed a leadership role and I enjoyed following her.

However, she was not completely at ease at the school or with me. She never removed her coat and scarf. She always said, "No, thank you. I will keep it on because I cannot stay too long this time," yet she stayed at least an hour each time. When she indicated that it was time to go, I tried to end the session by planning for the next one. "We will see each other next week same time and same station." Also, I wrote her name and the time of the next session in a notebook and put an asterisk by it with a comment, "I will be here waiting for you; see you next week." She liked the special attention and the feeling of importance that I tried to create. I tried to convey the message that on a particular day, at a particular time, my only concern was to see her—everything else was secondary.

Her concern about her "importance" and her "impression on me" was apparent at our fourth session, the first held in her home. I arrived early in the midst of her cleaning. She was apologetic for not having the house in order. I told her, "I understand about the house not being tidy. I am a member of a large family too." We both chuckled as she moved various articles from a chair to give me a seat. Yet almost by an unconscious time mechanism, she communicated that my visit here, too, was to last for one hour. "My, it is almost time for Judy to go to school, and I have not even started to get her ready. I got to fix lunch for my children." She also communicated this nonverbally: her hand twisting, looking out the window, turning the TV on and adjusting it many times, and making frequent comments to her children about their behavior. As I left, I wrote her name in my notebook, the time I would return, and the big asterisk. I hoped to convey the same message of significance and importance.

After a few more visits in her home, I learned each of her children's names and something about them in order to fix their names and individualities in my memory. Whenever family members were present, which was usually the case, I always chatted with them before starting the session.

Because chores had such a high priority, Mrs. Higgins' kitchen became the focal spot for our conversations. While we talked, she prepared lunch, ironed, and tended the children. She impressed me as a warm person who was overwhelmed by her family and its many problems. But when she came to talk about these problems, she became defensive and talked as if she were an outsider looking in.

I discovered at the end of the first home visit that Mr. Higgins had been sent out of the house, not to return until 12 noon, after I had left. For this reason, I decided that I should always call before coming to the house. I found out why when I met Mr. Higgins.

The Unseen Other Force

Mrs. Higgins' restless behavior and her side remarks about Mr. Higgins led me to wonder about her fear of him and her fear of his disapproval of my being there.

I met Mr. Higgins on my fifth visit. He looked me up and down, from head to foot. I stood up to acknowledge his presence, extended my hand, and he shook it. Mrs. Higgins fell silent when he entered. He took the aggressive leadership role, and seemed hostile. "What you here for, and how long you be here?" I responded: "I am here because I want to help you with some of the problems you are having. I think I can be of some help, and I hope you will allow me to try. I will leave at any time you suggest, but I am hoping you will allow me to stay in your home so that we can work together."

He fired more questions at me: "Where are you from? About how old are you? Who told you about us? Who do you work for?" I answered each question truthfully and fully. After I had responded to his barrage of questions, he voluntarily began to talk about himself. By the end of the session, he had relaxed and was less defensive. He invited me to come again and we shook hands when I left. Having met him, I felt I could win his trust and confidence as well as continue coming back to the home. He was concerned about the family name, about what the neighbors would think if they learned he was not "man" enough to handle his own family. I assured him his family would not be discussed with anyone but my colleagues.

Mr. Higgins always asked about my little blue book (of process notes). I told him the notes were recorded and shared with my teacher. I offered to share the notes with him or any member of the family who chose to read them. They never read them, but occasionally he would ask, "How the notes coming?"

He was also suspicious of his wife's telephone conversations with me. One morning I called to say I would be late because of bad weather and Mr. Higgins, who answered the phone, advised me to stay home. I did not go.

One reason for the lack of trust on the part of both parents was my age. Mrs. Higgins had difficulty in perceiving me as a person with ability to be therapeutically helpful because she had a daughter as old as I. Her daughter was not helpful to her; therefore, she associated youth with immaturity, lack of knowledge, and understanding.

It took about five weeks and ten visits to establish myself in their confidence as a decent and genuine human being as well as a competent member of the therapy team.

Four Crises

During my five months' work with the family, four crises developed, any one of which could have destroyed the already tenuous family unit and produced new problems for the "uninvolved" members.

The first crisis involved Bill, the seventh child, a hefty 10-year-old who prided himself on being "the toughest kid in the neighborhood." Bill was already being seen by another member of the health team.

The center of another crisis was Judy, the fourth child, a shy 15-year-old whose assets were seen in her interest in cooking and in tending to the younger children. She became an unwed mother during the period of intervention.

Mary, the fifth child, an obedient but hostile 13-year-old, was described as "fast and selfish" with no interest in home responsibilities.

The onset of menses produced another problem as Mary threatened to have sexual relations with her boy friend, which started a power struggle between her mother as to who was to set the limits for night hours.

The fourth crisis involved Mrs. Higgins herself when she sought and accepted employment. Her step toward economic independence threatened the weak ego structure of her unemployed husband as well as the traditional family role pattern.

Crisis One

Bill had broken into the school building during the weekend with a group of boys who lived in the neighborhood. He had been taken, with the others, to the district police station for questioning. Bill did not mention the incident to his parents, but another neighborhood boy did. The parents completely denied the neighbor boy's statement and said nothing to Bill.

The principal told Mrs. Higgins about the incident when she came to school to keep her appointment with me the following week. During our session Mrs. Higgins cried, then we sat in silence for a long time. When Mrs. Higgins did speak, she expressed guilt and a feeling of failure. "Maybe I could have helped my little boy more than I did." The guilt was explored to some extent by allowing Mrs. Higgins to talk about her feelings concerning Bill. She tried to place blame on her husband as the cause of all the family's misfortunes and failures: "My husband could help too. I have everything to do. Jim will not cooperate." But her attempt to absolve herself was not successful because, as she talked, she grew progressively sadder in expression, her voice became softer, her hand twisting increased, and she shifted positions in her chair many times. When the session ended, we agreed to meet at her home the following week, at which time we would focus on Bill, as we had agreed to during previous sessions.

Mr. Higgins was present when I arrived, and much of my time was spent answering questions he posed concerning myself and my credentials: "Where are you from? Where do you go to school? How long have you been in the city? Is your family here, or do you live alone?" Mr. Higgins showed anger toward and impatience with his son, frequently referring to Bill as being "bull-headed" and "a toughie" who was trying to "get away with everything." He boasted that he punished Bill by beating him with the cord of an electric iron. In fact, he said, "I am the best beater that you have ever seen."

Before the police incident could be completely explored by Mrs. Higgins and me, it was compounded by Bill's attack on a teacher at school. Apparently the teacher had irritated Bill, and he swung at her. Several male teachers were needed to subdue him. The mother was not at home when the principal called, but Mr. Higgins was. He went to the school and returned in a rage, cursing, slamming doors, threatening any available family member, and kicking furniture.

In the meanwhile, the entire family were affected by the parents' attitude toward Bill. Mr. Higgins had instructed Bill to remain quiet in the household. He was to have small portions of food and was not permitted to make the slightest complaint. He was screamed at not only by the parents, but by other brothers and sisters as well. He was laughed at and called names by his brothers and sisters. Both the mother and Bill's therapist agreed in their reporting that Bill was becoming hostile and withdrawn.

During the sessions in the home Mr. Higgins showed his helpless rage toward Bill. He began to compare Bill with Hitler: "He wants to push people around—he wants to have his way." He described to me how he beat Bill. I listened to the outburst of hostility and recognized that the entire household was angry with Bill. Although she was on the verge of tears, the mother was not able to express her feelings, but Mr. Higgins continued loudly and clearly: "That boy is no good. He has caused me nothing but worry and trouble. I am getting tired of him." When the parents were asked about Bill's desirable qualities, Mr. Higgins could recognize none, but Mrs. Higgins mentioned that he was "dutiful" in that he helped to care for the younger children and helped to clean the house.

I helped the parents look at methods they had used in communicating with Bill that might have caused him to become angry and unable to control his aggression. For example, feelings of rejection were being experienced by Bill because of his aggression toward the teacher and fear of some type of punishment by the father and teacher. Every one in the family could feel free to humiliate him.

Methods of punishment were discussed. I pointed out that the methods used by the father apparently were not the answer. Mr. Higgins said he would try another method, but he assured me that he was "very skilled at beating." He added, "If beating is what he needs, that is what he will get." The three of us concluded that since Bill liked to attend the social center at school, restricting him from doing so might be a more effective method of punishment when punishment was justified. I suggested that identifying the activities that made the parents and the other family members intolerant of Bill might be the most useful method of working with the negative feelings they were experiencing toward him.

Finally, I pointed out that Bill's behavior was not necessarily abnormal or odd, but a struggle on his part to be understood. It was apparent that the family was not aware of the struggle Bill was having.

I emphasized that Bill's problems were created by a lack of understanding and communication within the family. Contributing to his problems was his particular phase of growth and development, pre-adolescence. I explained that the pre-adolescent phase is accompanied by emotional and physiological changes, among which are interest in status in peer groups and rebellion through restlessness, hostility, and irritability. Helping Bill successfully complete this phase of development should aid him in becoming more successful in the other phases of growth and development.

EVALUATION   After I assessed the situation, it was clear to me that the crisis was Bill's inability to control basic impulses, aggression and anger, which, in turn, created undesirable behavior that could not be accepted by other family members. In other words, the crisis was a complex problem brought about by Bill's encounter with the police, his aggressive attack on the teacher, and his family's response to his behavior. Bill seemed to be responding to hostility within the family structure by becoming even more aggressive and more hostile. Since all efforts at self-expression were thwarted in the home, Bill took his pent-up frustrations and conflicts with him to the community.

The tension seemed to increase considerably immediately after Bill struck the teacher, and intervention seemed to be most effective at this point. Intervention included:

1. Helping the family members understand how they were contributing to Bill's aggression and hostility.
2. Having the father express reasons for his negative attitude toward Bill.
3. Helping the family understand some of the feelings Bill may be experiencing.
4. Identifying other methods to be used in setting limits.
5. Identifying the activities that made the family intolerant of Bill.
6. Discussing the struggle inherent in the pre-adolescent phase of growth and development.

My effectiveness was dependent on the family's willingness to accept my guidance, support, and clarification. Since they were in a state of crisis, they allowed somewhat tentatively for my intervention.

Crisis Two

While there was an abatement in the intensity of feelings, as well as some success in solving the problems that brought about the first crisis, a second crisis was in process. Mrs. Higgins contacted me by phone over the weekend and said that she had received a certificate of merit for having completed a nurses' aide course. She wanted to display the certificate, but Mr. Higgins refused to let it be shown in the household. She expressed her need and desire for beginning a job as nursing assistant at a general hospital, but said Mr. Higgins disapproved. They had had a violent argument two hours before she called me.

Mrs. Higgins enrolled in a four-week course for nursing assistants and completed it, and Mr. Higgins did not object to her attending school. In fact, he told me that he was attending school for interior designing. Within this framework of confusion, the children could not decide whom to support or not to support.

On my ninth visit to the home, several of the children were in the living room listening to records or watching television. The apartment was noisy. The physical setting reflected the family's depression. The apartment was dark, although it was but 10 a.m.; curtains were drawn, and several of the family members were in pajamas. After Mrs. Higgins came into the living room, the family members lowered the hi-fi and television, but they remained seated. Mr. Higgins, however, began wandering in and out of the living room. In between his pacing, he muttered, "Finishing school is a good and a bad sign." On the next go-around he questioned, "Will she leave us now that she has completed school? Will she think she is better than we are?" Mrs. Higgins talked with me very softly and frequently interrupted our conversation to set limits for Cathy, her youngest child, and Ophelia, her grandchild. Though little verbalization took place, much nonverbal communication went on, and a shifting back and forth within chairs took place. The family members stared at me and talked among themselves, not including Mrs. Higgins or me in the conversation. I feared that the amount of tension and anxiety being experienced by the family, in addition to my verbalization of present problems, would irritate the situation, thus leading to no productive end. I left because the family was too upset to discuss their problems with me. I was feeling uncomfortable also.

The following week, during my tenth meeting in the home, tension and anxiety were still present. Mr. Higgins was home again. He and Mrs. Higgins said that I had helped them, that they could talk with me about the problem within the family without worrying about the neighbors knowing "their business." We began discussing Mr. Higgins' feelings about Mrs. Higgins' coming job. He sounded very jealous of her progress, "She thinks she is better than anyone else. She thinks she is getting too good for me and the children." He stated his concern about the household activities being neglected if Mrs. Higgins should go to work, and emphatically pointed out that she would still be responsible for all household tasks as well as for maintaining her job if *he* decided to *allow* her to work. Mrs. Higgins accepted the job at a nearby hospital one week later.

After I suggested that Mrs. Higgins' duties be shared among other family members so that she could keep her job, the family members began to listen. They wanted to know what I meant, how I thought it would work out: "Who would be doing the work?" We discussed tasks that could be performed by other members of the household: the older ones cooking breakfast, Mrs. Higgins preparing lunch for younger children, Judy and Mary getting Cathy ready for kindergarten, and so on. All family members were to come home immediately after school so that none of the younger children would be at home alone. Mr. Higgins would not accept any responsibility in the household, mainly because he insisted that he was employed. This was refuted by Mrs. Higgins as well as by other family members. However, he did encourage the other children to "help their mother out around the home." Mr. Higgins did not object to the planning, and Mrs. Higgins beamed when he did not object verbally. I constantly asked him for suggestions and criticism.

When the plans were concluded, Mr. Higgins talked about a social worker who had visited his home and questioned his role as a father, challenged him about his unemployment, and told him that his family was living in deplorable circumstances. As he poured out his feelings of humiliation, he talked quickly, occasionally stuttering. He also fancied what he would do if another social worker or anyone else intruded. He threatened to literally "throw the social worker out of his house" if she ever came again. I heard all of this as an expression of his feelings of failure and unworthiness, his need to be recognized as the authority figure in his family, all brought about by Mrs. Higgins' attempt to make a decision without consulting him.

After Mrs. Higgins became employed, the family had to accept a smaller welfare check which meant less total income. I encouraged her in her attempt to have self-respect and to be self-sufficient even though necessities were hard to obtain. I told her and the family about a new food stamp program that would allow Mrs. Higgins to purchase approximately one hundred dollars worth of food for eighty dollars. Mr. Higgins volunteered to purchase the food stamps, but Mrs. Higgins was reluctant to give him the money as she was afraid of his ever-present need to socialize with his neighborhood drinking friends. However, Mr. Higgins said he would like to help do things around the house, to help Mrs. Higgins with some of her duties. He was trying to assume more responsibility and earn respect within his family and community.

EVALUATION   The crisis identified was the inability of family members to adjust to a transitional role—a working mother. Mrs. Higgins found it very difficult to communicate to her family her need for a job and to cope with the problems resulting from her aggressive steps into a new role as a nursing assistant in a nearby hospital. Anxiety, tension, fear, and hostility developed quickly, but family members were unable to express the reasons for their feelings.

On the ninth visit, I too felt their anxieties and fears, and the threats to their shaky family structure. This made intervention impossible until the family had reached that point when their emotional turmoil had calmed and we could be rational and sensible in dealing with the problem.

Intervention included:

1. Allowing the mother to express fears over the telephone.
2. Postponing active intervention until the family was more amenable to therapeutic help.
3. Allowing Mr. Higgins to verbalize his feelings about Mrs. Higgins' intended employment.
4. Providing Mr. Higgins with an opportunity to express negative feelings about a recent social worker's visit; listening to him express his need for a feeling of worthiness and respect.
5. Discussing with the family members ways of getting household tasks done by reassigning roles to various family members.
6. Providing information about food stamps.

The basic structure of the family was weak and consequently easily affected by any change in traditional roles. The family had rather poor interpersonal relationships: feelings, ideas, information, behavior, and messages were not discussed freely within the family. The family was amenable to help when I intervened and gave direction and support. In this crisis, because of the timing of the intervention, equilibrium was restored temporarily.

Crisis Three

In the midst of the second crisis, I heard a baby crying. When I asked about the weak cry, Mrs. Higgins hedged about their keeping a neighbor's infant. She brought the baby to the living room, and I cuddled her and put her shoes on. No one disagreed with the mother's remark concerning the infant. It turned out that Patricia was not the child of a neighbor but of Judy, the 15-year-old daughter, a fact I learned through conference with my teammates. This shock wave of "upsetness" caused by Judy's becoming a mother out of wedlock became the third crisis that befell the family within this five-month period.

When I made the eleventh home visit, the house was very untidy. Judy was at home with her pajamas on. Mr. Higgins was in the back, and Mrs. Higgins was ironing. We talked first about her new job; she enjoyed being away from home, as well as being a wage earner again. We talked about Bill, who was doing "nicely," and the family members complimented Bill's therapist for his progress. As Mrs. Higgins ironed, I cuddled Patricia and gave her a bottle, I displayed warmth for the child in such a fashion that the other family members could observe my approach to the infant. I expressed no moral judgment, no ostracism.

Mr. Higgins appeared irritated. He stalked through the dining and living room areas, making frequent demands upon Mrs. Higgins. "It is time for me to eat. Send Ann to the store for a pop." I did not stay long because of the number of duties Mrs. Higgins was commanded to perform. I did not want to make another demand by my presence. Before I left, she assured me that she would call very soon.

During the weekend, Mrs. Higgins called me to tell me that the infant was Judy's baby. A few hours before she called, Mr. Higgins had come into the living room intoxicated and nude. He had begun to humiliate Judy. Mrs. Higgins reported his comments: "No good woman has a baby without a husband. Why aren't you married? You should not be in *my* house with the baby." All of the family members were embarrassed, shocked, and frightened, especially the females, who scurried into their bedrooms. The two older boys subdued the father and put him in a back room for the rest of the night. Mrs. Higgins planned to sleep in a chair in the living room with Judy and the infant in the front bedroom for security. Above the noise in the background, I learned that the family had begun to reject Judy because she had had a baby out of wedlock. In fact, they had become hostile toward her. Mrs. Higgins pleaded with me to come as soon as I could find the time.

Two days later, I went to the home. Again, the baby was crying. I cuddled the infant while Mr. and Mrs. Higgins, Judy, and Aaron slowly settled in the living room. Aaron, their second son, is mentally retarded. Everyone was quiet. The family apparently had wanted to keep Judy's pregnancy a secret because of Mr. Higgins' attitude. He was very concerned about what his friends would think. Mrs. Higgins said she was finding it difficult to talk about illegitimate pregnancies because her oldest child, Carmen, was born out of wedlock. Mrs. Higgins was experiencing an awakening of old conflicts, guilt, shame, and failure. Mrs. Higgins also said that Carmen, at the age of 19, had given birth to an illegitimate child who lived in the home at present.

My approach was to encourage the family to talk about how they felt concerning Judy and the infant. Mr. Higgins said he felt as though he had failed; he was ashamed and was feeling guilty. Then he fell silent. I broke the silence when I asked how they thought Judy was feeling. No one commented. She looked very remorseful, hands folded in lap and head bowed. I asked Judy about *her* reaction to having a baby and seeing the family become so disorganized and irritated. Judy responded, "I am tired from washing and ironing. I cannot go out of the house. My friends are having fun without me. My face is fat and big. The baby is so tiny—I am not sure if I can care for it. I have not seen my boy friend in a long time. I feel that I have disgraced my family."

The family members present said they were not aware of how Judy felt concerning her baby. They seemed to have overlooked the fact that Judy was experiencing mixed feelings about the infant, too. Mr. and Mrs. Higgins thought Judy enjoyed being a mother, especially since she was always so "dutiful" around the home with her younger sisters and brothers. I pointed out that Mr. Higgins' behavior may have caused Judy to "dislike herself," and pointed out that his attitude could have played a part in influencing the other family members to respond to Judy in a hostile, detached manner.

The next step was to try to get the family to help Judy through the crisis, as well as to restore the equilibrium within the family. Mr. Higgins began to soften a bit and asked for suggestions as to how things could be "quieted." I guided the members of the family who were present in identifying the constructive methods to resolve the crisis.

Some suggestions elicited were the following:

1. Responsibility for the care of the baby should be shared by the members of the family.
2. The family, along with Judy, should keep the infant at different times so that Judy could return to school.
3. Judy should continue to live in the home.
4. No derogatory behavior toward Judy should be permitted.
5. Talks about feelings of disappointment, shame, failure, and guilt should be carried on within the family structure.
6. Judy, the father of the child, and Mr. and Mrs. Higgins should be permitted to talk about marriage.
7. The infant should be accepted by other members of the family.
8. Judy should be permitted to participate in the core of family life as she had previously done.

I emphasized that Judy was experiencing mixed feelings concerning the baby, and that she needed their help more than ever before. At this comment, Judy's face seemed to light up. Mr. Higgins very loudly and clearly said that the family had his support. Mrs. Higgins challenged him, "He never does anything." I added that maybe he was trying to assume more responsibility and be a better father; why not give him a chance to improve?

I stayed a long time at the home, approximately three hours. Feeling that the session had been most profitable, I left with the satisfaction of having been helpful.

EVALUATION   The crisis (a family member, Judy, becoming a parent out of wedlock) was identified. The family viewed Judy's behavior as "disgraceful" and had begun to take steps to punish her within the family setting. As a consequence, Judy withdrew, and experienced feelings of shame, failure, unworthiness, and ugliness.

Had there been better interpersonal communication, the family might have been better equipped to deal more effectively with the birth of Judy's infant. The family was obsessively concerned about their reputation, their "image," their "impression on others." This was their reason for keeping the pregnancy a secret. They denied the parentage of the child, and decided to reject both the mother and child.

In this value judgment, I decided to focus upon Mr. Higgins as the law giver and injustice collector. Even though the family members were fond of Judy, they responded to his plans to "put her out," and, by her absence, thus restore the equilibrium to solve his status problem.

He seemed to have no understanding of any standard but his own—no feeling for the emotional trauma that Judy was experiencing—and thus no basis for reevaluating his actions to integrate or compromise for the sake of family unity.

Intervention included:

1. Displaying my acceptance of the child by cuddling her and feeding her.
2. Listening to the mother talk about frightening incidents over the telephone.
3. Being receptive to the family's expressions of failure, shame, guilt, and hostility.
4. Encouraging Mr. Higgins to look at his behavior and the responses it provoked within the family.
5. Encouraging Judy to express her feelings about giving birth to the infant.

6. Encouraging the family to be more accepting of and helpful to Judy through crisis and to permit her to live within the home, as well as to participate in family life.
7. Helping the family put their family love for Judy and her baby in a higher priority than the opinion of the neighbors.

Crisis Four

After the third crisis, I was not able to contact Mrs. Higgins for about three weeks. I called several times and was told by the child who answered the phone that Mrs. Higgins "was busy" or "not at home." I always left a message saying I had called, but she did not return the calls. No home visits were made because I could not contact any of the older family members.

After my many thwarted attempts to see the family again, Mrs. Higgins phoned me one afternoon. We talked about Bill, Judy, and her new job. Everything was working out nicely. She asked to see me again and we agreed to meet in her home the following week. When I arrived at the home, I talked for the first time with Mary, the 14-year-old daughter. She was pouting because her mother would not allow her to attend a two-week meeting for teen-age girls being cosponsored by a local university, and a YWCA. Mary was dressed like many adolescents—socks, slim skirt, and pony tail. Mrs. Higgins described her as "fast and fresh."

After Mary had left the room, Mrs. Higgins assembled her ironing equipment. Having finished several menial tasks, she settled down and began to talk about a "problem that may develop," namely, Mary's difficulty in adjusting to the beginning of adolescence. Mrs. Higgins said that Mary had threatened to "have a sexual affair" with her steady boy friend. She had told Mrs. Higgins about her "deep love" for her boy friend, which caused Mrs. Higgins to tell Mary about birth control methods. Although she cautioned her about becoming involved sexually before marriage, she added that Mary should use some form of contraceptive if she "just *must* become involved." She related that at some time earlier the boy had visited with Mary in the home, but the visits were embarrassing. Mr. Higgins argued with the boy friend or anyone available, used profane language, and disrupted the entire household. The house was crowded and noisy with the younger children. Privacy was impossible. Because of all this, Mary decided not to invite her date home again. Instead, she would go *out* with him.

I perceived this story as another potential crisis and planned to intervene before the entire household became upset. At the time of our discussion, other family members were not aware of the struggle that Mary and her mother were involved in. I, therefore, wanted to act quickly to forestall as much conflict as possible within the family, and, at the same time, give Mrs. Higgins and Mary freedom to solve their problems.

During this visit, Mrs. Higgins focused on sex education. She had told her other daughters the same thing she was telling Mary. To the boys, when they became of age (approximately thirteen), she said, "Be careful and always protect the girl." Mrs. Higgins thought this was extensive enough, valid and proper. To defend herself from criticism, she added, "That is what I was told."

Our session then focused upon the double message she was giving Mary. The two older girls had responded to the covert message, "Don't, but if you *do*, use a contraceptive." Yet she hoped Mary would not have a baby out of wedlock. Consequently, we decided that Mrs. Higgins should go into greater detail about the physiologic changes that accompany growing up, as well as healthier ways of relating to members of the opposite sex. Curfews should be set for Mary, and she should be expected to obey them. Family members should be told beforehand when Mary's guest would be coming into the home in order to allow for some privacy. I pointed out that Mary would need help in channeling her sexual behavior in socially acceptable ways. Her interests in dancing, dating, and "speaking a private language" were merely a phase in growth and development used as a means to explore and master her environment.

I stressed Mary's need to be able to talk about her problems. Mrs. Higgins agreed to make herself available to Mary whenever she indicated that she would like to talk. Her need for privacy should be respected by all the family. At the time of our discussion, she was keeping her "private things" in a suitcase under her bed.

Getting back to Mary's attending the two-week meeting for teenagers, Mrs. Higgins' reason for not allowing her to participate was that Mary did not have proper clothing. I suggested that she could take what she had, and launder it frequently. This suggestion was not accepted because of Mrs. Higgins' fear of embarrassment. I was not able to convince her that the meeting would no doubt prove to be helpful and educational for Mary.

EVALUATION   The crisis identified was a power struggle between mother and daughter over the daughter's method of adjusting to the adolescent phase of growth and development. The crisis was aborted because the mother identified the situation and sought help early. When I came to the home, chaos had not spread throughout the entire household as it had in previous crises. The problem was still limited to Mary and her mother.

Mary found this phase of growth and development especially difficult because of the type of sex education she received from her mother.

Initially, Mary's behavior was viewed by the mother as "fast," "selfish," and "fresh," and not as an attempt to grow up. The fear that Mary provoked within Mrs. Higgins was familiar, a fact that possibly motivated her to call me again. Having had two other daughters with babies out of wedlock was an appropriate reason for Mrs. Higgins to seek help when another daughter began to reach this period of development.

I intervened before the tension was at a peak, and when intervening, I tried to let Mrs. Higgins handle the problem. I wanted to give her guidance and support while she worked through the problem. Mary did not participate in the session, but I felt that Mrs. Higgins was the dominant force in the family and that helping her would be the best way to reach all of the family members. Intervention included:

1. Helping Mrs. Higgins understand Mary's struggle with the adolescent phase of growth and development.
2. Encouraging Mrs. Higgins to reexamine her methods of teaching sex education.
3. Assisting with devising methods of manipulating the environment when Mary had company.
4. Encouraging Mrs. Higgins to help other family members to understand Mary's need for privacy.

Conclusion

Termination after five months had been prepared for at the outset of my work with the Higgins family, because the date was determined by my plan to leave the area after completing the master's program. The thirty sessions had meant a great deal to me, not only because the Higgins home was less tense and family members seemed strengthened from having weathered these crises, but also because they had allowed me to be allied with them in their struggle with these crises.

References

Books

Ackerman, Nathan: The Psychodynamics of Family Life. New York, Basic Books, 1958.
Bellak, Leopold., Ed.: Community Psychiatry and Community Mental Health. New York, Grune and Stratton, 1964.

Berlo, D. K.: The Process of Communication. New York, Holt, Rinehart and Winston, 1960.

Caplan, Gerald: An Approach to Community Mental Health. New York, Grune and Stratton, 1961.

Caplan, Gerald, Ed.: Emotional Problems of Early Childhood. New York, Basic Books, 1955.

Caplan, Gerald: Principles of Preventive Psychiatry. New York, Basic Books, 1964.

Josselyn, Irene: Psychosocial Development of Children. New York, Family Service Association of America, 1948.

Kotinsky, Ruth, and Witmer, Helen E.: Community Programs for Mental Health. Cambridge, The Commonwealth Fund, Harvard University Press, 1955.

Lindemann, Erich: Symptomology and Management of Acute Grief. In Parad, H. J., Ed.: Crisis Intervention: Selected Readings, New York, Family Service Association of America, 1965.

Orlando, Ida Jean: The Dynamic Nurse-Patient Relationship. New York, G. P. Putnam's Sons, 1961.

Parad, H. J., and Caplan, Gerald: A Framework for Studying Families in Crisis. In Parad, H. J., Ed.: Crisis Intervention: Selected Readings. New York, Family Service Association of America, 1965.

Articles

Backscheider, Joan E.: The influence of sociocultural factors on the mentally ill patient. Perspect. Psychiatric Care, 3:12–16, #3, 1965.

Connolly, Mary Grace: Mental health and use of community resources. J. Psychiat. Nursing, 1:5–8, Jan., 1963.

Eller, Florence: A psychiatric nurse's experience in community nursing. Perspect. Psychiat. Care, 3:14–18, #6, 1965.

Harris, Faye G.: A psychiatric nursing experience with a troubled child in the community. Perspect. Psychiat. Care, 5:92–97, #2, 1967.

Harris, Faye G.: Psychiatric and Mental Health Nursing. Failure at Four. In ANA Regional Clinical Conferences (1969). New York, Appleton-Century-Crofts, 1970, pp. 259–265.

Harrison, Mary: Lindemann's crisis theory and Dabrowski's positive disintegration theory—a comparative analysis. Perspect. Psychiat. Care, 3:8–13, #6, 1965.

Mereness, Dorothy: The potential significant role of the nurse in community mental health services. Perspect. Psychiat. Care, 1:34–37, #3, 1963.

Norris, Catherine: The trend toward community mental health centers. Perspect. Psychiat. Care, 1:36–40, #1, Jan., 1963.

PSYCHOTROPIC
MEDICATIONS

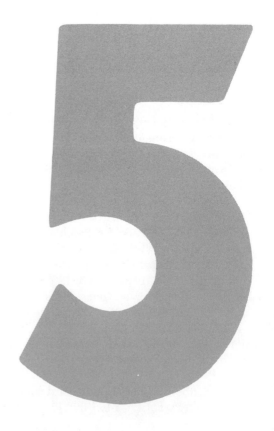

Introduction

Psychopharmacology is an area far too frequently avoided in the nursing literature. The reasons for this, while multifold, stem in part from the belief that all decisions regarding medications fall within the province of the physician/psychiatrist. While it is true that only the physician is legally empowered to prescribe medications, it is frequently the nurse who is in the best position to observe and evaluate the appropriateness and efficacy of the prescribed medications, by nature of her often daily interaction and relationship with the client. Additionally, the nurse must be aware of dosage ranges, expected and untoward side effects, the time lapse between initial administration and effect, as well as countless other components involved in the evaluation of the needs of clients taking medications. Thus, the nurse should be highly knowledgeable about the specific details of psychiatric medications. The image of Nurse Ratched in *One Flew Over the Cuckoo's Nest* standing behind a glass window dispensing drugs is an image which has no place in nursing. Without knowledge beyond the generic and trade names of medications (necessary for pouring and dispensing), the nurse cannot be involved in providing optimum care to her/his clients, nor can she/he be a fully contributing member of the health-care team. Frequently, it is only the nurse's understanding of why the medications are necessary and a belief in their usefulness that provides the necessary encouragement to her/his clients to ensure that they may derive the most benefit from their medication schedule.

Nursing intervention with clients taking psychotropic medications includes teaching and primary-level intervention. The nurse must be able to anticipate drug reactions and institute teaching to circumvent unnecessary reactions. Thus the nurse can help her clients who are taking Chlorpromazine (Thorazine) to understand why they must not go into direct sunlight; or she may relieve the anxiety of the client who suffers from drug-induced ejaculatory inhibition. Similarly, by telling her clients not to expect the tricyclics to take effect before two weeks' time, she may help to insure that they will continue to take the medication for at least that period without first giving up in despair. The teaching implications for the MAO inhibitors regarding the forbidden foods, and for Lithium Carbonate in terms of maintaining an adequate fluid balance are numerous. Of equal import for these two drugs are the knowledge of early warning signs of impending drug toxicity. These examples only skim the surface of the nursing implications of psychotropic drugs, but they illustrate the role which nurses should and must take in working with clients who are being maintained on this class of medications.

The unit consists of a two-part article which represents a comprehensive and concise presentation of the implications, cautions, dosage ranges, contraindications, side effects, and precautions for the entire class of psychiatric drugs. Although written for the general practitioner physician, it is an especially appropriate review for the nurse as well. The information is simply presented in an easy, reference-chart format, and the reader should be able to apply the data to nursing practice. Regardless of one's philosophy or feelings about psychotropic drugs, they remain a cornerstone of psychiatric treatment. For optimum client care, it is essential that the nurse be able to incorporate all this information into the foundation of her practice as well as to translate the information appropriately and accountably to her clients.

A COMPENDIUM OF PSYCHIATRIC DRUGS: PART I

Russell M. Cain, M.D.
Nancy N. Cain, M.D.

Introduction

THE NUMBER AND VARIED EFFECTS OF THE MEDICA-
TIONS used in psychiatric practice are sufficient to confuse any physician
who has not used them regularly. The old advice—to pick a few drugs of a
given type, know them well, and use them in practice—is still the best
rule. However, the clinician frequently sees patients who have been
placed on any of a wide range of medications by other physicians. This has
often been the authors' experience in emergency room, consultation, and
referral settings.

This drug compendium is designed to assist in organizing and using
current information about psychiatric drugs. Using this chart alone has
both the convenience and the drawbacks of "cookbook" medicine.
Further information is available in several excellent reviews of the clinical
use of these drugs, including: *Diagnosis and Drug Treatment of Psychiatric Disorders,* • *Modern Psychiatric Treatment,* † and *Clinical Use of
Psychotherapeutic Drugs.* ‡

Reprinted, with permission, from *Drug Therapy*, January 1975.

•Klein DF, Davis JM; *Diagnosis and Drug Treatment of Psychiatric Disorders.* Baltimore,
Williams and Wilkins, 1969.

†Detre DP, Jarecki HG: *Modern Psychiatric Treatment.* Philadelphia, JB Lippincott, 1971.

‡Hollister LF: *Clinical Use of Psychotherapeutic Drugs.* Springfield, Ill., Charles C
Thomas, 1973.

The drugs included are major tranquilizers (i.e., neuroleptic or anti-psychotic agents), minor tranquilizers, antidepressants (tricyclics, monoamine oxidase inhibitors), stimulants, and lithium carbonate. Information on dose precautions, side effects, interaction with other drugs, and effects on clinical tests is included. Dosages given are those used in adult psychiatric practice. Upper limits given are high and generally not used in outpatient settings. They should be exceeded only when the physician is aware of specific precautions and indications for doing so. The information about lethal doses refers only to situations where the drug in question was taken alone. Interactions that can significantly reduce the lethal dose may occur in multiple drug administration.

All except the neuroleptic drugs are arranged by chemical class. The neuroleptics are arranged according to the nature of their side effects and dose equivalence as antipsychotics. The more activating drugs at the top of the list are preferable in a number of situations where sedation is not desirable, while the more sedating compounds at the list's bottom are indicated with the more agitated patient. Low doses of neuroleptics are also finding use as an alternative to minor tranquilizers for situational and neurotic anxiety.

In depressions requiring drug treatment the tricyclic antidepressants should generally be used first. Monoamine oxidase inhibitors should be used—with particular caution—after tricyclics have proved ineffective. Stimulants such as amphetamines are to be avoided in management of depression, because the transient beneficial effects are outweighed by their high abuse potential.

Overdose is always a potential hazard, and patients who have taken an overdose of psychiatric drugs should be managed with a number of points in mind. Several of the more significant ones are listed here, but the detailed management of all the possible forms of overdose with these drugs is beyond the scope of this paper.

1. Ingestions are frequently multiple.
2. Recurrence is frequent.
3. If short-acting barbiturates are required to manage convulsions secondary to neuroleptic overdosage, the dosage should be reduced because of the potentiation of CNS depression.
4. Severe dystonias secondary to neuroleptic overdose should be managed with nonatropinizing anti-Parkinson agents, especially if tricyclic antidepressants are also taken, since neuroleptictrycyclic antidepressant combination can give an atropine psychosis.
5. Phenothiazine overdose may block effects of emetics.

6. Dialysis and forced diuresis are not effective for phenothiazine and tricyclic antidepressant overdose.

7. Tricyclic antidepressant overdose has significant atropinelike central nervous system effects and peripheral effects; the latter are particularly grave in relation to the cardiovascular system. Physostigmine salicylate (Antilirium) 1–3 mg. IV has been effective in managing both central and peripheral effects. Neostigmine (Prostigmin) and pyridostigmine (Mestinon) have been useful in managing the peripheral atropinelike effects.

8. There may be a "rebound" of symptoms of tricyclic antidepressant overdose 72 hours or more after initial satisfactory response to treatment. This includes cardiac effects.

9. Extreme caution is necessary when using sympathomimetics, stimulants, or sedatives in the management of monoamine oxidase inhibitor overdose.

10. Effects of phenothiazine overdose are maximum within 4–6 hours; with monoamine oxidase inhibitors, more than 24 hours may be required.

While the following charts are no substitute for thorough review, they will, we think, serve both office- and hospital-based physicians as a reminder of how the psychiatric drugs are used, and of the problems associated with using them. Handled in this way, we have found the charts enormously useful in our own practice.

MAJOR TRANQUILIZERS

BRAND NAME (GENERIC NAME)[1]	APPROX MG EQUIV (ORAL)[2]	COMPARATIVE RELATIONSHIP OF SIDE EFFECTS[3] (APPROX)	USUAL ORAL DOSAGE RANGE[4] (ANTIPSYCHOTIC)	FORMS AVAILABLE
Haldol (haloperidol) (B)	2		2–15 mg/day	tab: 0.5, 1, 2, 5, 10 mg, conc, IM
Navane (thiothixene) (T)	2		10–60 mg/day	cap: 1, 2, 5, 10, 20 mg, conc, IM
Prolixin, Permitil (fluphenazine) (P)(3)	2		5–20 mg/day	tab: 0.25, 1, 2.5, 5, 10 mg, conc, elixir, IM
Prolixin Decanoate (fluphenazine) (P)(3)			Injectable only; average dose: 25 mg q 2 wk; range: 12.5–100 mg q 1–3 wk	depo: IM or subcutaneous 25 mg/cc
Prolixin Enanthate (fluphenazine) (P)(3)			Injectable only; average dose: 25 mg q 2 wk; range: 12.5–100 mg q 1–3 wk	depo: IM or subcutaneous 25 mg/cc
Stelazine (trifluoperazine) (P)(3)	5		10–40 mg/day	tab: 1, 2, 5, 10 mg, conc, IM
Quide (piperacetazine) (P)(2)	10		40–160 mg/day	tab: 10, 25 mg, IM
Trilafon (perphenazine) (P)(3)	10		12–64 mg/day	tab: 2, 4, 8, 16 mg, conc. syrup, repetabs, IM, IV

Extrapyramidal syndromes (parkinsonian effects)

•

Above side effects tend to increase as you move up the chart

MAJOR TRANQUILIZERS (continued)

		Side effects below tend to increase as you move down the chart • Persistent sedation and depression / Adrenergic blocking / Orthostatic hypotension / Allergic responses / Seizures		
Repoise (butaperazine) (P)(3)	10		15–100 mg/day	tab: 5, 10, 25 mg
Compazine (prochlorperazine) (P)(3)	15		30–150 mg/day	tab: 5, 10, 25 mg, span, IV, IM, conc, suppos
Tindal (acetophenazine) (P)(3)	20		40–120 mg/day	tab: 20 mg
Proketazine (carphenazine) (P)(3)	25		25–400 mg/day	tab: 12.5, 25, 50 mg, conc
Vesprin (triflupromazine) (P)(1)	25		30–150 mg/day	tab: 10, 25, 50 mg, susp IM, IV
Serentil (mesoridazine) (P)(2)	70		150–400 mg/day	tab: 10, 25, 50, 100 mg, IM, conc
Sparine (promazine) (P)(1)	100		150–800 mg/day	tab: 10, 25, 50, 100, 200 mg, conc, syrup, IM, IV
Taractan (chlorprothixene) (T)	100		75–600 mg/day	tab: 10, 25, 50, 100 mg, conc, IM
Mellaril (thioridazine) (P)(2)	100		75–800 mg/day	tab: 10, 15, 25, 50, 100, 150, 200 mg, conc
Thorazine (chlorpromazine) (P)(1)	100		100–2000 mg/day	tab: 10, 25, 50, 100, 200 mg, conc, IV, IM, suppos, span, syrup

1. Drug categories related to chemical structures: (P) Phenothiazine (1) Aliphatic (2) Piperidine (3) Piperazine. (B) Butyrophenone (T) Thioxanthene
2. For example: 2 mg Haldol = 100 mg Thorazine
3. Be sure to see p 109 for full side effects discussion
4. Exceed maximum doses only when familiar with the specific drug

319

MAJOR TRANQUILIZERS: GENERAL CHARACTERISTICS

CAUTIONS	EFFECTS ON CLINICAL TESTS	DRUG INTERACTIONS
Contraindications	Alkaline phosphatase false ↑	DO NOT USE: epinephrine for hypotension and/or shock
Comatose states	Bilirubin (serum, urine) false ↑	USE: Neo-Synephrine (phenyl-ephrine) or Levophed (levarterenol) when vasoconstrictor needed
Presence of large amount of CNS depressants	CSF-protein false ↑ with Folin-Clocalteu reagent	
Bone marrow depression		Aminophylline not compatible in parenteral solution
Subcortical brain damage	Cholesterol possible false ↑	Antacid, may decrease phenothiazine absorption
Seriously impaired liver function	Diacetic acid, urine false ↑	
Hypersensitivity (may use drug from another class)	Estrogens, urine inaccurate readings	Anticoagulant, oral effect may be ↓
Uncontrolled epilepsy	Fasting glucose possible false ↑	Antihistamine effect ↑
Precautions	Frog pregnancy test, Hogben false +	Antihypertensives ↑ hypotension (however, guanethidine effect ↓)
Use cautiously with:	5 HIAA, urine false + or—	
Depressed patients	17-OH steroids, urine false +	Depressants: potentiated, eg, alcohol, minor tranquilizers, narcotics, major analgesics, sedatives and hypnotics
Allergy history	Phenylketonuria test, urine inaccurate readings	
Patients on anticonvulsants		
ECT		Hypoglycemics, oral effect may be ↑
Pregnancy		MAO inhibitors effect ↓
Respiratory disease		
Cardiovascular disorders, hypotension		
Use lower doses:		
In elderly patients		
With sedatives, narcotics, alcohol		

MAJOR TRANQUILIZERS: GENERAL CHARACTERISTICS (continued)

Warn patients about: Operating dangerous machinery or driving Use of depressants including alcohol (see drug interactions) Withdrawal: Occasionally occurs after long-term use (3 or more months with abrupt stop) SYMPTOMS OF WITHDRAWAL Nausea, malaise, vomiting, headaches, diaphoresis, tension, restlessness, insomnia Gradually decrease dose when stopping medication If on anti-Parkinson drug, continue 1 + wk *after* neuroleptic is stopped	PBI, radioiodine uptake inaccurate readings Porphyrins false ↑ Transaminase false ↑ Uric acid possible false + or— Urobilinogen false ↑	Reserpine (and related drugs) action ↑ Scopolamine (eg, overdose Compoz, Sominex) ↓ BP, shock Succinylcholine effect ↑ Diuretics (eg, Diuril, Dyazide) ↓ BP, shock Tricyclic antidepressants, sedative effect additive (caution, but not contra-indicated)

MAJOR TRANQUILIZERS: SIDE EFFECTS

SERIOUS ADVERSE EFFECTS (RARE) AND TREATMENT

Adverse effects	Treatment
Agranulocytosis	Stop medication; isolate from sources of infection; give antibiotics; hospitalize.
Progressive obstructive jaundice	Stop medication; may change to another phenothiazine immediately if necessary as cross-sensitivity is rare; bed rest; high protein/high carbohydrate diet.

Periodic white blood counts and liver batteries may actually be of little value in detecting above. The best procedure is to warn the patient to report immediately about sore throat, fever, severe itching, increased bruising, bleeding tendency.

Adverse effects	Treatment
"Extrapyramidal" crisis (Symptoms: profuse perspiration, drooling, dyspnea, cyanosis, fever, tachycardia, BP fluctuation, increasing anxiety)	Stop medication to prevent seizures, increasing fever, and death.

MILDER, MORE COMMON SIDE EFFECTS AND TREATMENT

Adverse effects	Treatment	Adverse effects	Treatment
Autonomic nervous system:		Cardiovascular:	
Blurred vision Flushing, pallor	Reassurance, frequently subsides in 2–6 wk	Peripheral edema Thrombosis	Must weigh benefit vs severity, consider stopping
Dry mouth	Rinse mouth frequently; if severe might try neostigmine 7.5–15 mg PO or pilocarpine nitrate 2.5 mg qid PO	Tachycardia Bradycardia	Decrease dose if possible
		Hypotensive crisis	Levophed IV or Ephedrine
		Syncope	
Hyperhidrosis Dysuria	Decrease dose if possible; if severe and cannot stop drug, use cholinergic drugs	Endocrine: Abnormal lactation, menstruation, and sex drive ↑ or ↓	Reassure patient, or try another class of drugs

Side Effect	Management
Aggravation of glaucoma	Concurrent tonometry, local cholinergics, and consultation
Fecal impaction	Mechanical aids
Paralytic ileus	Stop medication, hospitalize
Constipation	Mild laxative
Diarrhea	Atropine, belladonna
Nasal congestion	Neo-Synephrine nose drops
Inhibition of ejaculation	Try a less antiadrenergic drug
Postural hypotension	Advise patient to get up slowly; use surgical elastic hose, if necessary
Allergic: Dermatitis	Stop or change to another neuroleptic; systemic antihistamine
Photosensitivity	Protective clothes: sunscreen (eg, Pabafilm)
Behavioral: Impaired psychomotor function	Have patient avoid dangerous tasks
Drowsiness	Give single daily dose at bedtime
Weight gain	Watch diet
Edema	Reassure patient; diuretic if necessary; NO thiazide necessary
Central nervous system (CNS): Parkinson snydrome	Artane 4–15 mg, or Cogentin 2–8 mg PO daily in divided doses
Dyskinesia Dystonia Oculogyric crisis	Cogentin 2 mg IM or Benadryl 25 mg IV or 50 mg IM
Tardive dyskinesia	Use drugs only as absolutely necessary, try drug holidays with chronic patients Discontinue drug at earliest signs, or use drug most dissimilar chemically Use low doses in elderly
Akathisia	Stop or change to another neuroleptic
Seizures from lowered convulsive threshold	Stop or decrease if possible, or give anticonvulsant (eg, Dilantin 100 mg PO qid)
Respiratory depression	Stop or reduce dose

MAJOR TRANQUILIZERS: SIDE EFFECTS (continued)

MILDER, MORE COMMON SIDE EFFECTS AND TREATMENT

Adverse effects	Treatment	Adverse effects	Treatment
Fatigue Lethargy Weakness	Frequently decreases once patient gets up and gets moving	Disturbed body temperature	Avoid extreme temperatures Treat hyperthemias as heat stroke
Oversedation	Give small initial doses to test tolerance	Gastrointestinal: Anorexia	Stop medication or start frequent small feedings
Anxiety Depersonalization	Reduce dosage or change to another phenothiazine	Gastritis Nausea Vomiting	Stop medication, or symptomatic treatment; take medicine with milk after meals
Insomnia	Use more sedating neuroleptic and give at bedtime	Miscellaneous: Neuralgia SLE-like syndrome has been reported	Stop medication
Depression Increased dreams Hallucinations Aggravation of schizophrenic symptoms in borderline patients	Reduce dose or substitute another neuroleptic		

ANTIDEPRESSANTS-TRICYCLICS

BRAND NAME (GENERIC NAME)	USUAL ORAL DOSAGE RANGE*	ONSET	UNIQUE CHARACTERISTICS	SUPPLIED FORMS	ADULT LETHAL DOSE
Aventyl (nortriptyline)	75–100 mg/day	2–3 wk		cap: 10, 25 mg, liquid	Approximately 10–30 times daily dose
Elavil (amitriptyline)	75–300 mg/day	2–3 wk	More sedative than Tofranil	tab: 10, 25, 50 mg, IM	Same
Norpramin Pertofrane (desipramine)	75–200 mg/day	2–3 wk		tab: 25, 50 mg	Same
Sinequan Adapin (doxepin)	75–300 mg/day	2–3 wk	Not likely to inhibit guanethidine up to 150 mg/day	cap: 10, 25, 50, 100 mg, conc	Same
Tofranil Presamine (imipramine)	75–300 mg/day	2–3 wk		tab: 10, 25, 50 mg cap: 75, 150 mg, IM	Same
Vivactil (protriptyline)	15–60 mg/day	2–3 wk		tab: 5, 10 mg	Same

ANTIDEPRESSANTS-TRICYCLICS (continued)

Combinations

Triavil Etrafon (perphenazine and amitriptyline)	3–9 tab/day	20 days	tab: 2–10 mg 2–25 mg 4–10 mg 4–25 mg
Deprol (benactyzine 1 mg and meprobamate 400 mg)	3–6 tab/day	20 days Benactyzine nontricyclic; classified possibly effective	tab: 1–400 mg

*Exceed maximum doses only when familiar with the specific drug

ANTIDEPRESSANTS-TRICYCLICS: GENERAL CHARACTERISTICS

PRECAUTIONS	CONTRAINDICATIONS	DRUG INTERACTIONS	EFFECTS ON CLINICAL TESTS
Use very cautiously in patients with: Urinary retention	MAO inhibitors: stop tricyclic a minimum of 14 days before beginning a MAO inhibitor	Alcohol potentiates tricyclics Anticholinergic drugs: effect increased	(false increase or decrease) Alkaline phosphatase —may be ↑ Bilirubin— ↑ BSP retention— ↑
Narrow angle glaucoma Increased ocular pressure	Acute myocardial infarction Hypersensitivity	Anticonvulsants: increase CNS depression, but may need to increase to control seizures	Cholesterol—may be ↓ FBS—may be ↓ or ↑ Transaminase— ↑
Convulsive disorders (may need increased anticonvulsants) Cardiovascular disorders Thyroid disease Benign prostatic hypertrophy	DO NOT give barbiturates if MAO inhibitor and tricyclic are combined accidentally, as they will further depress respiration	Antiparkinsonian agents: potentiates anticholinergic properties; at tonic levels may produce syndrome of agitation, convulsion, hyperpyrexia Estrogen: interaction reported in several cases Guanethidine (Ismelin): inhibits Ismelin (except Sinequan under 150 mg/day)	

ANTIDEPRESSANTS-TRICYCLICS: GENERAL CHARACTERISTICS (continued)

Quiescent schizophrenia	Hypnotics and some tranquilizers: may affect tricyclic serum level (benzodiazepines do not)
Organic brain syndrome	
Warn patients about driving vehicles or operating dangerous machinery	MAO inhibitor: may potentiate both (see contraindications)
Safe use during pregnancy not yet established	Minor tranquilizers: additive effect
Seriously depressed patients may be suicide risks	Phenothiazines: sedative effects additive (caution, but not contraindicated)
Use caution in children under 12	Reserpine: inhibited
Withdraw gradually if patient has been on more than 150 mg/day for more than 2 mo	Sympathomimetic amines (epinephrine, norepinephrine, amphetamines, many over-the-counter cold, cough, and sinus remedies): effects increased
	Veratrum alkaloids: effect decreased

ANTIDEPRESSANTS-TRICYCLICS: SIDE EFFECTS

SERIOUS ADVERSE EFFECTS (RARE) AND TREATMENT

ADVERSE EFFECTS	TREATMENT
Agranulocytosis (most frequently occurs between the 2nd and 8th weeks)	Stop medication; isolate from sources of infection; give antibiotics, hospitalize.
Cholestatic jaundice	Stop medication, bed rest; high protein/high carbohydrate diet.
Leukocytosis, Leukopenia, Loeffler's syndrome, Eosinophilia, Purpura	Require immediate medical evaluation.
Paralytic ileus	Stop medication; hospitalize.

OTHER ADVERSE EFFECTS

ADVERSE EFFECTS	TREATMENT
Allergic:	
Rash, itching (rare)	Stop medication; use anti-histamine
Photosensitivity	Wear protective clothes or use sunscreen (eg, Pabafilm)
Autonomic nervous system:	
Flushing	Needs no treatment
Dry mouth*	Rinse mouth frequently; if

ADVERSE EFFECTS	TREATMENT
CNS:	
Drowsiness* (except Vivactil)	Give single daily dose at bedtime
Jitteriness*, Seizures, Twitching, Dysarthria, Paresthesia, Palsies, Ataxia, Sudden falls	Decrease dosage or switch to another drug
Muscle tremor	Use muscle relaxant

ANTIDEPRESSANTS-TRICYCLICS: SIDE EFFECTS (continued)

Side Effect	Treatment
	mine 7.5–15 mg PO or pilocarpine nitrate 2.5 mg PO qid
Blurred vision*	If severe and cannot decrease dosage, might try 1% pilocarpine nitrate eyedrops
Diaphoresis	Reassurance
Constipation*	Milk of magnesia
Urinary retention or frequency	Reassure; decrease dose
Aggravation of glaucoma	Concurrent tonometry, local cholinergics, and consultation
Cardiovascular: Hypertension	
Postural hypotension Dizziness Tachycardia Palpitations	Reassurance; avoid sudden changes in position; use surgical elastic hose if necessary
Arrhythmias Ankle edema	Evaluate cardiac status
Flattened T wave on EKG	Frequently benign but follow
Congestive heart failure, particularly over age 60	Stop medication, give digitalis, diuretics
Weakness Fatigue Headache	Reassurance
Insomnia	Give single daily dose in a.m.
Induced mania Activation of schizophrenia Visual hallucinations Delusions	Stop medication; treat as for any acute manic or schizophrenic state
Anger Agitation Vertigo	If severe, stop and/or change medication
Gastrointestinal: Nausea* Vomiting	Stop medication, or symptomatic treatment
Heartburn*	Take after meals
Anorexia	Stop medication, or frequent small feedings
Miscellaneous: Peripheral neuropathy Impotence Galactorrhea Tinnitus Bad taste in mouth Weight gain Weight loss Orbital edema Endocrine changes	Advisability of continuing medication must be weighed against the severity of symptoms

*Common side effects

ANTIDEPRESSANTS—MAO INHIBITORS*

BRAND NAME (GENERIC NAME)	USUAL ORAL DOSAGE RANGE†	ONSET	UNIQUE CHARACTERISTICS	SUPPLIED FORMS	ADULT LETHAL DOSE
Hydrazines					
Marplan (isocarboxazid)	Initial: 30 mg/day Maintenance: 10–20 mg/day	3–4 wk		tab: 10 mg	Approximately 10 times daily dose when taken alone, but data clouded
Nardil (phenelzine)	Initial: 45 mg/day Maintenance: 15 mg qd-qid	3–4 wk	See precautions and interactions below	tab: 15 mg	by the many serious reactions with other substances
Nonhydrazines					
Parnate (tranylcypromine)	Initial: 20–30 mg/day Maintenance: 10–20 mg/day	10 days		tab: 10 mg	Approximately 6 times daily dose Same hazards as hydrazines

*Reserve for cautious use in depressions that do not respond to tricyclics
†Exceed maximum doses only when familiar with the specific drug

ANTIDEPRESSANTS—MAO INHIBITORS: GENERAL CHARACTERISTICS

PRECAUTIONS	CONTRAINDICATIONS	DRUG INTERACTIONS
Warn patient to:	Tricyclic drugs	Alcohol: inhibits MAO inhibitor (possible hypertensive crisis if beverage contains tyramine)
Report headaches or unusual symptoms immediately	Stop MAO inhibitor minimum 14 days before beginning tricyclic	Amphetamine: potentiates amphetamine, risk of hypertensive crisis
Avoid self-medication (including over-the-counter drugs like cold and sinus drugs and analgesics)	Amphetamines	Anesthetics: increase CNS depression
	Sympathomimetic amines	Anticholinergics: effect increased
		Antiparkinsonian agents: potentiated
Avoid tyramine-containing foods—cheese, wine (especially sherry and Chianti), beer, pickled herring, yeast extracts, chicken liver, cream, chocolate, fava beans	Hypertension	Barbiturates: potentiated
	Cardiovascular disease	Chloral hydrate: potentiated
	Headaches	Cocaine: potentiated or hypertensive crisis
	Pheochromocytoma	Curare: effect increased
Avoid excess amount of caffeine	Liver or advanced renal disease	Foods with tyramine (see list under precautions): hypertensive crisis
Also avoid: Marmite, Bovril, yogurt, beestings	Quiescent schizophrenia	Insulin, oral: hypoglycemia; potentiated

ANTIDEPRESSANTS—MAO INHIBITORS: GENERAL CHARACTERISTICS (continued)

PRECAUTIONS	CONTRAINDICATIONS	DRUG INTERACTIONS
Use analgesics in lower doses if needed Taper off when stopping Safe use in pregnancy not yet established	Avoid combination with: Dopa, amphetamines, hypoglycemics alcohol, narcotics, diuretics, levodopa, meperidine, methyl-dopa, barbiturates, antiparkinsonian agents, insulin, guanethidine, sympathomimetic amines, reserpine, anticholinergics, antihypertensives, antihistaminics, hypnotics, other MAO inhibitors, anesthetics, phenothiazines tryptophane	Meperidine hypotension potentiated; may inhibit MAO Inhibitor Methyldopa (Aldomet): hypertension, excitation Minor tranquilizers: potentiated Other MAO Inhibitors: additive Phenothiazines: potentiated; may inhibit MAO inhibitor Reserpine: excitation Sympathomimetic: potentiated; extreme hypertension Thiazide diuretics: hypotension; potentiate MAO inhibitor Tricyclic antidepressants: potentiate both

ANTIDEPRESSANTS—MAO INHIBITORS: SIDE EFFECTS

SERIOUS ADVERSE EFFECTS

Severe headaches (may be first sign of pending hypertensive crisis)	Stop medication.
Hypertensive crisis	Prevent by giving detailed list of things to avoid; no specific antidote; to lower blood pressure give Regitine (phentolamine) 5 mg IV if available; if not, Thorazine 50–100 mg IM may be used as emergency measure.
CVA Hepatocellulr, toxic jaundice Leukopenia Anemia Shocklike coma Edema of glottis	Stop medication.

OTHER ADVERSE EFFECTS

(Many may be managed with treatment used for **Major Tranquilizer** adverse effects; however, check interactions before using medication.)

Autonomic nervous system:
Perspiration, dry mouth,* blurred vision, delayed micturition, orthostatic hypotension, constipation, * epigastric distress, delayed ejaculation, impotence, paroxysmal hypertension

Cardiovascular:
Hypotension, hypertension, tachycardia, palpitations, peripheral edema; may mask angina by suppressing pain

Gastrointestinal:
Nausea, diarrhea, anorexia, abdominal pain, constipation

CNS:
Insomnia, * drowsiness, overstimulation, * tremor, hyperreflexia, seizures, hypomania, mania, fatigue, dizziness, * weakness, headache, vertigo, ataxia, twitching, schizophrenic psychotic symptoms (anxiety, agitation, hallucinations), peripheral neuropathy, acute confusion with disorientation, mental clouding and illusions

Miscellaneous:
Rashes,
hyperpyrexia,
photosensitivity

*Most common

STIMULANT DRUGS
AVOID USE IN PSYCHIATRIC PRACTICE*

BRAND NAME (GENERIC NAME)	DOSAGE[†] (INITIAL)	ONSET	UNIQUE CHARACTERISTICS	FORMS SUPPLIED	ADULT MINIMUM LETHAL DOSE
Benzedrine (amphetamine)	10 mg/day	1 h		tab: 5, 10 mg span: 15 mg	Fatalities: doses over 100–500 mg
Dexedrine (dextroamphetamine)	10 mg/day	1 h	Letdown often	tab: 5 mg span: 5, 10, 15 mg elixir	See Benzedrine
Ritalin (methylphenidate)	20–30 mg/day	1 h	occurs after initial	tab: 5, 10, 20 mg	See Benzedrine
Deaner (deanol)	25–300 mg/day	1 h	relief of symptoms	tab: 25, 100 mg	See Benzedrine
Desoxyn Methedrine "speed" (methamphetamine)	5–10 mg/day	1 h		tab: 5, 10, 15mg	See Benzedrine

*Although these drugs should not be used as "antidepressants," they are often included in this group and are listed here for the reader's information

[†]Exceed maximum doses only when familiar with the specific drug

335

STIMULANT DRUGS: GENERAL CHARACTERISTICS

PRECAUTIONS	CONTRAINDICATIONS	DRUG INTERACTIONS
Danger of habituation	Marked agitation, severe anxiety	Cocaine: potentiation
Use cautiously in emotionally unstable or mildly agitated persons	Hypersensitivity	Furoxone (furazolidone): ↑ amphetamine effect after 4 days
	Glaucoma	Guanethidine: effect reduced
Hypertension	Epilepsy	Apresoline (hydralazine): ↓ hypotension
Insomnia		
Pregnancy	Severe depression	
	Chorea	MAO inhibitor: potentiated; possible hypertensive crisis and even death
	Advanced arteriosclerosis	
	Symptomatic cardiac disease	Pargyline (Eutonyl): cautions as with MAO inhibitors
	Hyperthyroidism	Vasopressors: potentiated

STIMULANT DRUGS: SIDE EFFECTS

Serious adverse effects:	Toxic manifestations (four phases)	Treatment of toxicity
High potential for abuse	1. Restlessness, irritability, insomnia, tremor, increased reflexes, sweating, mydriasis, flushing	Give Ipecac —if no coma or convulsions
Common adverse effects:		
Hypertension, tachycardia, overstimulation, increased tension, insomnia, headache, nervousness, dizziness, skin rash, dry mouth	2. ↑ Activity, confusion, ↑ BP, ↑ respiration, ↑ pulse, PVCs, fever, sweating	Thorazine IM— 1 mg/kg to 17 mg/kg
May aggravate psychosis in large doses	3. Delirium, mania, self-injury; excessively increased BP, pulse, and temperature; arrhythmias	Other support measures as needed
Rarely: cardiac arrhythmias, angina	4. Convulsions, coma, circulatory collapse, death	

A COMPENDIUM OF PSYCHIATRIC DRUGS PART II

Nancy N. Cain, M.D.

Russell M. Cain, M.D.

PART II REVIEWS THE MINOR TRANQUILIZERS—IE, THE benzodiazepines, the mephenesinlike compounds, the sedating anti-histamines—and lithium carbonate.

Certain observations should be made about using this chart:

Dosages given are for adults.

The upper dosage limits are high, above those generally used in out-patients, and should be exceeded only when the physician is aware of specific precautions and indications for higher doses, and familiar with the properties and action of the particular drug.

The information about lethal doses refers only to situations where the drug in question was taken alone. Physicians should remember that interactions can significantly lower the usual lethal dose of a drug.

The Chart in its entirety is a reference tool, and not a substitute for thorough review. For more detailed information, the reader can consult one of several excellent reviews on the use of psychiatric drugs.*

Reprinted, with permission, from *Drug Therapy*, February 1975.

*Klein DF, Davis JM: *Diagnosis and Drug Treatment of Psychiatric Disorders,*. Baltimore, Williams and Wilkins, 1969; Detre DP, Jarecki HD: *Modern Psychiatric Treatment,* Philadelphia, JB Lippincott, 1971. Hollister LE: *Clinical Use of Psychotherapeutic Drugs,* Springfield, Ill., Charles C Thomas, 1973.

MINOR TRANQUILIZERS-BENZODIAZEPINES

BRAND NAME (GENERIC NAME)	ORAL DOSAGE RANGE	FORMS SUPPLIED	UNIQUE CHARACTERISTICS	ADULT LETHAL DOSE
All Benzodiazepines			May increase anxiety in low-anxiety patient Physical dependence with high doses Prolonged use may cause attacks of anger and increased irritability	All less depressing than barbiturates; thus less suicide risk when taken alone Minimum uncombined fatal dose reported
Librium (chlordiazepoxide)	15–100 mg/day	cap: 5, 10, 25 mg tab: 5, 10, 25 mg IM, IV		Librium 750 mg
Serax (oxazepam)	30–120 mg/day	cap: 10, 15 30 mg tab: 15 mg		Serax as yet unknown
Valium (diazepam)	6–40 mg/day	tab: 2, 5, 10 mg injectable	Good muscle relaxant	Valium approximately 700 mg
Tranxene (clorazepate)	15–60 mg/day	cap: 3.75, 7.5, 15 mg		Tranxene as yet unknown

339

MINOR TRANQUILIZERS-MEPHENESINLIKE COMPOUNDS

BRAND NAME (GENERIC NAME)	ORAL DOSAGE RANGE	FORMS SUPPLIED	UNIQUE CHARACATERISTICS	ADULT LETHAL DOSE
Miltown, Equanil (meprobamate)	1200–2400 mg/day	tab: 200, 400 mg cap: 200, 400 mg PO liquid	Psychic and physical dependency; convulsions and delirium when stopped after prolonged use of high doses Inhibits other drug action by inducing drug-metabolizing enzymes	Uncertain (8400 mg reported fatal, but 40,000 mg reported taken with complete recovery)
Tybatran (tybamate)	1250–3000 mg/day	cap: 125, 250, 350 mg	Physiologic dependency and withdrawal signs claimed rare	

MINOR TRANQUILIZERS—BENZODIAZEPINES AND MEPHENESINLIKE COMPOUNDS

CLINICAL INTERACTIONS	CLINICAL INTERACTIONS	CAUTIONS
Mephenesinlike Compounds	**Benzodiazepines**	**Contraindications:**
Clinical interactions similar to those of the benzodiazepines	Anticonvulsant	Hypersensitivity
	Dose of standard anticonvulsant may require adjustment when Valium added	Porphyria: do not use mephenesin derivatives, eg, Miltown
Additional Interactions:		Glaucoma
MAO inhibitors— mutual potentiation	CNS depressants (including alcohol)— mutual potentiation	**Precautions:**
		Patient on oral anticoagulants, variable blood coagulation reported; however, can be used concurrently in most patients without difficulty
Oral anticoagulants (eg, coumarin)— decrease anti-coagulation	Sedatives and hypnotics— mutual potentiation	Addiction-prone individuals, dependence reported
	Major tranquilizers potentiation	Elderly: use smaller doses to prevent decreased BP, cardiac problems
Lab tests:	Tricyclic antidepressants mutual potentiation of sedation	Patient with history of allergies, hepatic disorders, or renal impairment
Urine 17-OH and 17-ketosteroids— unpredictable results		Breast feeding mothers; may be transferred via milk

MINOR TRANQUILIZERS–BENZODIAZEPINES AND MEPHENESINLIKE COMPOUNDS (continued)

Lab tests: Transaminase false ↑ Alkaline phosphatase possible false ↑ Bilirubin false ↑	Warn patients about: operating dangerous machinery or driving; the use of depressants, including alcohol (see drug interaction) Withdraw slowly when used long term Withdrawal symptoms: weakness, nervousness, insomnia, convulsions, delirum Pregnancy: safe use not yet established

Minor Tranquilizers–Benzodiazepines and Mephenesinlike Compounds

Adverse effects	Treatment
CNS:	
Drowsiness, * ataxia, * confusion, * slurred speech, * headache, * lethargy, * giddiness, * muscular incoordination, tremor, somnolence, dysarthria	Begin with initial low dose and increase over 3–4 days
Autonomic nervous system:	
Dizziness, * vertigo, * impaired visual accommodation, * salivation changes, incontinence, urinary retention, blurred vision	Reassurance or decrease dose, if severe
Cardiovascular:	
Hypertension, hypotension, syncope, hypotensive crisis rare, anaphylaxis	Begin with low dose initially and increase gradually
Behavioral:	
Euphoria, fatigue, weakness, depression, psychic dependency	Reassurance or decrease dose
Hematologic:	
Agranulocytosis, leukopenia, anemia, thrombocytopenic purpura	Stop medication
Hepatic:	
Jaundice, hepatic dysfunction	Stop medication
Gastrointestinal:	
Nausea, vomiting, constipation	Decrease dose
Dermatologic:	
Rash, urticaria, stomatitis, exfoliative dermatitis, Stevens-Johnson syndrome, erythema multiforme	Decrease dose / Stop medication
Endocrinologic:	
Menstrual irregularities, altered libido	Reassurance or stop medication

MINOR TRANQUILIZERS-BENZODIAZEPINES AND MEPHENOSINLIKE COMPOUNDS (continued)

Paradoxical reaction:
Acute excited states, anxiety, hallucinations, increased muscle
spasticity, insomnia, rage, convulsions, sleep disturbances, stimulation — Stop medication

Miscellaneous:
Chills, fever, paresthesias, edema, angioneurotic edema — Stop medication
*Most frequent side effects

MINOR TRANQUILIZERS-SEDATING ANTIHISTAMINES

BRAND NAME (GENERIC NAME)	ORAL DOSAGE RANGE	FORMS SUPPLIED	UNIQUE CHARACTERISTICS
Vistaril, Atarax (hydroxyzine)	75–400 mg/day	tab: 10, 25, 50, 100 mg; syrup	
Phenergan (promethazine) Benadryl (diphenhydramine)	Not generally used in psychiatric practice		Good sleep medication for elderly patients

CLINICAL INTERACTIONS	CONTRAINDICATIONS	ADVERSE EFFECTS	TREATMENT
	Hypersensitivity	Drowsiness, dry mouth	Reassurance or decrease dose
Lab tests: Catecholamines, plasma—false ↑ 17-OH steroids, urine—false ↓ ↑	Precautions: Caution about operating hazardous machinery or driving May potentiate action of CNS depression Pregnancy: safe use not yet established	Involuntary motor activity with rare tremors and convulsions	Begin with low doses initially— gradually increase

LITHIUM CARBONATE*

BRAND NAMES	DOSAGE	ONSET	UNIQUE CHARACTERISTICS	FORMS SUPPLIED	ADULT MINIMUM LETHAL DOSE
Eskalith	Initial: 600 mg tid (1200–1800 mg/day); this dosage is given until serum lithium level reaches	6–10 days	Ability to tolerate lithium is decreased after the acute mania subsides—thus dose should be decreased	cap: 300 mg	2–4 meq/liter toxic
Lithane	1.0–1.5 meq/liter and therapeutic effect seen Maintenance: 300 mg tid (600–1200 mg/day); maintain serum lithium level between 0.5–1.5 meq/liter	then → dose to maintenance level	Tolerance to lithium is decreased with marked sweating or diarrhea—thus may need to decrease dose during warm weather or illness	tab: 300 mg	5–7 meq/liter may be fatal
Lithonate			May have some prophylactic effect against both recurrent mania and depression in manic-depressive psychosis	cap: 300 mg	

*For control of acute mania in manic-depressive psychosis

LITHIUM CARBONATE: GENERAL CHARACTERISTICS

PRECAUTIONS	CONTRAINDICATIONS	INTERACTIONS
May precipitate depression May impair mental and physical abilities Warn patient about driving vehicles or operating dangerous machinery Use cautiously in: Pregnant patient Children under 12 Breast feeding Thyroid disease Mild kidney or heart disease Epilepsy Elderly patients (use lower doses) Caution patient to maintain an adequate salt and fluid intake Serum lithium levels should be done: (1) biweekly, while establishing dosage (2) weekly, when first beginning maintenance dosage (3) monthly, once a stable maintenance dosage is established	Significant: Renal disease Cardiovascular disease Evidence of brain damage Recommended evaluation prior to beginning lithium therapy: Physical examination: Urinalysis PBI　　　CBC T_3 uptake　　Electrolytes Thyroid scan EKG BUN　　Creatinine In patients with borderline renal function a test dose may be given to determine renal clearance	Diuretics: may potentiate Na and fluid depletion; thus lithium toxicity Tricyclics: (1) may interfere with prophylactic effects of lithium; (2) may lead to hypomania or mania; (3) may potentiate antithyroid effect; (4) however, they are sometimes needed in the treatment of an acute depression in a patient receiving lithium therapy Lab tests: FT_4 (mean free thyroxine) $\downarrow$ Glucose tolerance $\downarrow$ ^{131}I $\uparrow$ uptake PBI $\downarrow$ (erythrosine-B dye in gelatin cap of lithium may falsely $\uparrow$ PBI) Phenothiazines, butyrophenones, etc. may be given concomitantly

346

LITHIUM CARBONATE: SIDE EFFECTS

ADVERSE REACTIONS RELATED TO SERUM LEVELS	TREATMENT
Fine tremor of hands	Frequent even at low doses; often unpreventable. However, if pronounced enough to interfere with use of hands or jaw begins to tremble, stop medication until serum lithium level decreases
Allergic: Allergic vasculitis	Stop medication, at least temporarily; determine serum lithium level
Autonomic nervous system: Blurred vision, dry mouth	Symptoms usually disappear after several days
Cardiovascular: Cardiac arrhythmia, hypotension, peripheral circulatory collapse	Treatment may then be resumed, but the serum lithium should be maintained at a lower level
CNS: Blackout spells, epileptiform seizures, slurred speech, dizziness, vertigo, incontinence of urine and feces, somnolence, psychomotor retardation, restlessness, confusion, stupor, coma	To help prevent cardiac and renal symptoms of lithium intoxication, maintain adequate sodium and fluid intake
Dermatologic: Dry, thin hair, anesthesia of skin	
Gastrointestinal: Anorexia, nausea, vomiting, diarrhea	

LITHIUM CARBONATE: SIDE EFFECTS (continued)

Genitourinary:
   Albuminuria, oliguria, polyuria, glycosuria

Neuromuscular:
   Tremor, muscle hyperirritability (fasciculations, twitching, clonic movements of whole limbs), ataxia, choreoathetoid movements, hyperacitve DTs

Miscellaneous:
   Fatigue, lethargy, weight loss, transient scotomata, dehydration, giddiness

UNRELATED TO SERUM LEVELS

Thyroid toxicity:
   Goiter formation, hypothyroidism, myxedema   Follow; may need thyroxine

EEG changes:
   Diffuse slowing, widening of the frequency spectrum, potentiation and disorganization of background rhythm

EKG changes:
   Flattened, isoelectric, or inverted T waves   Reversible; no need to interrupt therapy, but should follow

Miscellaneous:
   Leg ulcers, headache, transient hyperglycemia, generalized pruritus with or without rash, swelling of ankles or wrists, metallic taste

SEVERE LITHIUM INTOXICATION—CLINICAL PICTURE
   Impaired consciousness or coma, hyperreflexia or hypertonicity, muscle tremor   Hemodialysis should be considered
   or fasciculations; hyperextension of arms and legs with grasping and opening of   Massive sodium therapy may not be help-
   the eyes; seizures may occur; anuria, kidney function, and EKG changes   ful when this point is reached
   moderate and reversible; death occurs from pneumonia or coma

348

CHANGE IN THE
SOCIAL SYSTEM
AND USE OF
THERAPEUTIC MILIEU

Introduction

Those of us who are involved in the practice of nursing today, whether we be students or licensed practitioners, are involved in the process of change within ourselves, within our clients, and within our profession and society. It seems crucial that if we as a profession are to continue to contribute to the health care and health privileges of our clients and to the continuation of nursing as a viable profession with a voice in planning and providing such health care, we need to look closely at our involvement in the processes of change. Nursing students, graduate nurse practitioners, nurse educators, and nurse administrators today may often find themselves in complex social systems where their basic focus of providing client-centered nursing care can very easily be redirected into channels of budget cuts, unresolved status and power disagreements, and professional and bureaucratic conflicts all of which can lead to their moving away from client contact and from nursing itself. The change-agent role in nursing then cannot be relegated to theory in a nursing school curriculum, but is a part of nursing present in our daily practice.

It is also from the daily practice of nursing that the concept of milieu therapy emerges. Nursing care is directed toward clients' daily living patterns in a hospital environment and/or home or community setting and does not necessarily end at 5 P.M.! Values that are inherent in milieu therapy, i.e., shared responsibilities among all staff for client care, clients' participation in their own care, and recognition of the environment as important, are values that nurses generally hold in terms of their own professional functioning. Hence, many nurse practitioners, in collaboration with other health team members, utilize this form of therapy as a treatment modality. One form of milieu therapy, the therapeutic community, presents some alternative approaches to traditional psychiatric treatment. It may or may not be feasible in any one particular setting. Here again, change-agent skills are vital for nurses involved in initiating this therapy. Through a selection of articles on the theory and process of change and on milieu therapy this chapter presents some ways in which nurses can utilize change theory and the environment in providing care for clients.

Rodgers (1973) considers various models of change as well as who the recipient of such change is—the client or the system. Reasons for resistance to change are reviewed and methods for dealing with such resistance are suggested. The problem-solving process and its relation to change is discussed, with specific delineation of the steps involved in this process. In conclusion, Rodgers looks at the function of power in the change process, and at how nurses can utilize this function in their role of change agent.

A description of how change was initiated in client care and in the organizational structure of a hospital unit is presented by Schuler and Campbell (1974). These two nurses, functioning as the Head Nurse and the Psychiatric-Nurse Clinical Specialist on an in-patient psychiatric unit, describe their planning for implementation of change. Involvement of nursing staff in the planning of change and nursing administration in support for change plans are some significant concepts which are discussed. Also of significance in the implementation of changes was the authors' continued collaboration as Head Nurse and Clinical Specialist. The article reviews the initiation of client groups and of a democratic milieu and therapeutic community, and concludes with an analysis of the effects of this change process on the client population and on the hospital staff.

Mitchell (1974) introduces the concept of the therapeutic community, describes how it differs from the hierarchial system of organization usually found in general hospitals, and provides ideas as to the values and problems of each of these models. The question he raises concerns the need of practitioners in psychiatry to ascertain where each model may be used most appropriately, and possibly as alternatives or options to existing treatment modalities.

The last two articles in this chapter pose some thought-provoking questions about the application of the concept of milieu therapy. Leone and Zahourek (1974) look at the emphasis on group interaction and interpersonal relationships in a therapeutic community and pose the question of how helpful this focus on group involvement is if many of the participating clients leave the hospital to return to solitary living situations? Staff involved in a therapeutic community with clients need to look at what happens to clients post-discharge and how the in-hospital treatment program relates to this.

In our desire to immediately "do" something therapeutic for clients admitted for short-term hospital care, Lewis and Selzer (1972) suggest that we may be utilizing milieu therapy without taking the time to adequately assess the needs of the individual client and form an appropriate treatment plan. Staff may become more involved with the conceptual aspects of milieu therapy, such as decision-making and communication processes, than with specific treatment plans for individual clients. The authors discuss five commonly encountered clinical problems in which staff really do need to know clearly the client's difficulties and how these clients' specific treatment plans were formulated. A summary of what the therapeutic milieu should provide for clients is presented.

This unit presents an overview of the nurse involved in change processes and in milieu therapy. As evidenced in other articles in this book (Fagin, Unit II, Brandner, Unit IV), change theory is an integral part of nursing practice. The treatment modality of milieu therapy still poses many questions and presents nurses with the challenge of how this treatment may be most effectively utilized by us to provide client care.

32 THEORETICAL CONSIDERATIONS INVOLVED IN THE PROCESS OF CHANGE

By Janet A. Rodgers, Ph.D., R.N.

IN AN AGE IN WHICH THE SINGLE CONSTANT is radical and rapid change, we all suffer in varying degrees from what Toffler calls "future shock." If we are to steer a course between disorganizing cognitive dissonance and reactive psychic and social inertia we need to increase our understanding of the nature and dynamics of change.

Who is the Client?

When examining the principles and strategies for changing social behavior, we frequently encounter the debate over who is the appropriate client: the individual or the social system? Schein reminds us that the issue is reminiscent of Koestler's distinction between the Yogi and the Commissar—between those who turn inward for insight and nirvana and those who turn outward for social salvation. (1:202) Put another way, it is the difference between those who look to self-actualization for ultimate social improvement and those who believe in the manipulation of external forces such as legal, technological, economic, and political. Sometimes the debate takes the guise of theoretical preferences—Freud versus Skinner or individualism versus statism.

The target of change is both the individual and the social system,

From *Nursing Forum*, Vol. XII, No. 2, 1973, pp. 160–174. Reprinted, with permission, from Nursing Publications, Inc., 194-B Kindermack Rd., Park Ridge, N.J. 07656.

usually a formal organization or some subdivision of it. The dynamics inherent in the change process are the same; the strategic differences lie in the complexity.

I am reminded of Ujhely's excellent paper " 'And' Instead of 'Either-or' or the 'Fallacy of False Opposition,' " (2:10–13) for certainly this is not an either-or phenomenon. Ujhely speaks on the seeming dichotomy of "social action" versus "working with individuals." After empathizing with the nurse's utter frustration at the multiplicity of problems in which patients are ensnared, and recognizing that nurses frequently would rather be active in other endeavors than witness the patient's plight, day in and day out, she says: . . .

. . . I am not sure at all that we have to either be with the patient or in the social arena. Is there any reason why we cannot do both? Is there any reason why, in the innumerable intolerable hospital situations we cannot help the patient by giving what little support we can. . . by aiding him. . . to survive in the sytem, while at the same time trying to alter his surrounding atmosphere by working with the staff and while also seeking power so that we can participate in top decision making with respect to his welfare? . . . Of course, it is much more difficult to keep involved in the patient's present situation while at the same time attempting to chip away at the walls that hold him bound. . . . It is not enough for him to know that you are trying to hoe a future exit out of his prison; he also needs someone who can be with him and help him bear the life he must lead now. (2:12)

Models of Change

Let me review the assumptions of three analytic models of change described by Chin: the system model, the developmental model, and the model for changing. (3:201–214)

The primary emphasis in a *system model* is on the manner in which stability is achieved. Change is derived from the structure and evolves out of the incompatabilities and conflicts in the system. The assumption is made that in an organization interdependency and integration exist among its parts, and that change is dependent upon how well the parts of the system fit together—or upon how well the system fits with other surrounding and interacting systems. The source of change is primarily structural stress, either externally induced or internally created. The process of change is one of tension reduction. The goals of change can be either internally or externally imposed and are set by vested interest groups. Stresses, strains, and tensions are the presenting symptoms, and adjustment and adaptation are the goals of intervention. Feedback mechanisms offer important inputs in restoring balance to the system. The change-agent's role is that of diagnostician and action initiator, and his position is, by necessity, external to the client system.

This "apartness" of the change-agent requires an expansion of the system model into an inter-systems model to account for the internal system of the change-agent. The connectives between the two interacting open systems may be either cohesive or divisive, and these relational issues are, as we all know, crucial factors in the promotion of, or resistance to, change. The intersystems model seems especially useful as a tool for studying problems of leadership, power, communication, organizational conflict, and intergroup relations of all sorts.

Underlying the *developmental model* is the assumption that there is constant change and development, and growth and decay of a system over time. The stability is that of a living organism, a progression—one stage giving way to another stage. Change is seen as "natural," rooted in the nature of the organism (social or biological), end-related and purposeful. Difficulties develop when a major blockage results in a gross discrepancy between potentiality and actuality. The change-agent's role in the developmental model is that of diagnostician, obstacle remover, and promoter of growth. His position is external to the client-system.

The change-agent in the developmental model has been compared to a horticulturist or midwife. A teacher, for example, may be seen as tending and cultivating the individual mind—feeding, watering, and weeding the student's intellectual garden to promote growth to full bloom or maturity. The psychotherapist aids the individual as he passes through various developmental phases, helping him to break loose and move forward if he has become "fixated" at a given stage. The midwife guides the delivery, removes any blockage, and aids the individual in giving "birth."

The third model—*a model for changing*—incorporates elements of the system model along with ideas from the developmental model into a framework in which the emphasis is on the forces producing change. In this model, stability is studied in order to unfreeze and move parts of the system. Change is induced and controlled, and built on rational choice. Goals are not fixed but instead are arrived at through a collaborative process. The change-agent is an active participant in the situation, playing the role of helper to the client-system.

Pace of Change

In examining the process of change we need to pause briefly to consider the pace of change. Lewin defines "no change" as a quasi-stationary equilibrium, ". . .a state comparable to that of a river which flows with a given velocity in a given direction during a certain time interval." (4:208) He describes a social change as comparable to a change in the velocity or direction of that river.

Earlier I referred to Toffler's concept of future shock, "the shattering stress and disorientation that we induce in individuals by subjecting them to too much change in too short a time." (5:4) Toffler's point is that the rate of change has implications quite apart from, and sometimes more important than, the direction of change. Physical and psychological distress arise from an overload of man's physical adaptive systems and his decision-making processes. Thomas Holmes and Richard Rahe have shown that change itself—not a specific change but the rate of change in one's life—is intimately related to physical health. Together they developed a life-change units scale for measuring the amount of change an individual had experienced in a given span of time and have found a positive correlation between high life-change scores and the frequency and severity of subsequent illness. (5:291–6)

The *psycho-physiological responses to novelty* are well known: pupils dilate, hearing becomes momentarily more acute, general muscle tone increases, brain wave patterns are altered. ACTH secretion is increased, peripheral blood vessels constrict, and respiratory and heart rates are altered. These changes are part of what is known as an alarm or orientation response. This response is one of man's key adaptive mechanisms, but it does exact a price in bodily wear and tear.

Change is essential to life but there are limits on one's adaptability. Just as environmental overstimulation causes physical damage, so does it affect one's ability to think and behave rationally. The combat soldier, the disaster victim, and the culturally dislocated traveler respond to overstimulation in strikingly parallel ways. With sensory overload comes confusion, disorientation, or a blurring of the lines between illusion and reality.

James Miller, Director of Mental Health Research Institute at the University of Michigan, suggests that information overload, like environmental overload, may be related to mental illness. He speculates that ". . .schizophrenia (by some as-yet unknown process, perhaps a metabolic fault which increases neural 'noise') lowers the capacities of channels involved in cognitive information processing. Schizophrenics consequently. . .have difficulties in coping with information inputs at standard rates like the difficulties experienced by normals at rapid rates. As a result, schizophrenics make errors at standard rates like those made by normals under fast, forced-input rates." (5:315)

Decision stress is another form of overstimulation. With the increasing tempo and complexity in our lives comes a great increase in the need for private and public decision making. The question becomes one of a delicate balance between "programmed" and "non-programmed decisions." As Toffler points out, each of us needs a blend of the two.

If this blend is too high in programmed decisions, we are not challenged; we find life boring and stultifying. We search for ways, even unconsciously, to introduce novelty into our lives, thereby altering the decision "mix." But if this mix is too high in nonprogrammed decisions, if we are hit by so many novel situations that programming becomes impossible, life becomes painfully disorganized, exhausting and anxiety-filled. Pushed to its extreme, the end-point is psychosis. (5:317)

Resistance to Change

In looking at the change process it is important that we examine the issue of resistance. Many people, perhaps most people, including the well-educated, find the idea of change so threatening they attempt to deny its necessity if not its existence. Because no one can change all his beliefs and still retain his sanity, people frequently prefer problems that are familiar to solutions that are not. (6:8) In a society in which every area of life is subject to change, we should not be surprised to find individuals, consciously or unconsciously digging in and hanging on to that which is familiar.

Stability in one area of life often enables a person to feel comfortable enough to risk or even seek change in other areas. It should come as no surprise that frequently the area of stability so tenaciously clung to is the work area. It is essential that a would-be change-agent recognize and take into account this likely possibility.

All psychiatric nurses are familiar with the phenomenon of resistance. When in the course of therapy a patient feels threatened by a painful awareness he balks, becomes silent, changes the subject, fills the interview with irrelevant chit chat, misses or comes late for appointments, or becomes angry with the therapist—all an effort to resist change and maintain the status quo. Similar resistance occurs when the target of change is a group or organization. Hostility, either overtly or covertly expressed, is a common defense against real or implied threats to an individual or group's self-image.

There are a number of conditions conducive to resistance to organizational change. For example, if the persons to be influenced by a proposed change are not given adequate information regarding the nature of the change, resistance can be expected. Moreover, personal idiosyncrasies and life experiences cause people to read different meanings into a proposed change. Adequate explanation, however, does not always assure that there will be no resistance to change. Explanations can be distorted, and information is not a panacea for the problem of implied threat to one's personal status or power position. Resistance may be expected when one feels pressured to make a change and will be decreased when one has a "say" in the nature or direction of the change. Resistance is also likely if a change is made on personal grounds rather than on impersonal requirements. And lastly, if the change ignores existing alliances within a group, resistance by the individuals in the group is a certainty. (7:543–8)

I do not want to leave the issue of resistance without commenting on its paradoxical form, namely, resistance to stability and order. Some people are so deeply attracted to an ever-changing, accelerated pace of life they feel tense, bored, and depressed when the pace is slow and the system relatively stable. They long to be "where the action is," without regard for whether the action is goal directed or not. For them, the goal is excitement, not constructive change. The hysterical personality and the fixated adolescent are classical examples.

They need a storm about them as a distraction from the essential emptiness or storm within. Though ostensibly dedicated to external change, these people are implacably resistant to internal change and are frequently an obstacle to external change because of the countertransference resistance they evoke in others.

Another obstacle to change, although not resistance *per se*, is relative satisfaction with the existing system. It is commonly agreed that most hospital personnel work very hard, are usually dedicated to their jobs, and are kept so busy within the present system they do not feel any particular pressure to make changes. If it doesn't hurt, that is, if a person is not dissatisfied, there is no motivation for changing the status quo: "if it doesn't itch, don't scratch." The important point to keep in mind here, however, is that though the hospital personnel may not itch, the patient may have a fulminating rash.

Process of Changing

The actual process of changing is described by Lewin as a three-step procedure: unfreezing, moving, and refreezing. (4:210–11) The first two stages are necessary conditions of change. The third, refreezing, ensures the stability of whatever change occurs. Unfreezing involves "breaking the habit"—disturbing the equilibrium. To break open a shell of complacency it is often necessary to deliberately cause an emotional disturbance.

An analogy that comes to mind is the act of giving up smoking. (I am tempted to refer to the process as an art rather than an act.) The point here is that breaking the habit (the step of unfreezing) is frequently accomplished only when there is a severe threat to the self-system. That shell of complacency is disturbed only when the threat is seen as a very real and present danger—not a problem that one might have to cope with at some vague point in the future.

In the unfreezing process the information which is introduced leaves the person feeling uncomfortable. It creates a sense of uneasiness, a disequilibrium. He feels frightened and sometimes guilty. As suggested earlier, he frequently reacts with anger, a defense against the loss of a previous form of stability. (The process of change has many parallels with the process of mourning.)

That the person not become too defensive or rigid, some type of psychological safety must be built into the situation, either by reducing the threat or removing some of the barriers to change. As the individual begins to feel safe, he will begin to seek new information about himself or his relationship to others. He may look for relevant cues from others around him or he may identify with some particular person whose beliefs seem to be viable. In other words, the changee may start to view himself from the perspective of another person or several other persons. As his frame of reference shifts, he will develop new beliefs which will lead to new feelings and responses. When these new feelings and responses become comfortable for the individual and are confirmed or reinforced by others, a kind of consolidation or freezing takes place. Thus, a degree of permanency is acquired. (1:275–76)

In essence, what I have been describing is the process of attitude change. An individual's core personality is deeply rooted in his formative years. However, the peripheral aspects of personality emerge at later developmental levels. When we attempt to introduce change, we are attempting to change the peripheral aspects of a person's personality. Thus, in order to initiate change it is important that we assess the attitudes and beliefs of those involved in the change. The characteristics that need to be looked at are the extremes of attitudes, the multiplicity of attitudes, their degree of consistency, the needs served, and the centrality of their related values. We also need to look at such general characteristics of the participants as level of intelligence, cognitive needs and style, personal ability, and group affiliations.

Need for a Theoretical Framework

In providing leadership in change it is essential that we move away from considering personal characteristics of the change-agent and toward a conceptual and operational framework. That is, although personal charisma may help some people effect change, knowledge is more reliable. Change theory must be derived from learning theory, communications theory, systems theory, and interpersonal theory.

In whatever type of work or community situation we find ourselves, once established, it is a system rather than a random collection of individuals. Thus, we need to understand the components of a system, the repetitive patterns of a system, our own part as a system representative, and the fact that any change attacks vested interests of system members and frequently changes their economic and social status. The issue of prestige allotments immediately points up the major, and at times seemingly insurmountable, difficulties in system change.

The Problem-Solving Process

The phases of the change process have been identified by such writers as Greiner (8:487–492) Foote and Cottrell (9:175–208) and Kolb and Frohman. (10:51–66) Intrinsic to each of these phase models is the concept of the problem-solving technique. That is, one needs to:

1. *Identify the problem.*—Enough pressure is exerted on the power structure to make it aware of the existence of a problem and of the possibility of change.
2. *Collect sufficient data to accurately diagnose the problem.*—This involves examining the components of the system and assessing the attitudes and beliefs of the system members.
3. *Make inferences and judgments.*—Look at for whom the present structure works and for whom it doesn't work. Assess the system's goals, one's own motivations and one's resources.
4. *Plan intervention on the basis of the above inferences and judgments.*—Formulate imaginative and creative proposals. Prepare alternatives. After developing effective solutions obtain commitment for implementing them. Select an appropriate place to start and the appropriate role of the change-agent.
5. *Intervene.*—Maximize the participation of personnel by involving people in the system in the change-making process. Give people adequate opportunity to express themselves. Use the leaders in the traditional setup and deal with resistances at all levels.
6. *Evaluate the change process and the solution*—Throughout the process the criteria of change should be clear, verbalized, and shared. Emphasis should be on growth as opposed to success or failure.

The Function of Power

Implicit throughout this discussion is the differentiation between planned change and other forms of change, since obviously not all change is planned. A major distinguishing feature involves the concept of power, or, "Who's in control of the change?" A primary feature of planned change is equal power distribution, that is, shared deliberations and goal setting. (11:154) Both indoctrinations (as practiced in many schools, prisons, and mental hospitals) and coercive change (thought control and brainwashing) are examples of an imbalanced power ratio, although indoctrinational change involves shared goal setting whereas coercive change does not.(11:154–55)

In the world of medicine and health-care delivery, power is generally sufficient to maintain things as they are. The role of the change-agent is to reorganize the distribution of power, either by encouraging the development of new sources of influence or by making old power centers more responsive to, and representative of, the structure as a whole. Both fragmentation of power and competitiveness, two related characteristics, profoundly affect the change process. A crucial task of the change-agent is to turn intergroup competition into intergroup collaboration. Successful change depends on a redistribution of power within the group system; usually, in the direction of greater shared power. The change-agent's power or influence within a system is derived from a combination of two sources: expert power and line power; (1:208–9) that is, the change-agent is seen as possessing expert skills and competencies or as occupying a certain position or holding a certain status in the system which legitimizes his influence.

Power is the means of access to all other values. However, as Deloughery points out, "Nurses, as a group, seem poorly equipped to recognize power, label it as such, and utilize it effectively, either in themselves or others." (12:127) It seems difficult for nurses to view power as other than a negative concept. The reasons for this are fairly obvious. Nurses have historically been a relatively powerless group. We have more frequently been the victims of power than the wielders of power. This is true in our roles as professionals and as women. Nursing is still a "feminine profession" and is likely to remain so within the foreseeable future. However, this fact in no way condemns nurses to traditional powerless and statusless roles.

Conclusions

There are a number of characteristics basic to the change-agent role. The change-agent is a professional who relies heavily on a body of knowledge to realize his aims. He is frequently a marginal individual without formal membership in the system. The role of the change-agent, a somewhat ambiguous one, involves certain risks, frequently drawing suspicion and hostility because of its ambiguity. At the same time, to be effective, any person intimately concerned with change needs to possess a tolerance for ambiguity. The role of the change agent is both insecure and risky. He may frequently be viewed as the most expendable person, and with the complexity of organizational change, unanticipated consequences of his actions can lead to totally undersirable outcomes. (1:217–8)

Probably the most singular skill of the successful change agent is that of *interpersonal competence*. Competence implies the capacity to meet and deal with a changing world, to formulate ends and to implement them. The interpersonally competent individual is healthy, intelligent, empathetic, autonomous, sound in his judgments and innovative. (9:36–60) He is the kind of individual who can size up a situation, maintain an awareness of the human factors involved, and develop a diagnostic sensitivity as well as behavioral flexibility in dealing with human problems.

References

1. Schein, Edgar H. and Bennis, Warren G., *Personal and Organizational Change through Group Methods: The Laboratory Approach*, New York: John Wiley & Sons, Inc., 1965, p.202.
2. Ujhely, Gertrud, " 'And' Instead of 'Either-Or' or 'The Fallacy of False Opposition,'" *Image* (Sigma Theta Tau), 4 (3): 10–13, 1970–71.
3. Chin, Robert, "The Utility of System Models and Developmental Models for Practitioners," in *The Planning of Change: Readings in the Applied Behavioral Sciences* (edited by Warren G. Bennis, Kenneth D. Benne and Robert Chin). New York: Holt, Rinehart and Winston, Inc., 1961, pp. 201–214.
4. Lewin, Kurt, "Group Decision and Social Change," in *Readings in Social Psychology* (edited by Eleanor E. Maccoby, Theodore M. Newcomb, and Eugene L. Hartley), New York: Holt, Rinehart and Winston, Inc., 1958, p. 208.
5. Toffler, Alvin, *Future Shock* New York: Random House, 1970, p. 4.
6. Postman, Neil and Weingartner, Charles, *The Soft Revolution*, New York: Dell Publishing Company, Inc., 1971, p, 8.
7. Zander, Alvin, "Resistance to Change—Its Analysis and Prevention," in *The Planning of Change: Readings in the Applied Be-*

havioral Sciences, (edited by Warren G. Bennis, Kenneth D. Benne, and Robert Chin). New York: Holt, Rinehart and Winston, Inc., 1961, pp. 543–548.

8. Greiner, Larry E., "Patterns of Organization Change," in *Interpersonal Behavior and Administration* (edited by Arthur N. Turner and George F. Lombard), New York: The Free Press, 1969, pp. 477–493.

9. Foote, Nelson N. and Cottrell, Leonard S. Jr., *Identity and Interpersonal Competence: A New Direction in Family Research,* Chicago: The University of Chicago Press, 1965.

10. Kolb, D. and Frohman, A., "An Organization Development Approach to Consulting," *Sloan Management Review* 12:51–66 (Fall) 1970.

11. Bennis, Warren G., "A Topology of Change Processes," in *The Planning of Change: Readings in the Applied Behavioral Sciences* (edited by Warren G. Bennis, Kenneth D. Benne, and Robert Chin), New York: Holt, Rinehart and Winston, Inc., 1961, p. 154.

12. Deloughery, Grace W., Gebbie, Kristine M., and Neuman, Betty M., *Consultation and Community Organization in Community Mental Health Nursing,* Baltimore: The Williams & Wilkins Company, 1971, p. 127.

THE THEME
IS CHANGE

Sandra Schuler, M.S.N., R.N.

Lenore B. Campbell, B.S.N., R.N.

NURSES TODAY ARE COMING INTO THE FIELD WITH
more and better educational preparation. From all apparent indices this
trend will continue as more attend undergraduate programs and receive
master's and doctorate degrees. Nursing schools, too, continue to experiment with and change their curriculums in an attempt to prepare better
qualified nurses. Teamwork among professionals continues to come more
to the forefront.

Expanded educational backgrounds and the interdisciplinary approach
to health care places a responsibility on professional nurses to take
leadership positions in clinical areas. Some important aspects of
leadership include the ability to make decisions, get pleasure from seeing
growth and change, and influence behavior in the direction of cooperative
work toward common goals. A leader needs a firm theoretical and
practical base in the profession, an understanding of management and a
liking for variety. Leadership requires knowledge of the profession, interpersonal and problem-solving skills, and administrative talent.

In the past year we, a Head Nurse and Psychiatric Nurse Clinical Specialist, have been actively involved as nurse leaders in organizational
change on a 39-bed psychiatric unit in a Medical-Surgical Veterans
Administration Hospital. Through a description of this change process we
hope to share some of our joy, frustration and overall sense of accomplish-

Reprinted, with permission, from *Journal of Psychiatric Nursing and Mental Health
Services*, July-August 1974.

ment. As nurses we were the catalysts in a move to update a hospital ward. We provided motivation to expand the role of the psychiatric nurse.

We shall first give a brief description of the ward as it was on July 1, 1972. Then we shall discuss our reasons for instituting the process of change, the effects of the change, and our future plans.

Why The Change?

The unit is a 39-bed, open psychiatric ward in a Medical-Surgical Veterans Administration Hospital. Built twenty years ago, the ward is typical of the custodial type care of that period. Paint is dull, little sunlight enters through old security screens, glass encloses the nurses' station and heavy brown doors with small windows open to all the rooms. The only facilities for patients to congregate are two solaria, a game room and the men's room. Conference and therapy rooms are nonexistent. All patients have access to other hospital facilities including the library, chapel, canteen, retail store, barbershop, and all medical-surgical services. Unless otherwise indicated, they eat in a general patient cafeteria.

The patients varied in age with the average between 40 and 45. The major diagnoses were alcoholism and depression. There were some cases of schizophrenia and drug abuse. Patients were generally from low to low-middle socioeconomic backgrounds. The average length of hospitalization was two months.

Staffing was barely adequate. There was one full-time Chief of Psychiatry who had responsibility for total inpatient care. His treatment philosophy was largely individual psychotherapy and drug therapy. His leadership was authoritarian in nature and he saw the nurse simply as carrying out his orders and keeping the ward "under control." He left in early November 1972. Since then, the two outpatient psychiatrists have been covering the ward on a six-week rotation basis.

The nursing staff consisted of three Registered Nurses, the Head Nurse, three Nursing Assistants, one Licensed Practical Nurse, and one part-time Psychiatric Mental Health Clinical Specialist who came in August 1972.

Other members of the Psychiatric Team included a Social Worker (three fifths of the time) who does individual and conjoint treatment; a psychologist, when available, two Occupational Therapists; a Physical Therapist, and a Clergyman. These people all had responsible duties throughout the hospital. They do not participate in psychiatry on a full-time basis.

The major treatment approaches were drug therapy, occupational therapy and supportive individual counseling. It was obvious from the ratio of professionals to patients that little could be done in the way of consistent individual psychotherapy. It became clear that the goal of individual psychotherapy was unrealistic. The use of drug therapy to keep patients "under control" was incongruent with the Head Nurse's and Clinical Specialist's philosophy of psychiatric care. Professional resources were scarce. All of this was taken into consideration in determining the need and direction of change.

Planning For Change

Instituting administrative changes is no easy task, especially when it is a first attempt. The Head Nurse and Clinical Specialist had taught Mental/Psychiatric Nursing and had learned a good deal about themselves, nursing, and mental health. Returning to the clinical area and being responsible for total patient care on a psychiatric ward were challenges.

It was apparent that much change was needed on the unit. Nurses needed to become more independent and self-directed. Patients needed to learn to change behavior patterns rather than merely "taking a rest." The goal was to help make the expanded role of the nurse a reality on this unit and help patients to better cope with their lives.

Because nursing was the only consistent group relating with patients on the floor, it became obvious that we as nurses were going to be the change agents on the unit. Not regularly having one doctor provided a good deal of freedom for nursing to expand and grow. It also resulted in some inconsistencies with each rotation.

It is obvious that changes in the physical set up were necessary. The administration was reluctant to make major changes due to budgetary restrictions and the lack of a physician. However, new screens were obtained so that the ward became a good deal brighter. An office for the Clinical Specialist was provided and this was used for individual counseling, change of shift report, and nursing staff meetings. A small examining room was converted to a nursing conference room where we kept books and files. This room was also used for seeing patients and their families. Plans for total renovation are now under way.

We based the establishment of a cohesive nursing group on some strongly held beliefs: (1) Learning is best developed in an environment of positive reinforcement with the provision for freedom to experiment, guidance and support; (2) People must be respected for their individuality and their own human needs; and (3) Nurses need to be more independent and self-directed.

Therapeutic and Administrative Planning

Conducting weekly nursing staff planning meetings was the *key* to creating a cohesive, motivated work group. It was at these meetings that we planned overall patient treatment. One of the highest priorities was to create and maintain a good work group. We firmly believe that in order to provide therapeutic care to patients, the staff must be supportive of each other and must be able to work well together. Greenblatt refers to this approach to organization as a "social interaction of human beings (based on) participation, consultation, cooperation, morale and consensus." He points out that leadership skills are necessary ". . . to give expression to group feeling."

One method used to maintain strong group feelings was individual monthly meetings with the Head Nurse. The purpose in doing this was to provide scheduled time with each staff member for the sharing of thoughts and feelings with the Head Nurse. This has helped staff relations greatly. There was a time when people felt the Head Nurse was seldom available to listen to them. These meetings have satisfied a need we all have: to be listened to.

Staff development was a major priority. The Head Nurse's goals for nursing staff beyond herself and a Clinical Specialist were for eight Registered Nurses; three day Nursing Assistants; two evening Assistants. The Head Nurse was to remain on day shifts Monday through Friday to provide for consistency and availability. Some necessary characteristics of the nursing staff were: (1) openness to change; (2) motivation; (3) basic knowledge of psychiatry; and (4) willingness to take risks. Nursing administration supported these goals and helped us in developing and maintaining them.

We were very much aware of our need for administrative support. Change is a most difficult process and we could easily expect much resistance from various sources including ourselves; we were already experiencing resistance from the psychiatrist. The Head Nurse was aware of herself as a role model for the other nurses on the unit. Consistent demonstration of independence as a person and as a nurse was necessary from the beginning. She often felt frustrated and discouraged after fighting resistance from the psychiatrist. The Chief Nurse provided a good deal of support when it was most needed and she encouraged a strong independent image of nursing. We were allowed to experiment and function independently while still getting needed direction in the area of administrative changes.

Another priority was to have clinical expertise available as a part of the administrative changes. Having a Clinical Specialist on the staff has been invaluable. It is difficult to define the specific contributions of the Clinical

Specialist to this particular change process as she and the Head Nurse worked so closely together. Generally she provided knowledge, direction, motivation and support to the Head Nurse as well as to the nursing staff group.

The administrative talents and clinical expertise meshed continuously and we believe they are both essential to the development of a cohesive work group, high quality nursing care, and the expanded role of the nurse.

Therapeutic Community

Initially we introduced the idea of a therapeutic community and this became our goal. This milieu would be one of involvement, sharing, openness and honesty. Increased patient and nursing responsibility and inpatient care would be particularly emphasized. Involvement and sharing here means staff with staff, staff with patients, and patients with patients. Maxwell Jones sees as a major objective in establishing a therapeutic social environment the creating of ". . .two-way communication involving as far as possible all personnel, both patients and staff." We also support Jones' belief in open communication and daily group discussions between patients and staff as a means to improve treatment modalities. From the beginning we stressed:

1. Staff and patient input into ward rules.
2. Respect for individuality among staff and patients.
3. Increased responsibility for patients with staff providing consistent limits and support.
4. Continuous staff input in the formulation of ward goals and patient care planning.
5. Weekly administrative planning.

We chose to use various types of groups to facilitate our goals. In the weekly nursing administrative staff meetings we identified our needs and established our goals. Reading material on "Therapeutic Community" was made available for all nursing personnel. The first month or two we concentrated on reading material related to our goals, getting basic ward tasks done, and establishing trust and rapport with the patients.

Groups

At this time the Head Nurse began therapy sessions three times per week. These paved the way for more nurse-led therapy groups. There are presently four inpatient groups all co-led by registered nurses and three outpatient groups co-led by one registered nurse and one person from the psychology department. One of the outpatient groups is specificaly for discharged psychiatric patients. All registered nurses do individual treatment as the need arises and some of us conduct individual meetings on a regular basis. A few see patients and family members for assessment and counseling as well as following individual patients after discharge on a weekly basis.

Democratic Mileu

With the addition of staff and the beginning of our cohesive work group, we began to have weekly ward meetings with patients. Our purpose was to open communication between staff and patients. At the first meeting, we explained various nursing roles and we discussed ward rules and regulations. Nurses led these meetings at first but encouraged patients to select officers to form a ward committee of patients who would provide for patient leadership. This was accomplished with some difficutly. The major problem was patient resistance to change for a number of reasons: (1) lack of trust; (2) fear of failure; (3) extreme dependence on staff; and (4) stereotyped perceptions of care. We found that the nurses present at the ward meetings had to project a sense of security in this approach to treatment. A good deal of support and direction was necessary during the initial meetings. These patients were accustomed to seeing nurses not as leaders but solely as helpers to the doctor. Since no other members of the psychiatric team attended these meetings, we had to guard against manipulation and be sure of our beliefs. Patients frequently challenged our approach to treatment and our right to use this approach. We had to be consistent in what we did and said as a nursing group. Constant assessment of our own beliefs and techniques was vital.

Patient independence and responsibility became evident with the growth and development of these ward meetings. The Head Nurse provided continuous support and direction to the patient officers at weekly "preward meetings." This group plans the agenda for the ward meetings. The total patient group recently voted to have the agenda posted one day in advance to provide for more awareness of plans. Patient communication is very effective now. Arguments are purposeful and most often result in mutual compromise. Parliamentary procedure has become more evident and is effective. A treasury has been established for the purpose of providing the ward with a coffee room as well as for occasional birthday and farewell parties. The patients also instituted a Welcoming Committee of two patients who orient new admissions to the ward.

A Patients' Relations Committee was established as the result of an interpatient conflict. The purpose of this group is to review grievances made by one person against another. The parties involved in the grievance, one registered nurse, and the committee members meet as a group. It is here that many conflicts are settled by mutual agreement. This has provided an alternative to fist fights and to useless, misdirected complaining on the unit. It also provides an opportunity for people to see themselves as others may see them and helps people to work out behavior problems interfering with their interpersonal relationship. This Committee evolved from patients' ideas and was patient-initiated.

One of the Nursing Assistants conducts Relaxation Therapy sessions for small groups of patients. Another aide has a daily exercise group. Nursing Assistants were included as co-leaders in group sessions for a time but this was discontinued due to their lack of training and education for this role. They now direct themselves to more task and goal-oriented group activities with the patients. They provide an important source of one-to-one support to the patients and act as liaisons between the patients and the registered nurses.

Two patients and one Nursing Assistant are responsible for recreational equipment and planning. Another patient works with the Nursing Assistant weekly to plan a patient "Work Detail." Ward jobs are listed and appropriate patients are given these responsibilities. At first, we made a list of work assignments and expected the patients to follow through. It soon became evident that we, as staff, needed to provide a minimal amount of support and back-up especially against peer pressure within the patient group. The present system is satisfying patient and staff goals.

Treatment Milieu

The weekly nursing staff meetings have resulted in many changes in the approach to nursing care. These include:

1. Problem-Oriented nursing notes and Kardex, based on Weed's Problem-Oriented Medical Record System.
2. An orientation file for new nurses containing the nursing philosophy and objectives, role, description, therapists and ward goals.
3. Team nursing.

In team nursing, patients are assigned to Team A or B. This is done on admission and the patients remain on that team throughout hospitalization. Assignment to a group is made by the members of the team. Registered nurses are responsible for individual therapy as needed with the patients in their group. Prior to doing team nursing, we each had five or six individual patients assigned to us. This presented problems with shift rotation and days off, and it also became difficult for us to maintain accurate and consistent communication among ourselves. The team approach and the tape recording of all our shift reports have helped us to communicate better with each other and with the patients.

An early means of implementing the goal of respect and sharing was the wearing of street clothes by staff and patients. We wrote up the rationale and objectives of such a change and submitted the request to the nursing administration. As staff, we were able to change into street clothes with more ease than were the patients in this hospital. Because of past experiences with psychiatric patients, doctors and hospital administrators wanted to move cautiously in this area of change. It was a few months and a number of committee meetings later before permission was granted for ten patients to wear street clothes on a two-month trial basis. After two months, twenty patients were given permission and presently all patients are expected to wear street clothes. Pajamas are worn only when there are therapeutic indications for it. To date, we have had no abuse of this privilege and people throughout the hospital are now much more accepting of this approach to treatment.

Inservice Education

In order to maintain this milieu approach to treatment, continuing inservice education has been provided. Since January, we have met every other week for two hours as a nursing staff group with a clinical psychologist for group supervision. He will now be coming every week for two hours. Prior to consultation from the clinical psychologist, we met weekly with the Clinical Specialist for group supervision. The Head Nurse and Clinical Specialist are now conducting a 20-hour course in basic principles and techniques for dealing with various behavior patterns.

An important aspect of our roles as nurse-leaders has been active involvement with nurses outside the unit. At weekly Head Nurse Administrative meetings we were responsible for changing the image of psychiatric nursing and contributed to the teaching of communication techniques and basic emotional needs of people. We are still involved in working on communication within nursing administration and on defining the role of the Head Nurse.

The Head Nurse and Clinical Specialist were also members of a smaller administrative planning group which included the Chief Nurse and the Psychology Consultant. The group met weekly for the purpose of discussing change and providing mutual support. A factor we have not stressed is the need for people involved in creating changes to have a source of support. These meetings helped us to deal with the process of change. Being actively involved in the Head Nurse meetings and the smaller administrative planning group were essential to the process of change on the ward and throughout the hospital.

The Effects of Change

The effects of this change were felt at all levels. The impact of change reached patients, nursing, and other professional staff throughout the hospital. The effects we have seen are qualitative observations made throughout the hospital.

Patient Population

Among the patient population, there are fewer malingerers, alcoholics and older recidivist patients. Both patient and staff comments bear this out. The major observable changes in patient behavior are:

1. Decrease in prn tranquilizers requested. In October 1972, ten or more given daily. It is rare if more than one is given now.
2. Decrease in acting-out and other attention-getting behavior.
3. Increase in self-direction and initiative. Patients themselves are initiating ideas for change and implementation as seen in ward meetings.
4. Increase in patient's responsibility for treatment. Patients now attend treatment sessions without resistance and question and decline in staff-patient inteaction.
5. Increase in patient's responsibility to other patients and to staff. Patients volunteer to help staff when staffing is short. Patients orient new patients to the unit, volunteer to help patients with physical problems and exert peer pressure to conform with the hospital and unit regulations. They are very conscious of their image as "psychiatric patients" throughout the hospital.
6. Change in patient attitudes toward the nurse's role. Patients now ask nurses for therapy and see them as independent professionals rather than mere transmitters of the doctor's orders.

Nursing Staff

There has been much positive change for the nursing staff on the psychiatric unit. Changes include:

1. Continued personal and professional growth.
2. More purposeful, directed therapy to individuals, groups, and families.
3. Feelings of accomplishment and self-worth; less dependence on the doctor.
4. Feelings of teamwork, closeness, intimacy and sharing with fellow nurses.
5. Feelings of involvement.

We, the authors, have experienced a sense of pride and accomplishment in seeing improved patient care brought about by the nursing service. We have experienced:

1. Increased self-confidence.
2. Strengthening of the belief in the treatment milieu.
3. Strengthening the belief that knowledge, skill, and a philosophy of nursing are essential to nurses assuming leadership.
4. Desire to continue to learn and effect change.
5. Respect for the time and effort necessary to effect change.

Other Professionals

We have seen the effects on other team members; *i.e.*, the doctors, social workers, psychologist, recreation director, and chaplains. They have become increasingly supportive of the treatment and more involved in this approach. They are asking for more meaningful input from nurses and they see us as valuable members of the team.

Finally, throughout this particular hospital, attitudes have been observably altered. Other nurses are seeing the role of the psychiatric nurse as more active and therapeutic. Change brought about by determined nursing leadership has become a reality. People are seeing the psychiatric patient in a more positive light. There is more respect for the staff nurse. Greater confidence is placed in the beliefs and decisions of nursing on the psychiatric unit.

We have listed some of the most obvious effects of this change to give the reader an idea of the far-reaching implication of changes initiated and implemented by nurses. The qualities and needs of the leadership which we feel made this change possible are:

1. Theoretical knowlege or ready access to it.
2. Clinical expertise.
3. Knowledge of the change process.

4. A nursing staff willing to make decisions and stand behind them.
5. Strong administrative support from the Chief Nurse in the form of encouragement to be independent and to experiment.

In this year of change what seems most striking is the impact nurses can have if they combine their administrative and clinical skills. The impact is widespread, including patients, other nurses, hospital administration, and all members of the health team.

Change as an Ongoing Process

With the anticipation of a permanent psychiatrist, the nursing staff is very anxious about the effects on the unit. Greenblatt states, "Management succession . . . can be responsible for . . . dramatic changes in human systems." Along with the anticipation of new leadership, we are dealing with termination and mourning for the present leadership. The Head Nurse and Clinical Specialist are both leaving. What is being done to lessen the effects of staff loss is to provide one month of orientation for the new Head Nurse and Clinical Specialist. The present Head and the new Head Nurse have established firm nursing goals and expectations with the hope of sharing these with the new doctor and planning for the changes together. The new Clinical Specialist will become familiar with the total hospital and ward, and together with this Clinical Specialist will be planning her own goals and sharing expectations with the nursing staff. Many new relationships will be developing as old ones are being lost. We frequently discuss the possible effects of these changes and share our feelings. We have found that the support we are able to give each other has helped us as we begin a new phase in the process of change.

Change is constant. This nursing staff will not take a backseat with the anticipated change approaching. Having lived through a very positive change process and having seen the possibilities for nurses they will insist on being an integral part of any new change process.

Acknowledgment

The authors wish to express sincere thanks to Alicebelle Rubotzky, Chief Nurse, and Henry Biller, Clinical Psychologist, for their assistance, support and help in the development and writing of this article.

34 THE THERAPEUTIC COMMUNITY v. TRADITIONAL PSYCHIATRY

Ross Mitchell, M.D.

TRADITIONALLY ILLNESS HAS BEEN TREATED BY DOCTORS AND nurses within hospitals. Gradually, the respective roles of 'doctor', 'nurse' and 'patient' have been worked out and defined. A doctor is a medical specialist who makes his skills and expertise available to the sick person, the patient. A nurse is also a medically qualified person but who works with the doctor and largely under his direction, although she has recognised areas of skills and competence in her own right. She, too, helps the patient. The patient is, by definition, a sick person who requires the skilled help that doctors and nurses can provide. It is the responsibility of doctors and nurses to provide help; it is the responsibility of patients to receive it.

There is therefore a clear-cut system in which each individual has his place, and, if he keeps within his defined role he will receive certain rewards—the doctor and the nurse receive the patient's gratitude and the satisfaction of a job well done, and the patient gets better, thankful to have been the recipient of medical skills. So long as each plays the game, each is rewarded and satisfied.

This is how it is supposed to be, but all kinds of things can happen to disturb this equilibrium: the doctor and nurse are often faced with the painful reality that they may not have any particular skill or expertise to help a given patient; not all people labelled as 'patient' by others are prepared to accept that role themselves; they may refuse to be treated, they

Reproduced, with permission, from *Nursing Times*, November 21, 1974.

may demand treatment that is not available, they may be highly critical of what is provided for them and so on.

This situation is further complicated by the fact that medicine has become increasingly technical. More and more people are added to the basic medical team of doctor and nurse—the social worker, the medical social worker, the psychologist, the physiotherapist, the laboratory technician, the X-ray technician, the EEG technician and ECG technician and so on.

The medical team has become less mobile and is now tied to vast hospitals which are needed to house the so-called 'hardware' of modern medical technology. A hospital with one thousand beds, attempting to cater for that number of in-patients requires as many personnel just to keep the machine working. This vast collection of people requires to be organised, and nature's natural organisation is the 'pecking order', that is a ranked system in which each person has a place, those above him to whom he is responsible and those below who are responsible to him.

There is a clear-cut chain of command with instructions being issued from the top downwards. Information is passed usually from the bottom upwards, so that successive ascending layers of administration can make the right decision with their competence, handing on for consideration and decisions, matters to the layer above.

Such hierarchies are to be found in all large organisations—the armed forces, the police, the prison service, public schools, religious orders, the established church, the law, education and so on.

Promotion for doctors and nurses is by a strict hierarchy system. The value of a hierarchy is its basic rigidity—everyone knows where they are: there is somebody above to hand matters over to, someone below to blame if necessary. Also, hierarchies maintain and defend traditional values.

Hard work and effort is rewarded by promotion, which brings not only greater responsibilities but theoretically greater rewards. However, as Peter has already pointed out in his famous principle, 'We all rise to our highest level of incompetence' - that is, the girl who is a 'good' nurse, gets on well with patients and knows her stuff, is promoted to sister where she has less contact with patients but more administration; then if she is a 'good' sister she will be promoted to a No. 7 and so on up the Salmon hierarchy, until she gets further and further away from the original area of her excellence—her clinical skills and contact with the patient.

Nevertheless, faced with the day to day emergencies, literally of life and death, and given the highly complicated and specialised technology through which medicine now expresses itself, there is no doubt that the only way in which many of these large hospital organisations can work is through a rigidly maintained and sustained hierarchy.

Psychiatry has inherited such an organizational hierarchy, as mental hospitals were really not all that different from general hospitals—doctors, nurses, psychologists, social workers, occupational therapists, arranged in a rigid hierarchy from the medical superintendent, down to the most junior nurse.

The difficulty for the so-called 'paramedical' professions has been to know where they fit in. Does a trained clinical psychologist equal four untrained nurses, or one and a half sisters? Does an occupational therapist stand closer to the nursing staff than, say to a social worker or a volunteer?

It began to be realised that whereas it made sense to put patients into bed in a general hospital and ask them for a time to deliver themselves up to the greater competence and skills of the medical staff, in psychiatry it seemed that what was wanted was not to take away responsibility for themselves from the patients, but in fact to give it back to them.

If psychiatric patients are not to be 'patients', that is relatively passive recipients of the skills of others, but were to take decisions for themselves, this means a challenge to the whole hierarchical system. The patient in fact comes to be invited to join the hierarchy, but not at the bottom; in a sense he may find himself at the top. The patient may be encouraged to think for himself and to make decisions, to be responsible for his actions, albeit guided by the 'professional team'.

Pushed to its logical conclusion the patient is encouraged to question and challenge the authority of the hierarchy, and this is very uncomfortable both for the staff and for the patient. Just how uncomfortable and threatening this can be, is well described by W. R. Bion in his book *Experiences in Groups* and by Denis Martin in his book *Adventure in Psychiatry* in which is described how a mental hospital decided to restructure its whole organisation in terms of a newer, more egalitarian pattern.

A new model which fitted this new philosophy had to be found, and it is enshrined in the concept of the 'therapeutic community'. Here, there is not a linear chain of command and information exchange, but more of a circle, with roles and command going round and round for ever, or a social matrix within which roles and responsibities are forever changing.

If the essence of a hierarchy is instruction and uncritical obedience, the essence of the therapeutic community is sharing, questioning and support. Within the therapeutic community, roles become less defined, and there is flattening of the so-called authority pyramid (a hierarchy with one 'chief' at the top and increasing numbers of 'executives' underneath down to an even greater number of 'slaves' at the bottom).

As an expression of this flattening of the authority structure, no one jumps just because a doctor says so; the doctor has got to justify giving anyone a command at all. Nurses may stop wearing their uniform, and call each other and the doctors and the patients by their first name. Outsiders visiting the therapeutic community may become quite upset because they cannot tell the difference between the staff and the patients.

Some may feel that this is the final accolade of a true therapeutic community, because in a sense all in the community are patients, that is, all have fears and worries, make mistakes, get 'hung up' about each other and suffer internally from anxiety and from depression. Similarly, all are 'staff' because all have experiences to share, insights into how life can be lived, and the capacity for a brief moment to help the one in trouble who is sitting next in the circle.

How different this is from the traditional psychiatric organisation where patients and staff are clearly distinguishable from each other, where the patients are truly patients because they are sick, have illnesses, 'are not themselves', and require and respond to the undoubted medical skills of the psychiatric team. This is a more comfortable model because each knows where he is and what is expected of him. There is a clear-cut structure within which everyone's anxieties can be contained and dissipated. There is a responsible person to tell others what to do, another to take over, and yet another to remain in control and see that things get done, to protect the weak, restrain the strong, see fair play according to the rules of the particular game which is being played.

In the therapeutic community everything seems to be the opposite: there is no clear-cut structure or organisation, and such organisation as there is, is in constant change. No one person is in command, each is required to be responsible for himself; anxiety, rather than being contained and dissipated, is generated and amplified; things can get out of control, the strong and the weak have to make out as best they can. And yet is it really as chaotic as all this?

A proper, as opposed to a pseudo or an aspiring, therapeutic community has this blue-print:

1. Frequent face to face meetings of all regular members of the community.

2. A social analysis made of all events which occur within the community.

3. All inter-personal tensions and conflicts dealt with by confrontation and working through, rather than by being repressed and treated as 'illness'.

4. A deliberate sharing of leadership within the membership of the community.

5. Each member encouraged to be himself and to express himself honestly, but within a responsibility for his actions, and for their repercussions on the other members of the community.

The work of the therapeutic community is done mainly in the daily community meeting which all members are obliged to attend. Any conflict between members or groups of members will be dealt with, in immediately called small groups of all involved, according to the principles of crisis intervention.

The therapeutic community aims to teach individuals, staff and patients alike, to be more aware of their behaviour and its effect on others. Members are encouraged to accept responsibility for themselves and not to escape into themselves and not to escape into concepts of 'illness', 'bad nerves', 'I couldn't help it', 'it wasn't me, they made me do it'. It aims to train people to stop thinking in terms of 'she upset me', to thinking in terms of 'I allowed her to upset me'.

The main critics of the therapeutic community movement say that it may well train people to live more effectively within the therapeutic community, but it does not help outside in the wider society where people do not relate to each other within an egalitarian democracy, but according to the rules of various merit-oriented hierarchies.

The trouble is that with all new or relatively new ventures, people tend to jump on the popular bandwagon and to go all out for what seems to be the 'in thing', without asking if this is the most appropriate model to their own needs and, more particularly, the needs of the patients which they seek to serve. Many so-called therapeutic community units have been set up without the architects necessarily asking themselves if their community really is therapeutic, or if it is only pretending to be so.

The traditional form of psychiatry is rooted in the well tried and well respected medical model: the therapeutic community is rooted in the less well tried, but no less potentially respectable sociological model. Each has its place, its values and its aims, rules and effects. Neither can nor should claim to contain within it the answer to all problems and all human dilemmas.

In given circumstances, one may be more appropriate to the other in pure culture. But here is the rub; some of the principles of the therapeutic community proper have been seen as possibly applicable in other contexts. It is suggested that a rigid hierarchical medical model can be humanised by being imbued with therapeutic community principles. Sociology can penetrate into medicine and can cast light upon it.

It is being asked by many if it is not possible for the medical model hierarchy to become softened, to be made more flexible with room for individual growth and initiative, to allow information to flow both upwards and downwards, to have responsibility shared between the various administrative levels, to allow a greater degree of mobility and mixing from one level to another, and to allow patients to have a greater say in what is going on and what is happening to them.

Can therapeutic community principles be applied, for example, to the busy short-stay multi-purpose admission ward, or in the sick bay, or in the psychiatric ward of the district general hospital, or in the ward which specialises in psychosomatic disorders?

The trouble may be that we cannot mix chalk with cheese or if we try to, each will be changed in the process. It seems as if some experiments of such mixing have led to a kind of illegitimate situation where the worst excesses of each model flourish and the best never manage to break through to the surface.

The dilemma that seems to face us at the moment in psychiatry, is to decide where each in its essence is more appropriate; that is, to see them as legitimate alternatives or options, and not as deadly enemies. And, further, to see to what extent the therapeutic community can shed light on the traditional model without destroying it altogether, and without having its own honourable repute called in question because it is strained to operate within a system in which it cannot flourish, and in which therefore almost inevitably it may be seen to have failed because it has been applied in a false way.

Further Reading

Bion, W. R. (1968) *Experiences in Groups,* Social Science Paperbacks. Tavistock Publications. London.

Clark, D. H. (1971) *Administrative Psychiatry.* Social Science Paperbacks. Tavistock Publications, London.

Jones, Maxwell (1968) *Social Psychiatry in Practice,* Penguin Books, London.

Martin, Denis (1962) *Adventure in Psychiatry,* Cassirer, Oxford.

Peter, Laurence (1969) *The Peter Principle.* Souvenir Press, London.

"ALONENESS" IN A THERAPEUTIC COMMUNITY

Dolores Leone M.S., R.N. and Rothlyn Zahourek M.S., R.N.

WITH THE INCREASING EMPHASIS ON GROUP INTERACTION AND interpersonal relationships in a therapeutic community setting, it appears that we have overlooked the positive values of patients spending time by themselves and using this time constructively. We need to be reminded that a large percentage of patients, when returned to their communities, live by themselves and spend much of their free time in solitude.

In one state institution, the Fort Logan Mental Health Center in Colorado, when records covering a five-year period were examined, it was found that out of the total patients discharged during that period 26 percent of the males and 17 percent of the females returned to solitary living arrangements in the community. Also, prior to admission, 57.3 percent of the total patients either lived alone or expected to live alone when discharged.

If these figures are typical of other hospital populations, it would appear that mental health workers should be made more aware of their patient's need to cope with aloneness. Does the therapeutic community, which provides an intensive group experience for patients, actually prepare them for less structured lives on discharge, often lives lived alone in the community?

From *Perspectives in Psychiatric Care*, Vol. XII, No. 2, 1974, pp. 60–63. Reprinted, with permission, from Nursing Publications, Inc., 194-B Kinderkamack Rd., Park Ridge, N.J. 07656.

Group psychotherapy, family therapy, and the therapeutic community are prime examples of how our culture's reliance on groups has been reflected in current methods of psychiatric treatment. One typical interdisciplinary team at Fort Logan Mental Health Center, employing the therapeutic community concepts of Maxwell Jones (1953) and Alan M. Kraft (1966), states part of its goal as achieving "an active, cooperative patient group striving to help themselves and others . . . with an emphasis on social and group interaction . . ."* In examining the schedule of treatment activities of this team, the group emphasis is striking: in a 40-hour week, patients spend approximately 83.7 percent of their time involved in formal and informal group activities.

We have no intention of condemning group treatment or the therapeutic community. Like other living things, patients vary a great deal, therefore, not all patients will benefit from the same treatment modality. However, any new and exciting method of treatment can be carried to an extreme, and staff, in its enthusiasm, may become forgetful of the needs of the individual patient.

If the goal of hospital treatment is to promote the successful return of a patient to the community, then we do question the efficacy of a heavy dose of group treatment for a patient who will be discharged to a solitary living situation. Would it not be possible to tailor and modify the therapeutic community to help such a patient to utilize solitary free time? Might not this approach reduce the "re-entry shock" when a patient is discharged and discovers he no longer has a cohesive group on which to depend? Might not an awareness of the problem of aloneness prevent some of the post-hospitalization loneliness and depression experienced by some patients? Might not this retailoring prevent some readmissions of "patients who can't seem to make it on the outside?"

In our readings, we have concluded that more attention has been given in the psychiatric literature to the negative connotations of isolation and withdrawn behavior in patients than to the positive aspects of aloneness and solitude. It appears that few, other than poets and philosophers, have recognized and written about man's need for aloneness and solitude.

Erich Fromm (1941) sees aloneness as both a constructive and destructive state. On the one hand, he emphasizes man's basic "need to avoid aloneness"; that a sense of complete aloneness or "moral aloneness" can lead to mental deterioration in which one is not only physically alone, but is unrelated to ideas, values, and social patterns that could give him a sense of relatedness. On the other hand, Fromm sees aloneness as

---

*Fort Logan Mental Health Center, Colorado, unpublished treatment philosophy of the Denver 6 team.

essential for the growth and development of a mature individual. He relates this to the awakening of a child's separateness, not only from his mother, but also from the entire world around him. "Growing aloneness" leads initially to anxiety, but the acceptance of this anxiety promotes individuation, and can result in a new inner strength and a new closeness and solidarity with others. Winnicott's (1958) term for this is "ego relatedness," where a person, although alone, maintains a sense of relationship with others.

Withdrawn behavior, however, is not synonymous with aloneness or solitude, and Schwartz and Shockley (1956) differentiate between the two: Solitude is when one takes time out to be alone to contemplate events that have occurred, or to become reacquainted with one's self. In a withdrawn state, the person is constantly by himself, and when approached is reluctant to interact. In a therapeutic community, a staff's attitude toward patient aloneness strongly influences the philosophies, goals, and methods of treatment. Based on the assumption that a capacity to deal both with others and with aloneness is important for mental health, we deemed patient capacity for "aloneness" as an important problem to study. Whether one lives alone or not, every person has time to himself, and if this time is not used in constructive relaxation, reflection, or activity, the pain of loneliness may be experienced.

Francel (1963) contends that "of all subjective states of mental illness, loneliness is the most productive of psychic pain." To Titus, (1960) loneliness is a reaction to uncontrollable circumstances and is characterized by a sense of loss, isolation, and feelings of frustration and sadness. Solitude, on the other hand, is a creative rather than a destructive force in life; it is sought and consciously desired.

Aloneness might then be defined as the actual physical state of being solitary — a state which has no positive or negative value. Solitude is the positive quality of the alone state in which a person experiences pleasure, psychic regeneration, or some other positive reaction to being alone. Withdrawal and loneliness are the negative qualities that may result from the alone state. Withdrawal is a behavioral reaction of physically pulling away and isolating one's self, usually because some threat exists. Loneliness, on the other hand, is a painful feeling (rather than a behavior) of isolation and unrelatedness. Both these qualities are characteristic of depression and other psychic maladies and disorders and, therefore, are not what we consider the positive qualities of, or reaction to, the alone state.

How then does the therapeutic community prepare patients to make positive and creative use of their time alone? To find out how this was done on one adult treatment team at Fort Logan, the authors devised and distributed an open-ended questionnaire to the thirteen team members. Nurses, technicians, recreational and occupational therapists, a psychologist, and a social worker comprised the team. A psychiatrist was not on the team on a full-time basis, and therefore was not included in the study. The questionnaire was designed to explore the following:

1. What the staff viewed as the most important treatment modality practiced on the team.
2. What the staff encouraged patients to do with their free time.
3. How many hours of free time the staff thought patients should have.
4. How the staff viewed a patient who was getting well.
5. What the staff thought it did that was most important in preparing a patient for return to the community.

Results

Consistent with the team philosophy, the responses showed that 100 percent of the subjects saw some form of group activity as the most valuable and therapeutic treatment modality. Looking at how the staff determined that a patient was "getting well," 60.7 percent of the responses made reference to the patient's increased participation in group and interpersonal activities; 28.8 percent of the responses indirectly referred to the patient's capacity for aloneness, and 10.5 percent referred to activities that show directly the patient's capacity to deal with aloneness as a sign of the patient's "getting well."

When the staff was asked how it viewed the patient who was alone during unstructured time, the results indicated that 60.7 percent viewed patient aloneness negatively, whereas 21.5 percent viewed it positively, and 17.8 percent said it depended on the patient and what he was doing. The staff also had difficulty distinguishing between the "withdrawn" and "solitary" patient. In viewing the patient who was alone, the staff frequently described him as "withdrawn," "isolated," "depressed," and "passive aggressive."

When asked how many hours of free or unstructured time a patient should be allowed in an 8-hour activity day, the staff's responses ranged from one to 4-hours, with a mean of 2.25 hours. Responses for allotment of free time in a 24-hour day ranged from 3 to 20 hours, with a mean of 10.75 hours.

When asked to list in order of therapeutic value what they encouraged patients to do during unstructured time — the activities "most valued" by staff for patients during unstructured time — 91.6 percent of the responses included group and interpersonal activities, and only 8.4

percent indicated such solitary activities as reading, personal grooming, and knitting.

Asked what is most important in preparing a patient for a return to life in the community, 53 percent of the staff listed activities that provide for the development of independence, 34.3 percent listed activities that help the patient with group and interpersonal relations. None indicated that the patient would need to utilize time alone.

Our preliminary investigation indicated that the most valued treatment modality of the team is group (both formal and informal), and the primary treatment goal is for the patient to improve his relationships with others. Furthermore, the staff most frequently views the patient who is alone in negative terms as "withdrawn," "depressed," "apathetic." However, when the staff considers the patient's return to his community, there is an indication of a beginning awareness of the patient's problem in coping with aloneness in the emphasis on the point that the patient must become independent, make his own plans, and forge his own place in the larger world outside the hospital.

Conclusions

Our investigation was, of course, limited to one setting, but the results are relevant, considering that a high percentage of patients do return to solitary living situations, and the staff emphasizes group treatment as most important.

We suggest that in each setting the staff look at what will happen to patients post-hospitalization and devise a treatment program that more realistically prepares their patients for re-entry into the community. Today, many hospitals implementing day care programs and transitional living situations are group oriented. Might there not be a decrease in the length of stay both in the hospital and in the transitional living situation if the patient's ability to cope with aloneness in all phases of treatment were considered? With the rising costs of hospitalization, this is no small issue to consider.

References

Francel, Claire G., "Loneliness," *Some Clinical Approaches to Psychiatric Nursing* (ed. Shirley Burd and Margaret A. Marshall), New York: Macmillan Company, 1963.

Fromm, Erich, *Escape From Freedom,* New York: Holt Rinehart and Winston, 1941.

Jones, Maxwell, M.D., *The Therapeutic Community, a Treatment Method in Psychiatry,* New York: Basic Books Inc., 1953.

Kraft, Alan M., "The Therapeutic Community," *American Handbook of Psychiatry,* Vol. III (ed. Silvano Arieti), New York: Russell Sage Foundation, 1966, pp. 542–551.

Schwartz, Morris S. and Emmy L. Shockley, *The Nurse and the Mental Patient,* New York: Russell Sage Foundation, 1956, p. 91.

Titus, Pauline Woodruff, *Never Be Lonely,* Englewood Cliffs, New Jersey: Prentice-Hall, Inc., 1960.

Winnicott, D. W., "The Capacity to be Alone," *International Journal of Psycho-Analysis,* XXXIX 1958, p. 417.

36 SOME NEGLECTED ISSUES IN MILIEU THERAPY

Alfred B. Lewis, Jr., M.D.

Michael Selzer, M.D.

MUCH HAS BEEN SAID ABOUT THE MERITS OF keeping a psychiatric hospitalization as short as possible, but not enough attention has been paid to what actually can be accomplished in a brief hospital stay. The emphasis on a short course of treatment followed by early discharge to the community has been labeled the "patch-and-dismiss" approach.[1] It is most effective in conditions that respond readily to somatic therapies, such as acute schizophrenic episodes and endogenous depressions.

Recent experience suggests that fewer newly hospitalized patients fall into these categories, and that an increasing proportion of cases can be classified as "borderline states" or "character disorders," which are unlikely to be helped significantly by somatic therapy. Evidence has also been advanced to show that while medication may control the symptoms of acute schizophrenia, the acute phase is often followed by a period of depression that is refractory to medication and difficult to manage.[2,3]

Reproduced, with permission, from *Hospital and Community Psychiatry*, Vol. 23 No. 10, October 1972.

[1] D. B. Rinsley, "Psychiatric Hospital Treatment With Special Reference to Children," *Archives of General Psychiatry*, Vol. 9, November 1963, pp. 489–496.

[2] M. B. Bowers, Jr., and B. M. Astrachan, "Depression in Acute Schizophrenic Psychosis," *American Journal of Psychiatry*, Vol. 123, February 1967, pp. 976–979.

[3] S. Roth, "The Seemingly Ubiquitous Depression Following Acute Schizophrenic Episodes: A Neglected Area of Clinical Discussion," *American Journal of Psychiatry*, Vol. 127, July 1970, pp. 51–58.

Therefore the real challenge in short-term hospital treatment is to provide effective therapy for chronic impairment, whether the underlying disorder be schizophrenia, borderline state, or character disorder.

The search for a practical therapeutic approach has led to the evolution of a variety of therapeutic communities and milieu therapy programs. They vary in sophistication from rather simplistic programs based on open doors, an attitude of permissiveness, and frequent community meetings to more elaborate programs that emphasize patient government or the involvement of patients and staff in interaction and confrontation. In some programs the patient group votes on privileges and passes for its members and in others patients present their case histories to their fellow patients.[4] Whatever the emphasis, most programs appear to be based on the rationale that participation in a democratic group experience in which free self-expression is encouraged will mobilize whatever ego strengths the patients have and promote their recovery.

The enthusiastic acceptance of the therapeutic community concept may have led to overconcern with how the milieu should be structured, especially with respect to the communication process and delegation of authority to the patient group. Hospital staffs are caught between the pressure to keep hospitalization as short as possible and the need to treat a population that includes an increasing proportion of chronic patients. Having the machinery of an elaborately structured milieu reduces the staff's anxiety; it gives them the sense of doing something for the patient without having to explore the psychopathology of the individual in depth, which can be both difficult and discouraging.

In a critique of the therapeutic community ideology, Nuttall has pointed out that there is a "tendency to pursue the idea of total communication as an end in itself (along with democratization, communalism, and other such concepts), surely a clear example of goal displacement."[5] In other words, the major task of milieu therapy has been obscured. Basically this task is to diagnose individual patients' needs in all their possible variations, and then to plan an individualized treatment approach that uses the patient's total environment to meet those needs. The basic question is, "What is it that this patient cannot do for himself, and how can we help him learn to do it?"

We will describe five commonly encountered clinical problems in which a clear diagnosis of the patient's needs led to a a rational plan of

---

[4]J. T. Quattlebaum, "A Therapeutic Community on a Short-Term Psychiatric Unit," *Hospital & Community Psychiatry*, Vol. 18, December 1967, pp. 353–360.

[5]K. Nuttall, "Communications in a Therapeutic Community," in *Progress in Community Mental Health*, edited by H. Freeman, Churchill, London, 1969, p. 229.

treatment: paranoid pathology, denial of affect, distancing behavior, identify diffusion, and hospital dependency. We will discuss some of the techniques used to arrive at the treatment plan, and we will identify some dangers of becoming overconcerned with the conceptual aspects of milieu therapy.

Paranoid Pathology

The first case involves a 50-year-old divorced woman with a diagnosis of paranoid reaction; she was admitted after six months of broadening paranoid delusions precipitated by her legal action against her former husband for support payments. The patient thought that people were talking about her, that her phone was tapped, and that her vitamin pills were being tampered with; she also felt that her former husband, in league with a group of ex-addicts, was trying to drive her crazy.

At a conference of unit personnel held a week after the woman's admission, several questions crystallized from the discussion. First, should the patient be encouraged to talk about her delusions, or should staff help her suppress them, and distract her whenever she brought them up? Second, if staff encouraged discussion of the delusional system, should they question its logic and try to inject doubt about it? Or should they comment on the underlying feelings of insecurity, loneliness, and fear that she must have experienced? Third, should they suggest that the patient might have similar fears about what was going on in the hospital, even though she had said she felt safe behind the locked doors?

To answer those questions rationally required an understanding of how the patient was using her symptoms. It appeared that she was unable to acknowledge the fear, isolation, and sense of rejection that her current existence gave her. Without that acknowledgement, she could not experience the pain of those feelings and, ultimately, put them into perspective. She avoided admitting the pain not only through her delusional system, which focused on what others were doing rather than what she was experiencing, but also by keeping everything private. Her uncommunicativeness prevented any reality testing and further rigidified the delusional system.

If staff routinely supported suppression of the delusions, the patient would perceive it as more reason not to share her thoughts. Conversely, to take her symptoms as a communication would be to use the potential bridge she offered to her underlying feelings, a necessary first step to therapeutic progress.

On the basis of this formulation, the staff decided to encourage her to talk about her delusions, and to interpret their implied affect rather than try to make her doubt their reality. For instance, they might say, "You must be frightened that there is so little safety for you." Thus they would indicate that the delusions had an internal emotional "logic" without agreeing that they were based on external reality. In addition, a staff member would be assigned to ask the patient at the end of each day whether she had questions about anything that had gone on during the day, to undercut any tendency she might have to incorporate the hospital or its personnel into her delusions. The goal was to establish a climate in which the patient could freely express her delusional ideas.

Another patient with the diagnosis of paranoid reaction, a 48-year-old man, had an elaborate delusion that the Mafia were gaining control of his thoughts and were going to make him kill his wife; the delusion occurred as he was increasingly aware of a wish to separate from her. Several weeks of treatment with phenothiazines, antidepressants, and individual psychotherapy brought about no change in the patient's delusional system or his behavior. He talked mechanically about the delusion, using set phrases, to staff and patients alike.

Improvement became noticeable only when staff realized that the patient was hiding behind his delusion to avoid relating to other people, as he had done at work and with friends before his hospitalization. They began to insist that he not talk about it; they concentrated instead on getting to know him as a person and on drawing him out about his interests and opinions.

These two paranoid patients presented opposite problems for milieu therapy, and different treatment plans were needed. Patients should be encouraged to express delusional material when their tendency is to be secretive about it. Conversely, they should be encouraged to suppress their delusions when they are using them for some kind of secondary gain, such as distancing themselves from others or reinforcing a definition of themselves as sick. The crucial issue is not the nature of the symptom but the use that is being made of it.

Denial of Affect

In another case, a 28-year-old woman diagnosed as paranoid schizophrenic had been hospitalized after a suicide attempt that occurred in the setting of a build-up of unexpressed anger toward her private psychiatrist. In the hospital she made no progress for several months because she persisted in denying her anger, even though it was clearly evident from her facial expression and attitude.

Her hospital therapist and the nursing staff decided that when staff saw that the patient was angry, they would ask her what her thoughts were.

Nurses and aides patiently and persistently followed that plan; for some time the patient continued to deny her anger, but she was finally able to acknowledge it, and to relate it to paranoid fears of her hospital therapist. This development was a turning point in her therapy.

Three aspects of staff-patient interaction are noteworthy here. First, the whole staff was used to make an interpretation to the patient that had been ineffective when made by the therapist alone. Both the consistency of the interpretation and the fact that it could be made precisely when the patient was obviously feeling angry contributed to its eventual impact. Second, the staff's approach conveyed the idea that they both wanted to know and could stand to hear the patient's feelings, no matter how intense and destructive they might seem to her. And third, the patient's denial of affect was extremely frustrating for therapist and staff alike. By clarifying the reasons for her behavior and developing an integrated approach to the problem, the staff were able to overcome their frustration and regain a sense of usefulness.

Distancing Behavior

The fourth case concerns a 23-year-old man with a diagnosis of a borderline personality. He adopted a very authoritarian attitude toward other patients, and at the same time he responded to staff only when their attitude was authoritarian. He seemed most comfortable when receiving or giving orders, and most uncomfortable when a kindly, permissive, or warm approach was used. He became upset when a nurse he had been close to went on vacation, but was unwilling to admit it.

While the nursing staff were making those observations, the therapist was exploring the patient's history; he elicited a pattern of severe early rejection that forced the patient to become independent at an early age. Information from both sources suggested that the patient was extremely fearful of intimacy. He guarded against it by internally structuring the world as a place in which people did things only because they were following someone else's orders.

On the basis of this formulation, a treatment plan was arrived at. First, the staff and therapist would avoid at all costs getting caught up in the patient's authoritarian way of relating, and would point out to him when he was using such techniques. Second, they would suggest, by explanation or, preferably, by interactional example, new ways of relating to others. Finally, they would continue to correlate the specifics of staff-patient interaction with therapy sessions.

There is a clear difference between the staff's role and the therapist's role, but the exercise of the two should be integrated through repeated consultation. The staff's emphasis is on identifying the problem for the patient, in the here-and-now, and suggesting alternative modes of behavior; the therapist focuses on the historical antecedents of the problem and on the patient's resistance to change. In a smoothly functioning unit, the continuing relationship between the patient and individual staff members provides material for psychotherapy and also gives the patient an opportunity to try out new behaviors. Dynamic psychotherapy and milieu therapy are thus integrated into an effective over-all treatment plan.

Identity Diffusion

The needs of another patient centered on her problem of identity diffusion. This 24-year-old schizophrenic girl was depressed, self-depreciatory, and subtly uncooperative with unit rules and routine. The staff described her as a patient who tended to "hide." No one knew her very well, and almost no one showed any interest in her. To one nurse, she was "not a real person." The validity of this feeling was confirmed by the therapist, who saw her as someone with a very vague sense of identity.

The patient responded to interpretations and confrontations by readily agreeing with everything that was said and then parroting it back. The staff gradually became aware that she actively sought out their comments as a way of avoiding self-definition. She maintained her "nonself" by consciously and unconsciously extracting from the world other people's definitions of her, which she could then present as herself.

It was therefore decided not to offer the patient definite interpretations or confrontation, but rather to concentrate on helping her define herself as a person. In their day-to-day contacts with her, nurses and aides would attempt to find out what kind of a person she already was. They would try to determine her interests, her background, her likes and dislikes, and her opinions on contemporary events. The staff's approach would be guided by the general proposition that "We won't tell you who you are, but *you* can tell us who you are."

If this approach is pursued in a steadfast, consistent manner, it teaches such a patient that she has something to offer to herself as well as to others, that she can be an initiator as well as a passive imitator, and that she can have constructive impact on others. Not uncommonly, such persons have had a parent figure who demanded the right to define them in exchange for doling out security. The patient may repeatedly try to reestablish that kind of relationship on the ward; only after considerable testing, during which the staff refuse to play the parent role, will the patient be convinced that things are now different and it is safe to grow.

This case illustrates one of the pitfalls of confrontation in milieu therapy. Patients with severe identity pathology are apt to show a chameleonlike tendency to conform their insight, their behavior, and even their feelings to the expectations of others. The nursing staff must avoid interpretative statements and instead ask questions designed to draw the patient out, insisting that he define himself.

Hospital Dependency

A common problem is the patient for whom the secondary gain of using the hospital as a refuge outweighs any motivation to return to outside living. Often such patients are elderly single women in straitened financial circumstances who become seriously depressed, disorganized, and suicidal. Within a few days after admission, much of the depression remits, and the patient makes a good adjustment to the hospital. Only when discharge is considered does it become apparent that the patient hopes to use the hospital as a permanent refuge. Though clinging to the hospital may take the form of a recurrence of symptoms, it more often appears as a helplessness in coping with the details of discharge planning: arranging living accommodations, seeking a job, dealing with welfare agencies, or even filling out forms or making appointments.

Sometimes such patients show an astonishing ability to blot out any thought of the future. A 69-year-old woman who was hospitalized because of depression and severe weight loss remained in the hospital for several months due to a series of physical problems resulting from malnutrition. When her physical condition was finally stable, she was asked about her plans. She appeared surprised at the question and insisted that she had never given a single thought to the future. She had denied the whole problem of future living arrangements and assumed that she could remain in the hospital indefinitely.

It is imperative to spot potentially hospital-dependent patients as early as possible. Characteristically they tend to feel threatened by any acknowledgement or discovery of their internal resources, because they view helplessness as a way of compelling others to provide them with security. They are often quite adept at provoking guilt in others. Their view of the future, insofar as they view it at all, is a polarized one in which they either stand absolutely alone or are totally dependent.

Therapy hinges on staff's acknowledging the anxiety associated with any successful step toward independence, and helping the patient develop a clearer sense of his future. However, merely gaining insight does not motivate him to plan constructively for the future. Three steps are important in the mobilization process.

First, immediately after the patient emerges from the acute disturbance that precipitated his admission, a discharge date must be set unequivocally, and the patient must be repeatedly reminded of it. Second, the highest priority must be given to encouraging self-reliance, the assumption of responsibility, and the making of independent decisions. The patient should be charged with responsibility for planning his own activities and handling dealings with public agencies, halfway houses, and clinics. At the same time, his tendency to polarize his view of the future should be acknowledged and discussed. Finally, hospital-dependent patients must be encouraged to talk about the future, not only with the therapist but also with the nursing staff, and most especially to talk about it in specific practical detail.

This kind of persistent focusing on the future may bring to light unrealistic fantasies even in those patients who do accept the inevitability of discharge. For example, a 62-year-old single secretary who had recently lost her job imagined that she would be taken into the household of her wealthy married sister. A family conference was held in which she was disabused of that idea, and referral to a welfare-supported residence was made. This is an example of how family therapy techniques can be utilized to help the overly dependent patient face the future more realistically.

Forming a Treatment Plan

The milieu therapy plans we have described evolved out of spontaneous discussion at unit meetings; they were based on operational diagnoses, collectively arrived at, of the patients' needs. Such a treatment program requires a level of staff cohesion and self-awareness that is by no means easy to achieve. To facilitate the freest possible discussion in unit conferences, staff should be encouraged to describe patients in non-clinical terms, supporting their descriptions with specific episodes and conversations reported in everyday language. And staff must report not only what the patient says and does but also their own responses, whether effective or not, and their own feelings.

If communication is free, and nurses and aides are confident that their information is potentially useful, the critical issues for the milieu therapy of the specific patient will emerge. When staff's information is combined with relevant information from the treating psychiatrist, a plan of treatment usually begins to take form. The staff's sense of usefulness will initially depend on how much of what they say goes in a visible way into the plan, as well as how much support and encouragement they receive to participate in its execution.

The treatment plan should be expressed in one or more simple statements about the problem; it will serve as a general guideline for nurses and aides in their daily contact with the patient. A typical statement might be, "This patient tends to deny anger and needs to be encouraged to accept his hostile feelings." Another might be, "This patient needs to develop a firmer sense of his own identity."

The statements should help define the goals of treatment rather than prescribe specific responses. Thus the nurse or aide is freer to use his own resources and personal style in moving toward the goals. And the statements must reflect the feelings and behavior observed by the staff rather than being tailored to fit the theoretical bias of the psychiatrist. Above all, they must be practical. Too often the tendency is to define goals or prescribe treatment in terms that are too abstract to be of practical use.

In establishing and carrying out a treatment plan, the patient's impact on the staff must also be taken into account. For example, no therapist should expect a patient to receive continuous warmth and attention from staff if he spends all his time being hostile. In individual sessions the therapist may be exposed to the lonely, frightened person underneath the hostility who, from the therapist's perspective, primarily needs nurturing. However, if on the ward the patient is experiencing recall of another aspect of his earlier situation—such as his rage at deprivation of nurturing—the ward staff may see a very different picture of him. Understandably, they may not respond as the therapist hopes.

The reverse situation can also occur: the staff may pick up personality assets or encouraging signs of change while the therapist remains the focus of the patient's negativism or rage. In either case, the conflicting pictures must be integrated through continuing free communication between the therapist and staff.

Milieu therapy must be viewed as a highly dynamic process, and the treatment plans for individual patients must be subject to continuous review and modification. A plan that is responsive to the needs of a disorganized patient will be irrelevant when that patient reorganizes. When a patient who must be confronted when he acts out begins to control his behavior and face his underlying depression, his needs become entirely different. As the patient changes, the staff must redefine their goals for him.

Some Pitfalls of Milieu Therapy

In the foregoing discussion we focused on structuring the interaction between the staff and the patient to promote constructive behavioral change. This is the essential task of milieu therapy. Unfortunately we may have lost sight of it in our preoccupation with such matters as democratizing the milieu, intensifying the ways patients may be confronted with their behavior, and delegating therapeutic responsibility to the patient community. The more pedestrian question of what staff members can actually say and do that will help patients move toward health tends to be neglected in our enthusiasm for structural innovation.

While almost any change may have a stimulating effect, we must recognize the danger of relying too much on innovative policies and procedures at the expense of good hard thinking about the specific problems of individual patients. Some of the innovations may be no more than gimmicks; although harmless in themselves, they may have the unnoticed effects of distracting staff from difficult problems of treatment and of encouraging complacency. Staff can fall into the error of thinking that because their unit is more innovative than traditionally operated units, it also must be more therapeutic.

There is another danger to which we must be alert. In a milieu therapy program, the behavior of staff as well as of patients is subjected to extremely close scrutiny. Individual nurses and aides are called on to deepen their understanding of behavioral dynamics and expand their repertoire of therapeutic responses. Having their performance exposed may prove too stressful, and insecure staff members may find a convenient hiding place in an elaborate program of ward meetings and patient committees. The staff as a group may take refuge in the principle of "all power to the patients," thus covertly abdicating responsibility for thoughtful treatment.

Milieu therapy programs have been based on certain basic concepts that can be built into a therapeutic environment. The most important of them appear to be free communication, participation in a democratic group process, the fostering of a cohesive community that can confront patients with their behavior and its social consequences, and the expectation that the patient participate actively in his own treatment instead of simply assuming the "sick" role. Those concepts can hardly be challenged. Their introduction has been associated with substantial progress in hospital treatment.

However, there is a risk that the old institutionalism of the state hospital may be giving way to a new institutionalism of the therapeutic community. To counter this possibility, we must refocus attention on the individual, and insist that the milieu be flexible enough to provide treatment programs tailored to the varied needs of individual patients. As a starting point, two questions about the newly admitted patient must be answered as soon as possible: what is this patient unable to do for himself, and how can we help him do it in a way that we may ultimately become unnecessary to him?

An effective milieu should be able to provide for the patient who is unaware of his emotions or unable to express them constructively, and for the patient who is unable to control emotions and is easily overwhelmed by them. It should be able to provide controls for the impulsive patient, flexibility for the constricted patient, confrontation for the patient with character pathology, and support for the patient in affective turmoil. The distrustful patient must be helped to feel secure, but the overly dependent patient must be firmly and rapidly mobilized. The patient who needs insight must receive appropriate interpretations, while the patient who conforms his behavior to the expectations of others must be nourished toward self-definition.

ISSUES,
CONTROVERSIES,
AND SOME
ALTERNATIVE
APPROACHES

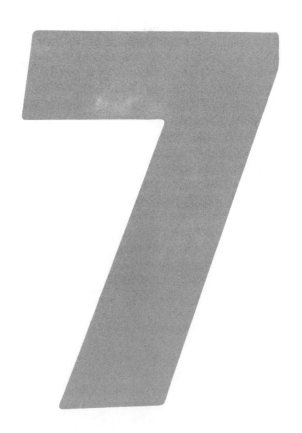

Introduction

What is "mental illness"? How well are we able to distinguish sanity from insanity, normal from abnormal? Do psychiatric diagnoses have any validity other than providing a set of labels for behavior we do not understand or agree with? For the final unit, we have selected several articles which question some of the assumptions underlying what happens in therapy sessions and psychiatric treatment settings. The authors' lack of agreement about possible answers may be discouraging to those who hope for definite guidelines and value-free diagnoses, but this is a field where practitioners must ultimately make their own moral and philosophical decisions.

In the first acticle Rosenhan (1973) describes a study in which "normal" people sought admission to mental hospitals; the results proved both controversial and disturbing. Following a thought-provoking discussion of the implications of the study for psychiatric diagnosis, Rosenhan presents an equally significant discussion of the experience of psychiatric hospitalization as recorded and reported by these "pseudopatients". Analyzing the data, Rosenhan attempts to identify sources of the powerlessness and depersonalization that characterized the patient experience in even the newest, best-staffed hospitals. His conclusions should prompt all readers to look more closely and critically at their attitudes towards clients.

The issues of labeling and psychiatric diagnosis are also the subject of the second article. Ventura (1975) attempts to answer three questions related to these issues: "First, is it useful to put clients in diagnostic categories? Secondly, how adequate are the diagnostic classification systems that we use today? Thirdly, what other alternatives are available?" As Ventura points out, there are definite advantages, as well as problems, which result from labeling behavior according to a system such as the American Psychiatric Association's *Diagnostic and Statistical Manual of Mental Disorders.* The DSM-II System is utilized to some extent at most agencies and hospitals which employ psychiatric nurses; consequently, nurses must be aware of the issues involved in the process of labeling whether or not they use the labels in their own work.

In the next article, Halleck (1971) calls our attention to political and moral implications of psychiatric-mental health practice. These issues are more noticeable when therapists work with prisoners, ghetto populations, and others living in oppressive social environments, but, Halleck contends, conflicts between the needs and goals of individual clients and their social environments are inevitable. The question is: when should the therapist direct her or his efforts toward changing the social milieu rather than toward helping the individual adjust to that milieu? Although Halleck's article is directed toward psychiatrists, and although some of his arguments reflect the student unrest of the Vietnam War period when the article was written, the concerns he raises are equally relevant today and also affect other mental health professionals.

Nurses, by virtue of their generalized preparation, have unique responsibility for considering the physical as well as emotional health needs of clients. Much progress has been made toward recognizing that clients do not leave their sexuality at the admissions office of an inpatient treatment setting, but this whole area is still too readily overlooked or avoided. Abernathy et al. (1976) deal directly with the problem of birth control for hospitalized psychiatric patients. In this article, the authors share their experiences in developng effective family planning programs in psychiatric hospitals, as well as their thinking about patients' rights and the risks and benefits of particular contraceptives for this client group.

In preceding units, articles concerning the use of operant conditioning, group therapy, and family systems approaches represent some of the philosophical and theoretical positions that now challenge the once dominant psychoanalytic and medical/disease models of practice. Transactional Analysis and Gestalt Therapy are additional examples of approaches that have gained considerable popularity, especially in outpatient treatment. Transactional Analysis, often called, "TA", may be familiar to many nurses and clients from popular books such as Berne's *Games People Play* and Harris's *I'm OK - You're OK.* The article by Babcock (1976) describes the basic concepts of TA and, with examples nures will recognize as all-too-familiar, illustrates how the TA system can help nurses understand and improve communications among themselves, as well as between themselves and clients. None of Babcock's examples concern identified psychiatric clients, but the same concepts are used in psychotherapy with individuals, groups, and families. Gestalt Therapy is described in the article by Resnick (1974). Like TA, Gestalt Therapy emphasizes the client's present experiences rather than the past, and, as the title indicates, attempts to help clients integrate and take responsibility for their own thoughts, feelings, and actions rather than attribute them to a disease process.

Depending on the point of view of the observer, control over the client's own behavior and environment in a psychiatric hospital may be regarded as a violation of individual autonomy or one of the most effective techniques for promoting healthy functioning. The token economy system employed on behavior modification units like the one described by Burley and Steiger (1972) is explicitly designed to change problem behaviors by controlling the consequences of those behaviors. Clients are paid for desired behaviors such as proper grooming with tokens that can be exchanged for "goodies"; undesired behaviors such as hitting someone result in the loss of tokens. This article focuses on a description of how the behavior modification system was implemented rather than on the ethical issues involved with such a treatment milieu, but the authors anticipate some questions which might be raised by explaining the theoretical rationale for this system and enumerating positive changes in staff and client behavior which they believe support this particular approach.

"Hour after hour, day after day, health and social service professionals are intimately involved with troubled human beings. What happens to people who work intensely with others, learning their psychological, social, or physical problems?" In the last article, Maslach (1976) provides some unsettling answers to that question, which is the core of her research on how persons in the helping professions cope with stress. Nurses, psychiatrists, poverty lawyers, social workers, and others are subject to similar stresses, and when the situation becomes overwhelming they may experience "burnout". In most settings, including psychiatric wards, the time said to be required for this emotional distancing was two years or less! Is "burnout" inevitable? Maslach does not think so, and her report indicates some factors which have potential for decreasing this appalling loss of human energy and concern.

This unit is an introduction to the issues, controversies, and alternative approaches in psychiatric-mental health nursing. A number of other approaches—such as primal scream therapy, encounter groups, community organization for change, other forms of behavior therapy, and the new sex therapies—have not been included in this collection of readings. The editors would like to caution readers not to interpret their absence as an indication that such approaches are not significant in contemporary psychiatric-mental health practice. Space limitations (compounded by the lack of reasonably neutral presentations of some approaches) restricted our selection to a few which we believe will provoke discontent with complacent acceptance of the status quo and stimulate curiosity about alternatives which may improve and expand our nursing practice.

37 ON BEING SANE IN INSANE PLACES

D. L. Rosenhan, Ph.D.

IF SANITY AND INSANITY EXIST, HOW SHALL WE know them?

The question is neither capricious nor itself insane. However much we may be personally convinced that we can tell the normal from the abnormal, the evidence is simply not compelling. It is commonplace, for example, to read about murder trials wherein eminent psychiatrists for the defense are contradicted by equally eminent psychiatrists for the prosecution on the matter of the defendant's sanity. More generally, there are a great deal of conflicting data on the reliability, utility, and meaning of such terms as "sanity," "insanity," "mental illness," and "schizophrenia" (1). Finally, as early as 1934, Benedict suggested that normality and abnormality are not universal (2). What is viewed as normal in one culture may be seen as quite aberrant in another. Thus, notions of normality and abnormality may not be quite as accurate as people believe they are.

To raise questions regarding normality and abnormality is in no way to question the fact that some behaviors are deviant or odd. Murder is deviant. So, too, are hallucinations. Nor does raising such questions deny the existence of the personal anguish that is often associated with "mental illness." Anxiety and depression exist. Psychological suffering exists. But normality and abnormality, sanity and insanity, and the diagnoses that flow from them may be less substantive than many believe them to be.

At its heart, the question of whether the sane can be distinguished from the insane (and whether degrees of insanity can be distinguished from each other) is a simple matter: do the salient characteristics that lead to diagnoses reside in the patients themselves or in the environments and contexts in which observers find them? From Bleuler, through Kretchmer, through the formulators of the recently revised *Diagnostic and Statistical Manual* of the American Psychiatric Association, the belief has been strong that patients present symptoms, that those symptoms can be categorized, and, implicitly, that the sane are distinguishable from the insane. More recently, however, this belief has been questioned. Based in part on theoretical and anthropological considerations, but also on philosophical, legal, and therapeutic ones, the view has grown that psychological categorization of mental illness is useless at best and downright harmful, misleading, and pejorative at worst. Psychiatric diagnoses, in this view, are in the minds of the observers and are not valid summaries of characteristics displayed by the observed (3-5).

Gains can be made in deciding which of these is more nearly accurate by getting normal people (that is, people who do not have, and have never suffered, symptoms of serious psychiatric disorders) admitted to psychiatric hospitals and then determining whether they were discovered to be sane and, if so, how. If the sanity of such pseudopatients were always detected, there would be prima facie evidence that a sane individual can be distinguished from the insane context in which he is found. Normality (and presumably abnormality) is distinct enough that it can be recognized wherever it occurs, for it is carried within the person. If, on the other hand, the sanity of the pseudopatients were never discovered, serious difficulties would arise for those who support traditional modes of psychiatric diagnosis. Given that the hospital staff was not incompetent, that the pseudopatient had been behaving as sanely as he had been outside of the hospital, and that it had never been previously suggested that he belonged in a psychiatric hospital, such an unlikely outcome would support the view that psychiatric diagnosis betrays little about the patient but much about the environment in which an observer finds him.

This article describes such an experiment. Eight sane people gained secret admission to 12 different hospitals (6). Their diagnostic experiences constitute the data of the first part of this article; the remainder is devoted to a description of their experiences in psychiatric institutions. Too few psychiatrists and psychologists, even those who have worked in such hospitals, know what the experience is like. They rarely talk about it with former patients, perhaps because they distrust information coming from the previously insane. Those who have worked in psychiatric hospitals are likely to have adapted so thoroughly to the settings that they are insensitive to the impact of that experience. And while there have been occasional reports of researchers who submitted themselves to psychiatric hospitalization (7), these researchers have commonly remained in the hospitals for short periods of time, often with the knowledge of the hospital staff. It is difficult to know the extent to which they were treated like patients or like research colleagues. Nevertheless, their reports about the inside of the psychiatric hospital have been valuable. This article extends those efforts.

Pseudopatients and Their Settings

The eight pseudopatients were a varied group. One was a psychology graduate student in his 20's. The remaining seven were older and "established." Among them were three psychologists, a pediatrician, a psychiatrist, a painter, and a housewife. Three pseudopatients were women, five were men. All of them employed pseudonyms, lest their alleged diagnoses embarrass them later. Those who were in mental health professions alleged another occupation in order to avoid the special attentions that might be accorded by staff, as a matter of courtesy or caution, to ailing colleagues (8). With the exception of myself (I was the first pseudopatient and my presence was known to the hospital administrator and chief psychologist and, so far as I can tell, to them alone), the presence of pseudopatients and the nature of the research program was not known to the hospital staffs (9).

The settings were similarly varied. In order to generalize the findings, admission into a variety of hospitals was sought. The 12 hospitals in the sample were located in five different states on the East and West coasts. Some were old and shabby, some were quite new. Some were research-oriented, others not. Some had good staff-patient ratios, others were quite understaffed. Only one was a strictly private hospital. All of the others were supported by state or federal funds or, in one instance, by university funds.

After calling the hospital for an appointment, the pseudopatient arrived at the admissions office complaining that he had been hearing voices. Asked what the voices said, he replied that they were often unclear, but as far as he could tell they said "empty," "hollow," and "thud." The voices were unfamiliar and were of the same sex as the pseudopatient. The choice of these symptoms was occasioned by their apparent similarity to existential symptoms. Such symptoms are alleged to arise from painful concerns about the perceived meaninglessness of one's life. It is as if the hallucinating person were saying, "My life is empty and hollow." The choice of these symptoms was also determined by the *absence* of a single report of existential psychoses in the literature.

Beyond alleging the symptoms and falsifying name, vocation, and employment, no further alterations of person, history, or circumstances were made. The significant events of the pseudopatient's life history were presented as they had actually occurred. Relationships with parents and siblings, with spouse and children, with people at work and in school, consistent with the aforementioned exceptions, were described as they were or had been. Frustrations and upsets were described along with joys and satisfactions. These facts are important to remember. If anything, they strongly biased the subsequent results in favor of detecting sanity, since none of their histories or current behaviors were seriously pathological in any way.

Immediately upon admission to the psychiatric ward, the pseudopatient ceased simulating *any* symptoms of abnormality. In some cases, there was a brief period of mild nervousness and anxiety, since none of the pseudopatients really believed that they would be admitted so easily. Indeed, their shared fear was that they would be immediately exposed as frauds and greatly embarrassed. Moreover, many of them had never visited a psychiatric ward; even those who had, nevertheless had some genuine fears about what might happen to them. Their nervousness, then, was quite appropriate to the novelty of the hospital setting, and it abated rapidly.

Apart from that short-lived nervousness, the pseudopatient behaved on the ward as he "normally" behaved. The pseudopatient spoke to patients and staff as he might ordinarily. Because there is uncommonly little to do on a psychiatric ward, he attempted to engage others in conversation. When asked by staff how he was feeling, he indicated that he was fine, that he no longer experienced symptoms. He responded to instructions from attendants, to calls for medication (which was not swallowed), and to dining-hall instructions. Beyond such activities as were available to him on the admissions ward, he spent his time writing down his observations about the ward, its patients, and the staff. Initially these notes were written "secretly," but as it soon became clear that no one much cared, they were subsequently written on standard tablets of paper in such public places as the dayroom. No secret was made of these activities.

The pseudopatient, very much as a true psychiatric patient, entered a hospital with no foreknowledge of when he would be discharged. Each was told that he would have to get out by his own devices, essentially by convincing the staff that he was sane. The psychological stresses associated with hospitalization were considerable, and all but one of the pseudopatients desired to be discharged almost immediately after being admitted. They were, therefore, motivated not only to behave sanely, but to be paragons of cooperation. That their behavior was in no way disruptive is confirmed by nursing reports, which have been obtained on most of the patients. These reports uniformly indicate that the patients were "friendly," "cooperative," and "exhibited no abnormal indications."

The Normal Are Not Detectably Sane

Despite their public "show" of sanity, the pseudopatients were never detected. Admitted, except in one case, with a diagnosis of schizophrenia (10), each was discharged with a diagnosis of schizophrenia "in remission." The label "in remission" should in no way be dismissed as a formality, for at no time during any hospitalization had any question been raised about any pseudopatient's simulation. Nor are there any indications in the hospital records that the pseudopatient's status was suspect. Rather, the evidence is strong that, once labeled schizophrenic, the pseudopatient was stuck with that label. If the pseudopatient was to be discharged, he must naturally be "in remission"; but he was not sane, nor, in the institution's view, had he ever been sane.

The uniform failure to recognize sanity cannot be attributed to the quality of the hospitals, for, although there were considerable variations among them, several are considered excellent. Nor can it be alleged that there was simply not enough time to observe the pseudopatients. Length of hospitalization ranged from 7 to 52 days, with an average of 19 days. The pseudopatients were not, in fact, carefully observed, but this failure clearly speaks more to traditions within psychiatric hospitals than to lack of opportunity.

Finally, it cannot be said that the failure to recognize the pseudopatients' sanity was due to the fact that they were not behaving sanely. While there was clearly some tension present in all of them, their daily visitors could detect no serious behavioral consequences—nor, indeed, could other patients. It was quite common for the patients to "detect" the pseudopatients' sanity. During the first three hospitalizations, when accurate counts were kept, 35 of a total of 118 patients on the admissions ward voiced their suspicions, some vigorously. "You're not crazy. You're a journalist, or a professor [referring to the continual note-taking]. You're checking up on the hospital." While most of the patients were reassured by the pseudopatient's insistence that he had been sick before he came in but was fine now, some continued to believe that the pseudopatient was sane throughout his hospitalization (11). The fact that the patients often recognized normality when staff did not raises important questions.

Failure to detect sanity during the course of hospitalization may be due to the fact that physicians operate with a strong bias toward what statisticians call the type 2 error (5). This is to say that physicians are more inclined to call a healthy person sick (a false positive, type 2) than a sick person healthy (a false negative, type 1). The reasons for this are not hard to find: it is clearly more dangerous to misdiagnose illness than health. Better to err on the side of caution, to suspect illness even among the healthy.

But what holds for medicine does not hold equally well for psychiatry. Medical illnesses, while unfortunate, are not commonly pejorative. Psychiatric diagnoses, on the contrary, carry with them personal, legal, and social stigmas (12). It was therefore important to see whether the tendency toward diagnosing the sane insane could be reversed. The following experiment was arranged at a research and teaching hospital whose staff had heard these findings but doubted that such an error could occur in their hospital. The staff was informed that at some time during the following 3 months, one or more pseudopatients would attempt to be admitted into the psychiatric hospital. Each staff member was asked to rate each patient who presented himself at admissions or on the ward according to the likelihood that the patient was a pseudopatient. A 10-point scale was used, with a 1 and 2 reflecting high confidence that the patient was a pseudopatient.

Judgments were obtained on 193 patients who were admitted for psychiatric treatment. All staff who had had sustained contact with or primary responsibility for the patient—attendants, nurses, psychiatrists, physicians, and psychologists—were asked to make judgments. Forty-one patients were alleged, with high confidence, to be pseudopatients by at least one member of the staff. Twenty-three were considered suspect by at least one psychiatrist. Nineteen were suspected by one psychiatrist *and* one other staff member. Actually, no genuine pseudopatient (at least from my group) presented himself during this period.

The experiment is instructive. It indicates that the tendency to designate sane people as insane can be reversed when the stakes (in this case, prestige and diagnostic acumen) are high. But what can be said of the 19 people who were suspected of being "sane" by one psychiatrist and another staff member? Were these people truly "sane," or was it rather the case that in the course of avoiding the type 2 error the staff tended to make more errors of the first sort—calling the crazy "sane"? There is no way of knowing. But one thing is certain: any diagnostic process that lends itself so readily to massive errors of this sort cannot be a very reliable one.

The Stickiness of Psychodiagnostic Labels

Beyond the tendency to call the healthy sick—a tendency that accounts better for diagnostic behavior on admission than it does for such behavior after a lengthy period of exposure—the data speak to the massive role of labeling in psychiatric assessment. Having once been labeled schizophrenic, there is nothing the pseudopatient can do to overcome the tag. The tag profoundly colors others' perceptions of him and his behavior.

From one viewpoint, these data are hardly surprising, for it has long been known that elements are given meaning by the context in which they occur. Gestalt psychology made this point vigorously, and Asch (13) demonstrated that there are "central" personality traits (such as "warm" versus "cold") which are so powerful that they remarkably color the meaning of other information in forming an impression of a given personality (14). "Insane," "schizophrenic," "manic-depressive," and "crazy" are probably among the most powerful of such central traits. Once a person is designated abnormal, all of his other behaviors and characteristics are colored by that label. Indeed, that label is so powerful that many of the pseudopatients' normal behaviors were overlooked entirely or profoundly misinterpreted. Some examples may clarify this issue.

Earlier I indicated that there were no changes in the pseudopatient's personal history and current status beyond those of name, employment, and, where necessary, vocation. Otherwise, a veridical description of personal history and circumstances was offered. Those circumstances were not psychotic. How were they made consonant with the diagnosis of psychosis? Or were those diagnoses modified in such a way as to bring them into accord with the circumstances of the pseudopatient's life, as described by him?

As far as I can determine, diagnoses were in no way affected by the relative health of the circumstances of a pseudopatient's life. Rather, the reverse occurred: the perception of his circumstances was shaped entirely by the diagnosis. A clear example of such translation is found in the case of a pseudopatient who had had a close relationship with his mother but was rather remote from his father during his early childhood. During adolescence and beyond, however, his father became a close friend, while his relationship with his mother cooled. His present relationship with his wife was characteristically close and warm. Apart from occasional angry exchanges, friction was minimal. The children had rarely been spanked. Surely there is nothing especially pathological about such a history. Indeed, many readers may see a similar pattern in their own experiences, with no markedly deleterious consequences. Observe, however, how such a history was translated in the psychopathological context, this from the case summary prepared after the patient was discharged.

This white 39-year-old male . . . manifests a long history of considerable ambivalence in close relationships, which begins in

early childhood. A warm relationship with his mother cools during
his adolescence. A distant relationship to his father is described as
becoming very intense. Affective stability is absent. His attempts to
control emotionality with his wife and children are punctuated by
angry outbursts and, in the case of the children, spankings. And
while he says that he has several good friends, one senses considerable ambivalence embedded in those relationships also. . . .

The facts of the case were unintentionally distorted by the staff to
achieve consistency with a popular theory of the dynamics of a
schizophrenic reaction (15). Nothing of an ambivalent nature had been
described in relations with parents, spouse, or friends. To the extent that
ambivalence could be inferred, it was probably not greater than is found
in all human relationships. It is true the pseudopatient's relationships
with his parents changed over time, but in the ordinary context that
would hardly be remarkable—indeed, it might very well be expected.
Clearly, the meaning ascribed to his verbalizations (that is, ambivalence,
affective instability) was determined by the diagnosis: schizophrenia. An
entirely different meaning would have been ascribed if it were known that
the man was "normal."

All pseudopatients took extensive notes publicly. Under ordinary circumstances, such behavior would have raised questions in the minds of
observers, as, in fact, it did among patients. Indeed, it seemed so certain
that the notes would elicit suspicion that elaborate precautions were
taken to remove them from the ward each day. But the precautions
proved needless. The closest any staff member came to questioning these
notes occurred when one pseudopatient asked his physician what kind of
medication he was receiving and began to write down the response. "You
needn't write it," he was told gently. "If you have trouble remembering,
just ask me again."

If no questions were asked of the pseudopatients, how was their writing interpreted? Nursing records for three patients indicate that the writing was seen as an aspect of their pathological behavior. "Patient engages
in writing behavior" was the daily nursing comment on one of the
pseudopatients who was never questioned about his writing. Given that
the patient is in the hospital, he must be psychologically disturbed. And
given that he is disturbed, continuous writing must be a behavioral
manifestation of that disturbance, perhaps a subset of the compulsive behaviors that are sometimes correlated with schizophrenia.

One tacit characteristic of psychiatric diagnosis is that it locates the
sources of aberration within the individual and only rarely within the

complex of stimuli that surrounds him. Consequently, behaviors that are stimulated by the environment are commonly misattributed to the patient's disorder. For example, one kindly nurse found a pseudopatient pacing the long hospital corridors. "Nervous, Mr. X?" she asked. "No, bored," he said.

The notes kept by pseudopatients are full of patient behaviors that were misinterpreted by well-intentioned staff. Often enough, a patient would go "berserk" because he had, wittingly or unwittingly, been mistreated by, say, an attendant. A nurse coming upon the scene would rarely inquire even cursorily into the environmental stimuli of the patient's behavior. Rather, she assumed that his upset derived from his pathology, not from his present interactions with other staff members. Occasionally, the staff might assume that the patient's family (especially when they had recently visited) or other patients had stimulated the outburst. But never were the staff found to assume that one of themselves or the structure of the hospital had anything to do with a patient's behavior. One psychiatrist pointed to a group of patients who were sitting outside the cafeteria entrance half an hour before lunchtime. To a group of young residents he indicated that such behavior was characteristic of the oral-acquisitive nature of the syndrome. It seemed not to occur to him that there were very few things to anticipate in a psychiatric hospital besides eating.

A psychiatric label has a life and an influence of its own. Once the impression has been formed that the patient is schizophrenic, the expectation is that he will continue to be schizophrenic. When a sufficient amount of time has passed, during which the patient has done nothing bizarre, he is considered to be in remission and available for discharge. But the label endures beyond discharge, with the unconfirmed expectation that he will behave as a schizophrenic again. Such labels, conferred by mental health professionals, are as influential on the patient as they are on his relatives and friends, and it should not surprise anyone that the diagnosis acts on all of them as a self-fulfilling prophecy. Eventually, the patient himself accepts the diagnosis, with all of its surplus meanings and expectations, and behaves accordingly (5).

The inferences to be made from these matters are quite simple. Much as Zigler and Phillips have demonstrated that there is enormous overlap in the symptoms presented by patients who have been variously diagnosed (16), so there is enormous overlap in the behaviors of the sane and the insane. The sane are not "sane" all of the time. We lose our tempers "for no good reason." We are occasionally depressed or anxious, again for no good reason. And we may find it difficult to get along with one or another person—again for no reason that we can specify. Similarly, the insane are not always insane. Indeed, it was the impression of the pseudopatients while living with them that they were sane for long periods of time—that the bizarre behaviors upon which their diagnoses were allegedly predicted constituted only a small fraction of their total behavior. If it makes no sense to label ourselves permanently depressed on the basis of an occasional depression, then it takes better evidence than is presently available to label all patients insane or schizophrenic on the basis of bizarre behaviors or cognitions. It seems more useful, as Mischel (17) has pointed out, to limit our discussions to *behaviors*, the stimuli that provoke them, and their correlates.

It is not known why powerful impressions of personality traits, such as "crazy" or "insane," arise. Conceivably, when the origins of and stimuli that give rise to a behavior are remote or unknown, or when the behavior strikes us as immutable, trait labels regarding the *behaver* arise. When, on the other hand, the origins and stimuli are known and available, discourse is limited to the behavior itself. Thus, I may hallucinate because I am sleeping, or I may hallucinate because I have ingested a peculiar drug. These are termed sleep-induced hallucinations, or dreams, and drug-induced hallucinations, respectively. But when the stimuli to my hallucinations are unknown, that is called craziness, or schizophrenia—as if that inference were somehow as illuminating as the others.

The Experience of Psychiatric Hospitalization

The term "mental illness" is of recent origin. It was coined by people who were humane in their inclinations and who wanted very much to raise the station of (and the public's sympathies toward) the psychologically disturbed from that of witches and "crazies" to one that was akin to the physically ill. And they were at least partially successful, for the treatment of the mentally ill *has* improved considerably over the years. But while treatment has improved, it is doubtful that people really regard the mentally ill in the same way that they view the physically ill. A broken leg is something one recovers from, but mental illness allegedly endures forever (18). A broken leg does not threaten the observer, but a crazy schizophrenic? There is by now a host of evidence that attitudes toward the mentally ill are characterized by fear, hostility, aloofness, suspicion, and dread (19). The mentally ill are society's lepers.

That such attitudes infect the general population is perhaps not surprising, only upsetting. But that they affect the professionals—attendants, nurses, physicians, psychologists, and social workers—who treat and deal with the mentally ill is more disconcerting, both because such attitudes are self-evidently pernicious and because they are unwitting. Most mental health professionals would insist that they are sympathetic toward the mentally ill, that they are neither avoidant nor hostile. But it is more likely that an exquisite ambivalence characterizes their relations with psychiatric patients, such that their avowed impulses are only part of their entire attitude. Negative attitudes are there too and can easily be detected. Such attitudes should not surprise us. They are the natural offspring of the labels patients wear and the places in which they are found.

Consider the structure of the typical psychiatric hospital. Staff and patients are strictly segregated. Staff have their own living space, including their dining facilities, bathrooms, and assembly places. The glassed quarters that contain the professional staff, which the pseudopatients came to call "the cage," sit out on every dayroom. The staff emerge primarily for caretaking purposes—to give medication, to conduct a therapy or group meeting, to instruct or reprimand a patient. Otherwise, staff keep to themselves, almost as if the disorder that afflicts their charges is somehow catching.

So much is patient-staff segregation the rule that, for four public hospitals in which an attempt was made to measure the degree to which staff and patients mingle, it was necessary to use "time out of the staff cage" as the operational measure. While it was not the case that all time spent out of the cage was spent mingling with patients (attendants, for example, would occasionally emerge to watch television in the dayroom), it was the only way in which one could gather reliable data on time for measuring.

The average amount of time spent by attendants outside of the cage was 11.3 percent (range, 3 to 52 percent). This figure does not represent only time spent mingling with patients, but also includes time spent on such chores as folding laundry, supervising patients while they shave, directing ward cleanup, and sending patients to off-ward activities. It was the relatively rare attendant who spent time talking with patients or playing games with them. It proved impossible to obtain a "percent mingling time" for nurses, since the amount of time they spent out of the cage was too brief. Rather, we counted instances of emergence from the cage. On the average, daytime nurses emerged from the cage 11.5 times per shift, including instances when they left the ward entirely (range, 4 to 39 times). Late afternoon and night nurses were even less available, emerging on the average 9.4 times per shift (range, 4 to 41 times). Data on early morning nurses, who arrived usually after midnight and departed at 8 a.m., are not available because patients were asleep during most of this period.

Physicians, especially psychiatrists, were even less available. They were rarely seen on the wards. Quite commonly, they would be seen only when they arrived and departed, with the remaining time being spent in their offices or in the cage. On the average, physicians emerged on the ward 6.7 times per day (range, 1 to 17 times). It proved difficult to make an accurate estimate in this regard, since physicians often maintained hours that allowed them to come and go at different times.

The hierarchial organization of the psychiatric hospital has been commented on before (20), but the latent meaning of that kind of organization is worth noting again. Those with the most power have least to do with patients, and those with the least power are most involved with them. Recall, however, that the acquisition of role-appropriate behaviors occurs mainly through the observation of others, with the most powerful having the most influence. Consequently, it is understandable that attendants not only spend more time with patients than do any other members of the staff—that is required by their station in the hierarchy—but also, insofar as they learn from their superiors' behavior, spend as little time with patients as they can. Attendants are seen mainly in the cage, which is where the models, the action, and the power are.

I turn now to a different set of studies, these dealing with staff response to patient-initiated contact. It has long been known that the amount of time a person spends with you can be an index of your significance to him. If he initiates and maintains eye contact, there is reason to believe that he is considering your requests and needs. If he pauses to chat or actually stops and talks, there is added reason to infer that he is individuating you. In four hospitals, the pseudopatient approached the staff member with a request which took the following form: "Pardon me, Mr. [or Dr. or Mrs.] X, could you tell me when I will be eligible for grounds privileges?" (or " . . . when I will be presented at the staff meeting?" or " . . . when I am likely to be discharged?"). While the content of the question varied according to the appropriateness of the target and the pseudopatient's (apparent) current needs the form was always a courteous and relevant request for information. Care was taken never to approach a particular member of the staff more than once a day, lest the staff member become suspicious or irritated. In examining these data, remember that the behavior of the pseudopatients was neither bizarre nor disruptive. One could indeed engage in good conversation with them.

The data for these experiments are shown in Table 1, separately for physicians (column 1) and for nurses and attendants (column 2). Minor differences between these four institutions were overwhelmed by the degree to which staff avoided continuing contacts that patients had initiated. By far, their most common response consisted of either a brief response to the question, offered while they were "on the move" and with head averted, or no response at all.

TABLE 1. SELF-INITIATED CONTACT BY PSEUDOPATIENTS WITH PSYCHIATRISTS AND NURSES AND ATTENDANTS, COMPARED TO CONTACT WITH OTHER GROUPS.

| | PSYCHIATRIC HOSPITALS | | UNIVERSITY CAMPUS (NONMEDICAL) | UNIVERSITY MEDICAL CENTER | | |
| | | | | PHYSICIANS | | |
CONTACT	(1) PSYCHI-ATRISTS	(2) NURSES AND ATTENDANTS	(3) FACULTY	(4) "LOOKING FOR A PSYCHIATRIST"	(5) "LOOKING FOR AN INTERNIST"	(6) NO ADDITIONAL COMMENT
Responses						
Moves on, head averted (%)	71	88	0	0	0	0
Makes eye contact (%)	23	10	0	11	0	0
Pauses and chats (%)	2	2	0	11	0	10
Stops and talks (%)	4	0.5	100	78	100	90
Mean number of questions answered (out of 6)	*	*	6	3.8	4.8	4.5
Respondents (No.)	13	47	14	18	15	10
Attempts (No.)	185	1283	14	18	15	10

*Not applicable.

417

The encounter frequently took the following bizarre form: (pseudopatient) "Pardon me, Dr. X. Could you tell me when I am eligible for grounds privileges?" (physician) "Good morning, Dave. How are you today?" (Moves off without waiting for a response.)

It is instructive to compare these data with data recently obtained at Stanford University. It has been alleged that large and eminent universities are characterized by faculty who are so busy that they have no time for students. For this comparison, a young lady approached individual faculty members who seemed to be walking purposefully to some meeting or teaching engagement and asked them the following six questions.

1) "Pardon me, could you direct me to Encina Hall?" (at the medical school: " . . . to the Clinical Research Center?").

2) "Do you know where Fish Annex is?" (there is no Fish Annex at Stanford).

3) "Do you teach here?"

4) "How does one apply for admission to the college?" (at the medical school: " . . . to the medical school?").

5) "Is it difficult to get in?"

6) "Is there financial aid?"

Without exception, as can be seen in Table 1 (column 3), all of the questions were answered. No matter how rushed they were, all respondents not only maintained eye contact, but stopped to talk. Indeed, many of the respondents went out of their way to direct or take the questioner to the office she was seeking, to try to locate "Fish Annex," or to discuss with her the possibilities of being admitted to the university.

Similar data, also shown in Table 1 (columns 4, 5, and 6), were obtained in the hospital. Here too, the young lady came prepared with six questions. After the first question, however, she remarked to 18 of her respondents (column 4), "I'm looking for a psychiatrist," and to 15 others (column 5), "I'm looking for an internist." Ten other respondents received no inserted comment (column 6). The general degree of cooperative responses is considerably higher for these university groups than it was for pseudopatients in psychiatric hospitals. Even so, differences are apparent within the medical school setting. Once having indicated that she was looking for a psychiatrist, the degree of cooperation elicited was less than when she sought an internist.

Powerlessness and Depersonalization

Eye contact and verbal contact reflect concern and individuation; their absence, avoidance and depersonalization. The data I have presented do not do justice to the rich daily encounters that grew up around matters of depersonalization and avoidance. I have records of patients who were beaten by staff for the sin of having initiated verbal contact. During my own experience, for example, one patient was beaten in the presence of other patients for having approached an attendant and told him, "I like you." Occasionally, punishment meted out to patients for misdemeanors seemed so excessive that is could not be justified by the most radical interpretations of psychiatric canon. Nevertheless, they appeared to go unquestioned. Tempers were often short. A patient who had not heard a call for medication would be roundly excoriated, and the morning attendants would often wake patients with, "Come on, you m-----f-----s, out of bed!"

Neither anecdotal nor "hard" data can convey the overwhelming sense of powerlessness which invades the individual as he is continually exposed to the depersonalization of the psychiatric hospital. It hardly matters *which* psychiatric hospital—the excellent public ones and the very plush private hospital were better than the rural and shabby ones in this regard, but, again, the features that psychiatric hospitals had in common overwhelmed by far their apparent differences.

Powerlessness was evident everywhere. The patient is deprived of many of his legal rights by dint of his psychiatric commitment (21). He is shorn of credibility by virtue of his psychiatric label. His freedom of movement is restricted. He cannot initiate contact with the staff, but may only respond to such overtures as they make. Personal privacy is minimal. Patient quarters and possessions can be entered and examined by any staff member, for whatever reason. His personal history and anguish is available to any staff member (often including the "grey lady" and "candy striper" volunteer) who chooses to read his folder, regardless of their therapeutic relationship to him. His personal hygiene and waste evacuation are often monitered. The water closets may have no doors.

At times, depersonalization reached such proportions that pseudopatients had the sense that they were invisible, or at least unworthy of account. Upon being admitted, I and other pseudopatients took the initial physical examinations in a semipublic room, where staff members went about their own business as if we were not there.

On the ward, attendants delivered verbal and occasionally serious physical abuse to patients in the presence of other observing patients, some of whom (the pseudopatients) were writing it all down. Abusive behavior, on the other hand, terminated quite abruptly when other staff members were known to be coming. Staff are credible witnesses. Patients are not.

A nurse unbuttoned her uniform to adjust her brassiere in the presence of an entire ward of viewing men. One did not have the sense that she was being seductive. Rather, she didn't notice us. A group of staff persons might point to a patient in the dayroom and discuss him animatedly, as if he were not there.

One illuminating instance of depersonalization and invisibility occurred with regard to medications. All told, the pseudopatients were administered nearly 2100 pills, including Elavil, Stelazine, Compazine, and Thorazine, to name but a few. (That such a variety of medications should have been administered to patients presenting identical symptoms is itself worthy of note.) Only two were swallowed. The rest were either pocketed or deposited in the toilet. The pseudopatients were not alone in this. Although I have no precise records on how many patients rejected their medications, the pseudopatients frequently found the medications of other patients in the toilet before they deposited their own. As long as they were cooperative, their behavior and the pseudopatients' own in this matter, as in other important matters, went unnoticed throughout.

Reactions to such depersonalization among pseudopatients were intense. Although they had come to the hospital as participant observers and were fully aware that they did not "belong," they nevertheless found themselves caught up in and fighting the process of depersonalization. Some examples: a graduate student in psychology asked his wife to bring his textbooks to the hospital so he could "catch up on his homework"—this despite the elaborate precautions taken to conceal his professional association. The same student, who had trained for quite some time to get into the hospital, and who had looked forward to the experience, "remembered" some drag races that he had wanted to see on the weekend and insisted that he be discharged by that time. Another pseudopatient attempted a romance with a nurse. Subsequently, he informed the staff that he was applying for admission to graduate school in psychology and was very likely to be admitted, since a graduate professor was one of his regular hospital visitors. The same person began to engage in psychotherapy with other patients—all of this as a way of becoming a person in an impersonal environment.

The Sources of Depersonalization

What are the origins of depersonalization? I have already mentioned two. First are attitudes held by all of us toward the mentally ill—including those who treat them—attitudes characterized by fear, distrust, and horrible expectations on the one hand, and benevolent intentions on the other. Our ambivalence leads, in this instance as in others, to avoidance.

Second, and not entirely separate, the hierarchical structure of the psychiatric hospital facilitates depersonalization. Those who are at the top have least to do with patients, and their behavior inspires the rest of the staff. Average daily contact with psychiatrists, psychologists, residents, and physicians combined ranged from 3.9 to 25.1 minutes, with an overall mean of 6.8 (six pseudopatients over a total of 129 days of hospitalization). Included in this average are time spent in the admissions interview, ward meetings in the presence of a senior staff member, group and individual psychotherapy contacts, case presentation conferences, and discharge meetings. Clearly, patients do not spend much time in interpersonal contact with doctoral staff. And doctoral staff serve as models for nurses and attendants.

There are probably other sources. Psychiatric installations are presently in serious financial straits. Staff shortages are pervasive, staff time at a premium. Something has to give, and that something is patient contact. Yet, while financial stresses are realities, too much can be made of them. I have the impression that the psychological forces that result in depersonalization are much stronger than the fiscal ones and that the addition of more staff would not correspondingly improve patient care in this regard. The incidence of staff meetings and the enormous amount of record-keeping on patients, for example, have not been as substantially reduced as has patient contact. Priorities exist, even during hard times. Patient contact is not a significant priority in the traditional psychiatric hospital, and fiscal pressures do not account for this. Avoidance and depersonalization may.

Heavy reliance upon psychotropic medication tacitly contributes to depersonalization by convincing staff that treatment is indeed being conducted and that further patient contact may not be necessary. Even here, however, caution needs to be exercised in understanding the role of psychotropic drugs. If patients were powerful rather than powerless, if they were viewed as interesting individuals rather than diagnostic entities, if they were socially significant rather than social lepers, if their anguish truly and wholly compelled our sympathies and concerns, would we not *seek* contact with them, despite the availability of medications? Perhaps for the pleasure of it all?

The Consequences of Labeling and Depersonalization

Whenever the ratio of what is known to what needs to be known approaches zero, we tend to invent "knowledge" and assume that we understand more than we actually do. We seem unable to acknowledge that we simply don't know. The needs for diagnosis and remediation of behavioral and emotional problems are enormous. But rather than acknowledge that we are just embarking on understanding, we continue to label patients "schizophrenic," "manic-depressive," and "insane," as if in those words we had captured the essence of understanding. The facts of the matter are that we have known for a long time that diagnoses are often not useful or reliable, but we have nevertheless continued to use them. We now know that we cannot distinguish insanity from sanity. It is depressing to consider how that information will be used.

Not merely depressing, but frightening. How many people, one wonders, are sane but not recognized as such in our psychiatric institutions? How many have been needlessly stripped of their privileges of citizenship, from the right to vote and drive to that of handling their own accounts? How many have feigned insanity in order to avoid the criminal consequences of their behavior, and, conversely, how many would rather stand trial than live interminably in a psychiatric hospital—but are wrongly thought to be mentally ill? How many have been stigmatized by well-intentioned, but nevertheless erroneous, diagnoses? On the last point, recall again that a "type 2 error" in psychiatric diagnosis does not have the same consequences it does in medical diagnosis. A diagnosis of cancer that has been found to be in error is cause for celebration. But psychiatric diagnoses are rarely found to be in error. The label sticks, a mark of inadequacy forever.

Finally, how many patients might be "sane" outside the psychiatric hospital but seem insane in it—not because craziness resides in them, as it were, but because they are responding to a bizarre setting, one that may be unique to institutions which harbor nether people? Goffman (4) calls the process of socialization to such institutions "mortification"—an apt metaphor that includes the processes of depersonalization that have been described here. And while it is impossible to know whether the pseudopatients' responses to these processes are characteristic of all inmates—they were, after all, not real patients—it is difficult to believe that these processes of socialization to a psychiatric hospital provide useful attitudes or habits of response for living in the "real world."

Summary and Conclusions

It is clear that we cannot distinguish the sane from the insane in psychiatric hospitals. The hospital itself imposes a special environment in which the meanings of behavior can easily be misunderstood. The consequences to patients hospitalized in such an environment—the powerlessness, depersonalization, segregation, mortification, and self-labeling—seem undoubtedly countertherapeutic.

I do not, even now, understand this problem well enough to perceive solutions. But two matters seem to have some promise. The first concerns

the proliferation of community mental health facilities, of crisis intervention centers, of the human potential movement, and of behavior therapies
that, for all of their own problems, tend to avoid psychiatric labels, to
focus on specific problems and behaviors, and to retain the individual in a
relatively nonpejorative environment. Clearly, to the extent that we re-
frain from sending the distressed to insane places, our impressions of
them are less likely to be distorted. (The risk of distorted perceptions, it
seems to me, is always present, since we are much more sensitive to an
individual's behaviors and verbalizations than we are to the subtle
contextual stimuli that often promote them. At issue here is a matter of
magnitude. And, as I have shown, the magnitude of distortion is exceedingly high in the extreme context that is a psychiatric hospital.)

The second matter that might prove promising speaks to the need to
increase the sensitivity of mental health workers and researchers to the
Catch 22 position of psychiatric patients. Simply reading materials in this
area will be of help to some such workers and researchers. For others,
directly experiencing the impact of psychiatric hospitalization will be of
enormous use. Clearly, further research into the social psychology of such
total institutions will both facilitate treatment and deepen understanding.

I and the other pseudopatients in the psychiatric setting had distinctly
negative reactions. We do not pretend to describe the subjective
experiences of true patients. Theirs may be different from ours, particularly with the passage of time and the necessary process of adaptation to
one's environment. But we can and do speak to the relatively more objective indices of treatment within the hospital. It could be a mistake, and a
very unfortunate one, to consider that what happened to us derived from
malice or stupidity on the part of the staff. Quite the contrary, our
overwhelming impression of them was of people who really cared, who
were committed and who were uncommonly intelligent. Where they
failed, as they sometimes did painfully, it would be more accurate to attribute those failures to the environment in which they, too, found
themselves than to personal callousness. Their perceptions and behavior
were controlled by the situation, rather than being motivated by a mali-
cious disposition. In a more benign environment, one that was less attached to global diagnosis, their behaviors and judgments might have
been more benign and effective.

References and Notes

1. P. Ash, *J. Abnorm. Soc. Psychol.* **44**, 272 (1949); A. T. Becker,
    Amer. J. Psychiat. **119**, 210 (1962); A. T. Boisen, *Psychiatry* **2**, 233

(1938); N. Kreitman, *J. Ment. Sci.* **107**, 876 (1961); N. Kreitman, P. Sainsbury, J. Morrisey, J. Towers, J. Scrivener, *ibid.*, p. 887; H. O. Schmitt and C. P. Fonda, *J. Abnorm. Soc. Psychol.* **52**, 262 (1956); W. Seeman, *J. Nerv. Ment. Dis.* **118**, 541 (1953). For an analysis of these artifacts and summaries of the disputes, see J. Zubin, *Annu. Rev. Psychol.* **18**, 373 (1967); L. Phillips and J. G. Draguns, *ibid.* **22**, 447 (1971).

2. R. Benedict, *J. Gen. Psychol.* **10**, 59 (1934).
3. See in this regard H. Becker, *Outsiders: Studies in the Sociology of Deviance* (Free Press, New York, 1963); B. M. Bragnisky, D. D. Braginsky, K. Ring, *Methods of Madness: The Mental Hospital as a Last Resort* (Holt, Rinehart & Winston, New York, 1969); G. M. Crocetti and P. V. Lemkau, *Amer. Sociol. Rev.* **30**, 557 (1965); E. Goffman, *Behavior in Public Places* (Free Press, New York, 1964); R. D. Laing, *The Divided Self: A Study of Sanity and Madness* (Quadrangle, Chicago, 1960); D. L. Phillips, *Amer. Sociol. Rev.* **28**, 963 (1963); T. R. Sarbin, *Psychol. Today* **6**, 18 (1972); E. Schur, *Amer. J. Sociol.* **75**, 309 (1969); T. Szasz, *Law, Liberty and Psychiatry* (Macmillan, New York, 1963); *The Myth of Mental Illness: Foundations of a Theory of Mental Illness* (Hoeber-Harper, New York, 1963). For a critique of some of these views, see W. R. Gove, *Amer. Sociol. Rev.* **35**, 837 (1970).
4. E. Goffman, *Asylums* (Doubleday, Garden City, N.Y., 1961).
5. T. J. Scheff, *Being Mentally Ill: A Sociological Theory* (Aldine, Chicago, 1966).
6. Data from a ninth pseudopatient are not incorporated in this report because, although his sanity went undetected, he falsified aspects of his personal history, including his maritial status and parental relationships. His experimental behaviors therefore were not identical to those of the other pseudopatients.
7. A. Barry, *Bellevue Is a State of Mind* (Harcourt Brace Jovanovich, New York, 1971); I. Belknap, *Human Problems of a State Mental Hospital* (McGraw-Hill, New York, 1956); W. Caudill, F. C. Redlich, H. R. Gilmore, E. B. Brody, *Amer. J. Orthopsychiat.* **22**, 314 (1952); A. R. Goldman, R. H. Bohr, T. A. Steinberg, *Prof. Psychol.* **1**, 427 (1970); unauthored, *Roche Report* **1** (No. 13), 8 (1971).
8. Beyond the personal difficulties that the pseudopatient is likely to experience in the hospital, there are legal and social ones that, combined, require considerable attention before entry. For example, once admitted to a psychiatric institution, it is difficult, if not impossible, to be discharged on short notice, state law to the

contrary notwithstanding. I was not sensitive to these difficulties at the outset of the project, nor to the personal and situational emergencies that can arise, but later a writ of habeas corpus was prepared for each of the entering pseudopatients and an attorney was kept "on call" during every hospitalization. I am grateful to John Kaplan and Robert Bartels for legal advice and assistance in these matters.

9. However distasteful such concealment is, it was a necessary first step to examining these questions. Without concealment, there would have been no way to know how valid these experiences were; nor was there any way of knowing whether whatever detections occurred were a tribute to the diagnostic acumen of the staff or to the hospital's rumor network. Obviously, since my concerns are general ones that cut across individual hospitals and staffs, I have respected their anonymity and have eliminated clues that might lead to their identification.

10. Interestingly, of the 12 admissions, 11 were diagnosed as schizophrenic and one, with the identical symptomatology, as manic-depressive psychosis. This diagnosis has a more favorable prognosis, and it was given by the only private hospital in our sample. On the relations between social class and psychiatric diagnosis, see A. deB. Hollingshead and F. C. Redlich, *Social Class and Mental Illness: A Community Study* (Wiley, New York, 1958).

11. It is possible, of course, that patients have quite broad latitudes in diagnosis and therefore are inclined to call many people sane, even those whose behavior is patently aberrant. However, although we have no hard data on this matter, it was our distinct impression that this was not the case. In many instances, patients not only singled us out for attention, but came to imitate our behaviors and styles.

12. J. Cumming and E. Cumming, *Community Ment. Health* 1, 135 (1965); A. Farina and K. Ring, *J. Abnorm. Psychol.* 70, 47 (1965); H. E. Freeman and O. G. Simmons, *The Mental Patient Comes Home* (Wiley, New York, 1963); W. J. Johannsen, *Ment. Hygiene* 53, 218 (1969); A. S. Linsky, *Soc. Psychiat.* 5, 166 (1970).

13. S. E. Asch, *J. Abnorm. Soc. Psychol.* 41, 258 (1946); *Social Psychology* (Prentice-Hall, New York, 1952).

14. See also I. N. Mensh and J. Wishner, *J. Personality* 16, 188 (1947); J. Wishner, *Psychol. Rev.* 67, 96 (1960); J. S. Bruner and R. Tagiuri, in *Handbook of Social Psychology*, G. Lindzey, Ed. (Addison-Wesley, Cambridge, Mass., 1954), vol. 2, pp. 634–654; J. S. Bruner, D. Shapiro, R. Tagiuiri, in *Person Perception and In-*

terpersonal Behavior, R. Tagiuri and L. Petrullo, Eds. (Stanford Univ. Press, Stanford, Calif., 1958), pp. 227–288.

15. For an example of a similar self-fulfilling prophecy, in this instance dealing with the "central" trait of intelligence, see R. Rosenthal and L. Jacobson, *Pygmalion in the Classroom* (Holt, Rinehart & Winston, New York, 1968).

16. E. Zigler and L. Phillips, *J. Abnorm. Soc. Psychol.* **63,** 69 (1961). See also R. K. Freudenberg and J. P. Robertson, *A.M.A. Arch. Neurol. Psychiatr.* **76,** 14 (1956).

17. W. Mischel, *Personality and Assessment* (Wiley, New York, 1968).

18. The most recent and unfortunate instance of this tenet is that of Senator Thomas Eagleton.

19. T. R. Sarbin and J. C. Mancuso, *J. Clin. Consult. Psychol.* **35,** 159 (1970); T. R. Sarbin, *ibid.* **31,** 447 (1967); J. C. Nunnally, Jr., *Popular Conceptions of Mental Health* (Holt, Rinehart & Winston, New York, 1961).

20. A. H. Stanton and M. S. Schwartz, *The Mental Hospital: A Study of Institutional Participation in Psychiatric Illness and Treatment* (Basic, New York, 1954).

21. D. B. Wexler and S. E. Scoville, *Ariz. Law Rev.* **13,** 1 (1971).

22. I thank W. Mischel, E. Orne, and M. S. Rosenhan for comments on an earlier draft of this manuscript.

38 THE DYSFUNCTION OF DSM-II*

Marlene S. Ventura, B.S., M.A., M.S.

MAN'S INCLINATION SINCE TIME IMMEMORIAL TO ORDER AND classify things in harmony needs little elaboration. There has always been a search to find words that take on a special meaning. Man's efforts to extend this desire to a development of a classification system of mental illness has been evident throughout the history of mental health starting with Kraepelin and culminating in 1952,[1] in the publication of the Diagnostic and Statistical Manual, Mental Disorders (DSM-I) and in 1968, with its revision, DSM-II.

Three main questions come to mind when receiving a nosology. First, is it useful to put clients in diagnostic categories as developed? Secondly, how adequate are the diagnostic classification systems that we use today? Thirdly, what other alternatives are available?

General Introduction for Using and Not Using a Nosology

Some reasons for using a diagnostic classification system in the area of mental health are as follows:

It aids in
1. grouping patients for a common purpose
2. making administrative decisions

Reprinted, with permission, from *Journal of Psychiatric Nursing and Mental Health Services*, January-February 1975.

*Diagnostic and Statistical Manual of Mental Disorders—1968 prepared by the committee on Nomenclature and Statistics of the American Psychiatric Association.

3. conducting research
4. reporting of statistical data
5. planning treatment modalities
6. Interfacing with the World Health Organization International Classification of Diseases (ICD-8)
7. working in primary prevention
8. communicating among professional and non-professional personnel providing health care services.

One disadvantage in using a diagnostic classification system is that the uniqueness of the individual seeking treatment in a mental health facility may be lost. One of the assumptions involved in using a nosology is that clients in a particular category have similar histories, similar characteristics and will generally respond to similar treatment modalities. This assumption may be an incorrect one. Similar symptoms such as anxiety, sleep disturbance, i.e., may be associated with several categories listed in a classification system. Since we don't understand, in detail, the causes of mental disorders there are varying opinions as to how they should be treated. For example, an elderly, depressed woman who has some suicidal ideation can be faced with treatment including medication, electroconvulsive therapy and/or extensive psychotherapy. Siegel, et al.[2] found that within a hospitalized population, older persons with less education were referred in disproportionate numbers for electroconvulsive therapy and responded more favorably to this treatment modality.

Critics of the current psychiatric diagnostic classification system are concerned over the system's questionable reliability.[3,4] Experienced psychiatrists frequently differ among themselves on which diagnostic labels should be associated with which set of symptoms. Some clinicians may also diagnose the same disease differently on several occasions. Most individuals have a wide range of behavioral responses and move along a continuum of normality. This concept of normality may differ under certain circumstances such as war, peace, cultural influences, etc.[5] Enright and Jaeckle[6] have investigated empirically the distortion occurring in a situation in which the American Psychiatric Association Standard Diagnostic Nomenclature was applied to individuals from different non-Western backgrounds. The author's objection, in this particular article, is that the diagnostic system is based on the symptom of patients from one general cultural background, namely Western European. In this study, patient groups from two different non-Western ethnic backgrounds, defined as psychiatrically identical by the American Psychiatric Association diagnostic system showed distinct differences in the frequency of occurrence of concrete symptoms. So long as the criterion of assessment is largely dependent on the psychiatrist's subjective integration of a different set of facts for each subject, non-uniform results can be anticipated.

Another disadvantage in utilizing a nosology is that putting a person in a particular category may unfavorably effect what happens to him and how other people feel about him.[7] In 1958, Hollingshead and Redlich[8] reported relationships between social class diagnosis, and treatment of persons with mental disorders in a community survey in New Haven, Conn. Some psychiatrists are hesitant to label clients who seek psychiatric treatment and may, at times, list their diagnosis as an "emotional disorder." Others make no attempt to label clients at all, but attempt to understand the symptomatology in terms of the patients' psychodynamic makeup.

The Northern New England Psychiatric Society which represents more than six hundred and fifty psychiatrists in Massachusetts and New Hampshire adopted a position paper,[9] in February 1972 to end legal and employment discrimination against homosexuals and to end legal restrictions on sexual acts between consenting adults, and has suggested that the term "Homosexuality" be replaced in the American Psychiatric Association Diagnostic Nomenclature by the term "sexual dysfunction." "Present evidence," according to the statement, "indicates that many homosexuals are functioning in a way that cannot be considered an illness." In recommending an end to all legal discrimination against homosexuals, the Society says that it believes there is a wide consensus within the American Psychiatric Association that "there is no proper medical basis to accord homosexuals less than full and equal protection under the laws."

The Stanford University Gender Identity Team has relegated the term "transexualism" to obsolescence, reported Dr. Norm Fish.[10] The term "Gender Dysphoria Syndrome" has been formally accepted to cover the various conditions that would lead to an evaluation for surgery. Dr. Fish stated that the use of this term called GDS for short, has corrected problems incurred by the arbitrary label of transexualism. The merit of this term has been recognized by those who dislike labeling people for any reason. It has been reported that patients themselves prefer it.

A classification scheme can also be very rigid. If it maintains a labeling procedure it may have little flexibility within its conceptual framework, although the option does exist for modifying it. The disadvantage of labeling also presents some speculation for further study on identifying social situations in which the self-fulfilling prophecy operates.

The Diagnostic and Statistical Manual of Mental Disorders assumes acceptance of the medical model. The medical model views emotional disorder like diseases wherein the person is "sick." This is the dominant model used today and it is reflected in our use of terminology such as "mental illness." One limitation is that we can't point to specific causes, or specific treatments for mental disorders, in the same way as we can in a particular disease such as rheumatic fever and pneumonia. Other models to be considered in contrast to the medical model, are the "normal model" and the "interpersonal relations model." Thomas Szasz[11] has attempted to show that the notion of mental illness has outlived the usefulness it might have had, and that it now functions merely as a convenient myth. Sustained adherence to the myth of mental illness allows people the option of avoiding the problem, namely what to do with themselves. It also allows people who believe that mental health is conceived as the absence of mental illness, to continue to believe that mental health automatically insures the making of right and safe choices in one's life.

Some professionals in the field of mental health feel that use of DSM-II is geared to the psychiatric client rather than to the person seen by other agencies such as juvenile court, family counseling centers and schools.

Bahn[12] says "DSM is essentially a 'single entry' system and cannot adequately describe etiology, intra-psychic dynamics, stage of illness, precipitating stress, psychological symptoms and behavior, physical health status, role functioning, familial control and prognosis."

DSM-II cannot also be used adequately to determine change in an individual's condition. Furthermore, child psychiatrists consider it inadequate for use with children and adolescents and have attempted separate classifications for these age groups. [13,14]

Other Alternatives to DSM-II Classification

With considerable reluctance, one might add to the confusion of proposing still other classifications of presenting problems. However it is hoped that these are devoid of any diagnostic intent.

First, a client may express problems in terms of his general mode of relating to other persons. Karen Horney[15] suggests that individuals tend to adopt one of several of the following three general strategies of coping with others: they may *move toward* other persons; against them, or away from them.

In movement toward people, "one accepts his own helplessness, and in spite of his estrangement and fears tries to win the affection of others and lean upon them."[16] Often this pattern is called dependency.

In the area of movement against people one accepts and takes for granted the hostility around him and determines consciously or unconsciously, to fight. He or she implicitly distrusts the feelings of others toward himself.[17]

In movement away from people he "keeps apart." He feels that he has not much in common with people and they do not understand him anyhow.[18] Horney often refers to this mode of coping as isolation or detachment.

Another alternative to classifying clients in a psychiatric setting is to look at the presenting problem rather than a specific diagnosis. For example this refers to developing a therapeutic approach to deal with an assaultive client rather than dealing with a chronic schizophrenic. This approach is not unlike some of the ones presently being used in other fields of medicine and particularly nursing where the focus of attention is with a patient with a respiratory problem rather than pneumonia. It is an attempt to be much more of a generalist dealing with concepts and relationships.

Still another approach is to view clients seeking help in the mental health field as individuals having disturbances in the "cognitive," "affective" and "motor" areas. Problems in the cognitive area may refer to disturbances in the intellectual process which are manifested in altered perceptions and/or ideas. Problems in the affective area relate to those specifically that deal with the client's feelings and emotions. Last, problems in the motor area are those that relate to disturbances of muscular action. There is a considerable amount of overlap here between categories. A problem in one area may also deal with all three orientations at once. Nonetheless, any given presenting complaint or statement can be classified according to the orientation which seems most problematic.

The New York Heart Association[19] has attempted through a classification of psychosocial functionings to develop levels used in the provision of health care based on the heart's ability to perform work.

The last alternative to a diagnostic classification system is one that was presented by Kaduskin[20] in a book on outpatient psychiatric care. It has been derived from Talcott Parson's theory of action,[21] with some modification by the above mentioned author. The major divisions of classification system are:

1. biosocial problems which include those of a physical nature.
2. inner emotional problems which include cognitive, catechetic and evaluative problems.
3. social problems—relating to primary work groups and the total social system.

The approach as related above is an attempt to look at problems from obvious viewpoints, namely, man's adjustment to his body, to his inner feelings and lastly, to his social surroundings. Just as it was mentioned before, there can be considerable interrelationship between the presenting problem and outcome areas.

Summary

The task of seeking alternatives to a classification system such as DSM-II that will maximize its benefits and minimize its limitations is a complex and arduous one.

There are no clear-cut answers. Certain issues had been elaborated on here. The task at hand is one that must be approached on a multi-professional basis seeking to integrate a variety of theoretical bases into a functional conceptual framework that will accomplish the purpose of a classification scheme. There is also need to conduct systematic data collection in an effort to determine operational definitions related to the phenomenon that is being studied. There is a movement by some professionals to have more emphasis placed on the social functioning level of the individual and his significant others. If a concerted effort is not begun to look at this problem it will remain unchanged for the most part or other interested professionals will have changed it with little impact from nursing.

References

1. Brill, H.: Classification in Psychiatry, Chapter 14 In Freedman and Kaplan's *Comprehensive Textbook of Psychiatry*. Baltimore, Md.: Williams and Wilkins Co., 1967.
2. Siegel, N. et al.: Social Class, Diagnosis and Treatment in Three Hospitals, *Social Problems* 10:191–196, 1967.
3. Zigler, E. Phillips, L.: Psychiatric Diagnosis: A Critique, *Journal Abnormal and Social Psychology* 1961, Vol. 63, No. 3, 607–618.
4. Blum, Richard: Case Identification in Psychiatric Epidemiology. Methods and Problems. *The Milbank Memorial Fund Quarterly* 40 (1962) 253–288.
5. Murphy, H. et. al.: A Cross-Cultural Survey of Schizophrenia Symptomatology, *Journal of Social Psychiatry* 9:237–249, 1963.
6. Enright, J. and Jaeckle, W.: Psychiatric Symptoms and Diagnosis in Two Subcultures, *International Journal of Social Psychiatry* 9: 12–17, 1963.
7. Simmons, O. et al.: Interpersonal Strains in Release from a Mental Hospital. *Social Problems* 4:21–8, 1956.
8. Hollingshead, A. and Redlich F.: *Social Class and Mental Illness: A Community Study*. New York: John Wiley and Sons, 1958.

9. ———: District Branch Urge Revised Labeling for Homosexuality. *Psychiatric News* — Official Newspaper of the American Psychiatric Association, Vol. 8, No. 6, March 21, 1973.

10. *Erickson, Educational Foundation Newsletter,* Vol. 6, No. 1, Spring 1973 (Baton Rouge, Louisiana).

11. Szasz, T.: The Myth of Mental Illness. *American Psychologist* 15:113–118, 1960.

12. Bahn, Anita: A Multi-Disciplinary Psychosocial Classification Scheme. *American Journal of Orthopsychiatry,* 41(5) 830–838, 1971.

13. Group for the Advancement of Psychiatry, 1966. Proposed classification of psychopathological disorders in childhood. GAP Committee on Child Psychiatry (mimeo).

14. Prugh, D.: 1970 Psychosocial Disorders in Childhood and Adolescence: Theoretical Considerations and An Attempt At Classification. Appendix A in Crisis in Child Mental Health: Challenge for the 1970's *Report of the Joint Commission on Mental Health of Children.* New York: Harper and Row.

15. Horney, Karen: *Our Inner Conflicts: A Construction Theory of Neurosis.* New York: W. W. Norton, 1945.

16. *Ibid.* p. 42.

17. *Ibid.* p. 43.

18. *Ibid.* p. 43.

19. New York Heart Association: *Diseases of the Heart and Blood Vessels: Nomenclature and Criteria for Diagnosis.* 6th edition. Boston: Little, Brown, 1964.

20. Kaduskin, Charles: *Why People Go To Psychiatrists.* New York: Atherton Press, 1969.

21. Parsons, Talcott and Shils, E.A. (eds): *Toward a General Theory of Action.* Cambridge: Harvard University Press, 1951.

39 THERAPY IS THE HANDMAIDEN OF THE STATUS QUO

Seymour L. Halleck, M.D.

THE THESIS THAT ALL OF OUR CITIZENS ARE oppressed by current social institutions is certainly debatable, but there can be little doubt that many individuals the psychiatrist is asked to help are living in highly oppressive environments. When the psychiatrist works with such patients, he learns some bitter lessons. He learns how much more help he could provide if he were able to change the environment. And he learns that he helps his patients little—or perhaps even hurts them—if he ignores their environment.

My own experience in trying to help persons trapped in a severly oppressive environment came when I worked as a psychiatrist in a prison. For many years I used verbal reassurance or drugs in attempts to comfort those who broke down under the strain of the prison regimen. By clarifying the stresses in their lives, I helped some make less-painful adjustments to the realities of their prison sentences, and I helped a few learn to modify their behavior so they could stay out of trouble. I made very little effort to alter the oppressive environment of the prison itself. Occasionally, I would suggest changes that I hoped would make the environment more humane, but I never pressed too hard for fear that I would alienate myself from the prison administrators and lose whatever effectiveness I had.

Now, looking back, I am plagued by doubt as to whether I did enough, or, for that matter, whether it was moral for me to work in the prison at all. Suffering is general in prison; every confined person is depressed at least some of the time. Every one of my patients was in a vicious environ-

Excerpted and reprinted with permission from a chapter in *Politics of Therapy* by Seymour Halleck. Copyright 1971 Seymour Halleck, Jason Aronson Inc., Publishers.

ment that stripped him of dignity and enforced upon him life conditions that were antagonistic to the values of mental health. By participating in the punishment process, even as a healer, I lent a certain credibility to the correction system.

ACTIVISM.   I recently heard a prominent psychiatrist say of his work in a ghetto that if he did not help a welfare patient get larger welfare payments, he considered that he had done an inadequate job. He was in frequent contact with welfare offices in his efforts to get livable stipends for his patients. This is a kind of political activism–a major step for a psychiatrist. It goes beyond merely encouraging the individual to recognize and deal with environmental stress in his life. It requires the psychiatrist to go out and do something to change the patient's environment.

The focus here is on a few individuals. This raises the troubling question of the social utility of helping only those few who are miserable enough or fortunate enough to get a psychiatrist's help. In a social system that massively oppresses a large proportion of its members, the psychiatrist's efforts to get preferential treatment for a few will drain the capacity of that system to help the many. If the psychiatrist's welfare patient gets more money, there will be less welfare money for someone else. If I had persuaded prison authorities to provide special treatment programs for my patients, other inmates would have been deprived.

To justify preferential activism the psychiatrist must be convinced that his patients are more needy or more deserving than others. Or he must hope that patients thus privileged will do so well that those who run the system will offer equal privilege to others. In an oppressive environment, this is wishful thinking. Those in control may even harden in their positions if they can boast about the special care they provide for problem cases.

TRAP.   The psychiatrist who commits himself to changing social institutions must consider where the commitment might lead him. In my more recent work with students I have come to realize that their perceptions of the world are growing more and more like those of prisoners. When they envision their futures, when they perceive the injustices of their society, and when they contemplate the improbability of being able to lead honorable lives in that society, many feel that they are trapped in a world that cannot or will not satisfy their needs.

The unhappiness of the young is too widespread and commonplace to be viewed as a weakness or defect in young persons themselves. It is a mistake to place the whole blame for their restlessness on affluence or on the permissiveness with which they were reared, and it is not that they have failed to learn responsibility or that they are simply too willing to define minor states of psychological discomfort as illness. The young are being put under stress by society–by its failure to provide a future for them, by its emphasis on meaningless competition, by its unjust wars, by its technology that pollutes the environment. They fear that overpopulation will destroy their world or drastically worsen the quality of their lives. The young feel these pressures more powerfully than adults because they have longer futures to anticipate.

For several years now I have realized that it is futile–in fact, dishonest–to reassure students about the state of their external world. When I first began to appreciate the impact modern society was having upon youth, my message to students who became my patients was: Yes, our world is a mess, but you could tolerate that mess better, or you might even be able to do something about it, if you freed yourself of your neuroses. This approach sometimes helped the individual patient, but it left me again feeling much like the prison psychiatrist who helps to sustain his patient's sanity so that the patient can better tolerate the process of daily punishment.

DUTY.   My doubts about the social role of today's psychiatrist grew as I discovered that my patients and those of a colleague had almost universally desperate views of society. I became even more troubled when, as a teacher, I found the same pessimism in a large proportion, perhaps the majority, of educated young people. Students have some freedom to attack society; they have ready access to the psychiatrist and are adept at making him feel guilty about not doing more to change the society. I was persuaded that the psychiatrist who believes that stresses of the modern world won't let the young anticipate decent lives must consider whether he has some responsibility for trying to change that world. I am convinced that the psychiatrist must involve himself in efforts to change the society. I am also convinced that he must try to find an ideology–or if you prefer, a uniform set of values–that will guide him in his work. Psychiatry was never, even in more stable times, an ethically or politically neutral profession. Values systems, usually implicit, have always dominated the different schools of psychiatry. Every psychiatrist who ever treated a patient has had some notion of what kind of life would be best for that patient. And every patient who has benefited from psychiatry has incorporated some of his doctor's values. Furthermore, by the very nature of his practice the psychiatrist consistently takes positions on issues that involve the distribution of power within soical systems–issues that have political implications. A psychiatrist usually focuses on his patient's internal problems, presupposing that the patient's environment is adequate and not contributing to his misery. But the patient is part of a social system. Treatment that doesn't encourage the patient to examine or confront his environment strengthens the status quo. Treatment that emphasizes the oppressiveness of the patient's external environment or shows that patient how to change it may help alter the status quo. The psychiatrist either encourages the patient to accept existing distributions of power or encourages the patient to change them. Every encounter with any psychotherapist, therefore, has political implications.

While my specific concern is with my own discipline, these political responsibilities lie just as heavily on all other therapists.

By reinforcing the positions of those who hold power, the psychiatrist is committing a political act whether he intends to or not. Once this fact is appreciated, the psychiatrist's search for political neutrality begins to appear illusory.

USE. A few psychiatrists have recognized the political implications of psychiatric practice. Frederic Wertham has warned of the potential danger in psychiatry's being used as a sort of Praetorian Guard, dedicated to preserving the status quo. R.D. Laing has insisted that some forms of psychiatric treatment are best viewed as repressive political acts. Thomas Szasz maintains that the psychiatrist has become an agent of social control who identifies and immobilizes those with deviant ideas in much the way that Medieval inquisitors identified and tortured witches. All of these critics, however, have concentrated on the repressive uses of involuntary psychiatry; they have not acknowledged that even when psychiatric treatment is accepted voluntarily it has profound political consequences.

To those concerned with finding a humane and effective use of psychiatry, it makes a critical difference whether one sees all of psychiatry or only some of psychiatry as politically influential. Szasz, who is the most eloquent critic of the repressive use of psychiatry, believes that institutional psychiatry–that practiced by state-employed physicians with involuntary patients–is a formidable political weapon and that contractual psychiatry, in which patients contract for help, is not. I am convinced that this is a false distinction. Any psychiatric intervention into social systems can have liberating or repressive consequences for individual patients. It makes some difference whether the patient seeks this intervention, passively accepts it, or has it thrust upon him. But ultimately, the moral and political outcome of psychiatric treatment is determined by the way in which the psychiatrist goes about it.

BIND. At present, the psychiatrist is being pulled in two different political directions. On the one hand he is being asked by government agencies, prisons, military organizations and parents of alienated children to help people adjust to the world as it is. On the other hand, he is being asked by students, blacks, and members of other oppressed groups to help change some institutions.

Until the past decade psychiatrists were allowed to pursue their work in relative calm and consensus. The great majority of citizens who were capable of expressing their opinions approved of the basic institutions that shaped their society. Undoubtedly many black citizens and others would not have been so approving, but until the 1960s the black man was distressingly "invisible," and his voice was rarely heard by psychiatrists or anyone else.

In the 1960s those who had quietly tolerated oppression for centuries became restless. Psychiatrists, like most other citizens, gradually gained a sense of the unrest in our nation. Some, responding to the unrest, tried to involve themselves in political change. However, massive ambivalence has afflicted their involvement. They are reluctant to criticize institutions that have brought them to positions of relative affluence and power that they wish to retain, and they are concerned over whether it is ethical for a "politically neutral" healer to fight for reform.

The rapid growth of new militancy in many professions suggests that the Establishment is willing to tolerate a considerable amount of dissent from its care-givers, at least at the moment.

MYTH.   Primarily because of their belief that the art and science of healing must be nonpolitical, psychiatrists have failed to take full advantage of the freedom to dissent that they already have. It is now time to lay to rest the myth of psychiatric neutrality. Psychiatrists can and should be as active as other care-giving professionals in seeking to change the society. It is time for psychiatrists who wish to do something about our society to go to their own leaders and to community leaders and to say something like the following: Look, I cannot practice good psychiatry without being an activist. I am going to say things and do things that may irritate or may even enrage you. I will repeatedly question your values and will try to get you to engage in dialogue with oppressed people. Much of what I do in the practice of psychiatry will make you uncomfortable. I am sorry it has to be this way. But I believe you have the wisdom and the flexibility to tolerate my activity.

Some conditions in American society are conducive to creating misery among large groups of people. There is no reason why psychiatrists, as citizens and as professionals, should not devote themselves to changing them. Certainly our country's continued involvement in wars not vital to its self-defense causes great suffering among many of our citizens and among those upon whose land we fight. It is likely that the majority of psychiatrists view the Indochinese war as unjust, unwise or unnecessary. There is nothing to keep psychiatrists from involving themselves in anti-war causes and no reason why they should not try to get their professional organizations to take antiwar stands.

TARGETS.   Psychiatrists should also lead the fight against any oppression based on skin color, age, sex or harmless social deviation. Oppression in our ghettos, old people's homes, and prisons creates massive human misery, as do the more subtle social attitudes that isolate and deny privileges to minority or socially deviant groups. The psychiatrist could and should be more active than the average citizen in seeking remedies for these conditions.

OVERPOPULATION   is another problem that could be ameliorated slightly by psychiatric activism. Psychiatrists could help with population control by supporting ready birth-control information and free abortion. Finally, the psychiatrist along with his fellow physicians, must work more and harder for legislation and for reform of medical practices to get adequate health care for the poor as well as the rich.

SHOCK.   Psychiatrists should be committed to ongoing study of, and informed comment on, the effect that all forms of technology and technological progress have on the human condition. They should constantly increase public awareness of the emotional consequences of living in a technocracy, and of the shattering consequences of what Alvin Toffler has referred to as "future shock." Similar examination and critique of economic and political institutions can also be useful.

In any kind of reform, the political role of professional psychiatric organizations is especially important. Certainly organizations such as the American Psychiatric Association cannot take formal stands on every social issue that its members raise. But some social problems are so urgent that professional organizations would be justified in taking active stands on them. Those who seek neutrality must appreciate that our professional organizations already are deeply involved in politics. The American Psychiatric Association already tries to review mental-health legislation and either support or criticize it. As might be expected, the term "mental health" is interpreted broadly enough to justify intervention in a wide variety of social problems, such as crime, violence or drug abuse. In practice the only limits imposed on the American Psychiatric Association's political activities have been in lobbying and support of political candidates. Thus, I am not advocating a major change in the broad policies of psychiatric organizations. I am only advocating that the organization speak out more forcefully on a broader range of issues.

SEARCH.   Organized psychiatry could be a powerful political force if psychiatric organizations presented position papers and testified before legislative bodies on social issues. Organized psychiatry could expose the oppressiveness of institutions and use its influence to change them. Violence is ône issue upon which the American Psychiatric Association has proven to be socially responsive. Largely because of the urging of Milton H. Miller, professor and chairman of the department of psychiatry at the University of Wisconsin, the American Psychiatric Association has agreed to spend a major part of its efforts throughout 1971 and 1972 searching for alternatives to violence. The emphasis will be on finding ways in which people can confront each other, militantly if that is necessary, but nonviolently. Implicit in this search is the belief that polarization is evil and that lack of communication between groups with dissimilar perspectives ultimately leads to violent confrontation.

REFORM.   Many of psychiatry's practices, ideologies and training methods interfere with efforts to create a climate that is responsive to social needs. Here are my recommendations for reform:

1. Individual psychotherapy should, in addition to focusing on internal problems, help the patient achieve greater awareness of his external environment.
2. Therapists should spell out their own belief systems and values to their patients as clearly as possible.
3. Family therapy is an important technique for social change and its use should be expanded. Like the individual therapist, the family therapist must clarify his own values to his patients.
4. Group therapy can be a powerful tool for stabilizing or changing the status quo. Its practitioners are obligated to make their political intentions clear.
5. Except in emergencies, therapists should not use mind-altering drugs or behavior therapy to treat symptoms without investigating the patient's family and community relationships. When it is apparent that drugs or behavior therapy can have repressive consequences, the patient should have a clear understanding of what these consequences might be. Psychiatrists also have a responsibility to acquaint their fellow physicians with the political and moral implications of drug therapy.

6. Because community psychiatry can be used to achieve political goals, psychiatrists who work in communities should make their political intentions clear.

7. The community itself should play a major role in selecting its psychiatrists, if the community should have the power to get rid of them.

8. Psychiatrists should be more careful with psychiatric labels. Many patients are judged to be schizophrenic, psychopathic, paranoid or alcoholic on the basis of flimsy evidence. Putting a label on a patient can have repressive consequences for that person. The arbitrariness of many categories of psychiatric disturbance must be made clear to the public.

9. Psychiatrists must examine certain myths that they have accepted as facts and must stop perpetuating them in a manner that oppresses blacks, women, the elderly, the poor and those who have unconventional sexual tastes.

10. In an age that increasingly calls upon them to comment on moral issues, psychiatrists must realize that their public statements about almost anything will be exploited by advocates of various political viewpoints, and they must carefully distinguish between fact and speculation in their statements. When their statements are used irresponsibly by moral or political partisans, psychiatrists should publicly repudiate such usage.

11. The results of psychiatric research will often support one or another political viewpoint. There is nothing inherently wrong with this, but psychiatrists must accept responsibility for how their research findings, which are often equivocal, are used as evidence in moral or political issues.

12. Naive psychological analysis that deprecates prominent persons is a form of political commentary that is not justifiable. Psychiatrists should not make public statements regarding the mental stability of living public figures.

13. A request by an agency or an insurance company for information about a former patient should not be honored unless ignoring the request would hurt the patient. Such requests should be discouraged vigorously.

14. Too frequently, and usually unwisely, psychological tests are used to grant or deny privileges. Psychiatrists have some responsibility for preventing repressive use of psychological tests.

15. The practice of granting psychiatric excuses caters to an elite, forces the psychiatrist to be dishonest and contributes to social stagna-

tion. Energy invested in providing psychiatric reasons why a woman should have an abortion or why a young man should not be drafted would be better used in efforts to legalize abortion and to end unjust wars. Investment of the energy of psychiatrists in the courtroom should be redirected toward reforming the system of correctional justice.

16. Civil commitment should be based primarily on substantial evidence that a patient is dangerous to himself or to others. Psychiatrists should insist that their decisions regarding commitment be reviewed frequently by judicial agencies.

17. In spite of many improvements in the last 20 years, the level of psychiatric care in most of our public hospitals is inadequate. There is no way to justify any indeterminate commitment, either civil or specialized, to an institution that cannot provide humane and modern treatment. Psychiatrists should devote themselves again to raising the standards of care in our public mental hospitals.

18. In seeking to define the optimum human condition, psychiatric research should focus upon finding solutions to moral problems. Research that sheds light upon the human condition (or what L. Jolyon West refers to as "biosocial humanism") should have as high a priority as does research that is designed to find causes for socially deviant behavior.

CONFESS.   Many of my recommendations will not be carried out until psychiatrists frankly acknowledge that their use of the concept of mental illness is scientifically inaccurate and socially dangerous. Too many psychiatrists still communicate to their patients that mental illness is an affliction, visited upon them by an external force.

In their more sober moments, psychiatrists understand that the analogy between mental and physical disorders is tenuous, and they recognize moral and political implications of treating unhappy people as sick people. But they do not acknowledge these implications in their relationships with patients and they tend almost totally to obscure them in their relationship with the public.

Psychiatry will never be able to deal with the moral and political questions that are so critical to its future unless psychiatrists become more consistent in conceptualizing and publicizing their work. Psychiatrists must immediately stop all propaganda designed to convince the public that mental illness is "a disease just like any other disease." Instead, they should acknowledge publicly that there are some behavior disorders that resemble physical illness and others that do not.

ELITISM.   Still other kinds of reform are needed in psychiatry. Certain changes in psychiatric ideologies, practices and training could do a great deal to bring about a more equitable distribution of mental-health services. Competent psychotherapy–long- or short-term–is a luxury available primarily to a social elite. Psychoanalysts spend a great deal of their time treating psychiatrists, psychologists and social workers. Many of their other patients tend to be professionals, artists and highly success-ful businessmen. Other therapists also treat primarily middle- or upper-class patients. Even when service is free, therapists will select for a long-term therapy patients who are intellectually oriented, creative and usually of upper-middle-class background–in short, persons who are most like themselves. This behavior by therapists, which is well documented, shows little sign of changing even in an era of greater social awareness.

Training more professional therapists in the techniques of family and group therapy will help enormously in teaching more people. Even these techniques, however, are unlikely to let the psychiatrist help the mass of people who need his services. In groups, as in individual therapy, psy-chiatrists are most likely to treat patients who are most like themselves. Doubling or tripling the number of professionally trained therapists would not solve the problem.

DEGREE.   It is time to acknowledge what many psychiatrists already know: that it is not necessary to have a medical degree to practice good psychotherapy. Even much of the training involved in obtaining a degree in clinical psychology, counseling, guidance or social work may not be absolutely essential to the making of a good psychotherapist. There are many relatively uneducated but otherwise intelligent and sensitive per-sons in all strata of our society who could and would make excellent therapists if they were properly trained. There has been more disagreement over how much training is needed to make an intelligent and sensitive person into a good therapist than there has been study of the question, but there are enough data to suggest that it can be done.

I foresee a future in which one of the psychiatrist's major functions will be to train nonprofessional therapists to do psychotherapy. Talented people will have to have ready access to psychiatric educational facilities and to the best psychiatric teachers. Up to now the best training programs in the mental-health fields have been open primarily to phy-sicians. In certain circumstances, experienced clinicians teach and supervise psychologists and social workers, but even they generally find it hard to get good clinical training.

The creation of a new class of therapists without specific degrees or licenses will create many new problems: ethics, selection, evaluation of competence, pay. Should lay therapists form a new profession, or will professionalization create distance between them and those they treat? Lay therapists will need to be aware of and sensitive to the political and moral implications of their work.

Those physicians who would resist any tendency to dilute the medical or professional status of psychotherapy must appreciate that in the short run, at least, there is no other humane choice. In our current climate of need and distrust of professionalism, it seems certain that large numbers of nonprofessionals will start doing psychotherapy with or without training. Thousands of persons with little or no training already are trying to help others with encounter or sensitivity experiences and with counseling, formal and informal. Psychiatrists know that bad psychotherapy can hurt people. If they refuse to commit themselves substantially to the training of lay therapists, they will renege on an important obligation to their society.

CHANGE.   By giving younger psychiatrists more power in professional organizations and training centers, we could speed the process of orderly change in the psychiatric profession. The young readily accept innovations, but when change comes rapidly the older psychiatrist has great difficulty. In the 12 years since I have finished my residency, I have had to integrate into my basically psychoanalytical orientation new developments in behavior therapy, drug therapy, community therapy, communication therapy, general-systems theory, sensitivity training and family therapy.

Many of the psychiatrists I know are frustrated visionaries, men who dream of contributing to social reform but who are afraid that to act will be to violate some medical or social ethic. In their quest for scientific and social respectability, psychiatrists have shunted visionary dreams into remote corners, or felt ambivalence or guilt when they occasionally used their professional skills for political purposes. However, the experience of practicing psychiatry in a time of chaos is teaching psychiatrists that they can–indeed must–be helpers and reformers at the same time. While this new awareness enormously complicates psychiatric theories and practices, it also liberates. Psychiatrists can now free themselves from artificial and inauthentic neutrality. They can dream and search for ways to make realities of their dreams.

40 FAMILY PLANNING DURING PSYCHIATRIC HOSPITALIZATION

Virginia Abernethy, Ph.D.,

Henry Grunebaum, M.D.,

Louise Clough, R.N.,

Barbara Hunt, R.N.,

Bonnie Groover, B.S.

EVIDENCE SUGGESTING THAT WOMEN HOSPI-
TALIZED FOR PSYCHIATRIC ILLNESS are in need of family planning
assistance[1,2,4,6,9,13,17] has led to development of voluntary birth control
services at three Massachusetts state mental hospitals. Areas to which our
concern has been directed include ethical considerations involved in dealing with a mentally impaired population; establishment of cooperative
relationships with the hospital staff in order to reach a maximum number
of women; and assessment of the suitability of various contraceptive
methods for mentally ill women. A review of the special needs of this
patient population is followed by a discussion of points of resistance and
strategy related to development of services.

Reprinted with permission from the *American Journal of Orthopsychiatry*, Vol. 46, January,
1976.

The Need

It is estimated that approximately four million female psychiatric patients are of reproductive age, of whom nearly half a million are admitted to inpatient status yearly, while nearly as many are discharged.[2] It has been shown in independent studies[5,10] that the prevalence of serious mental illness is greatest in the lower classes, and that lower-class women are deprived in terms of access to family planning alternatives.[3,7] We believe that one of the major pockets of deprivation is to be found in the conjunction of these two categories: the poor and the mentally ill. Therefore, our obligation to these women and to society is development of a family planning program that meets their special needs.

It seems clear that while most sexually active, mentally ill women want to use effective contraception,[1,9] they do not usually have access to birth control services through private, community, or psychiatric hospital channels, even though organized family planning services have burgeoned over the last decade.[2] This may be due in part to impaired ability of mental patients to communicate their need. __ take effective action on their own behalf. It is also certain that few family planning programs have actively sought to recruit mental patients through their outreach programs. In addition, it has been assumed, incorrectly, that because such a large proportion of psychotic women are unmarried, they are not likely to be exposed to the risk of pregnancy and childbearing.[12,16]

The reproductive rate of mentally ill women in the United States appears to have risen markedly since the mid-1950s, concurrent with the widespread use of psychoactive drugs, declining reliance on mental hospitals as long-term custodial institutions, and a trend toward partial hospitalization, day care, rapid discharge and patient maintenance in the community.[2,6,15] Shearer *et al*[15] have documented that between 1935 and 1964 there was a 366% increase in the delivery rate of psychotic women while in Michigan's six major state mental hospitals, 63% of these births were to schizophrenic women.

Similarly, Erlenmeyer-Kimling[6] and her co-investigators concluded from analysis of nearly 3,000 case histories of schizophrenics that there was a large increase in marriage and reproduction rates both before and after onset of the disease in a 1954–1956 sample compared to a 1934–1936 sample, and that the increase in rates was relatively larger than for the general population over the same intervals.

However, the increasing availability of abortion may be altering this trend and even reversing it in some localities. Data from a group of young women (average age, 21) interviewed in the two hospitals where the program originated suggest that, although their conception rates are slightly higher than the national average, virtually all of their pregnancies were unplanned and unwanted, with nearly half terminating in abortion or miscarriage. Of live births, more than half resulted in a foster home placement.[1]

Childbearing may have deleterious consequences for the resulting children, as well as for the mental patient.[14] Not only are the children of the mentally ill often unwanted, they are sometimes seen by their parents—as well as by therapists—as precipitating recurrent psychotic decompensations in the mother.[9,13,17] Moreover, such children are themselves at high risk of becoming mentally ill both because of genetic predispositions and probable experiential deficits.[2]

Ethical Considerations

Underlying our approach to family planning is a commitment to voluntarism and informed consent. Overall, it appears that 1) exclusive use of reversible birth control methods, 2) separation of family planning from other hospital personnel, 3) emphasis on education as a major element in family planning counseling, and 4) staff commitment to voluntarism are the best means of insuring that the patients' informed right to give or withhold consent is well protected. The decision to practice birth control is made by the patient, and insofar as it is medically sound, the choice of contraception is hers. From a legal point of view, inpatients who sign a voluntary admission form have agreed to accept medical treatment under hospital auspices, but we consider that it is necessary to emphasize voluntarism in family planning well beyond this legalistic interpretation.

A workshop* organized by the authors to discuss the ethics of family planning for women seen in psychiatric hospitals tentatively concluded 1) that voluntarism should remain the guiding principle in the provision of services; 2) that whereas it was regrettable to have children born to chronically mentally impaired parents, the loss to society would be even greater if coercive measures were introduced; and 3) information given to the patient in helping her come to a decision about contraception could appropriately include the probabilities that she would be under pressure to accept an abortion, that the baby would be taken away from her, and that it might inherit her impairment of mental function. The total package of information approaches a threat, yet the various ethicists felt there was an essential difference: the agents of information-giving were different and organizationally separate from those who would be ordering the abortion or taking the child.[8]

---

*Funded through the Office of Economic Opportunity.

These conclusions do not confront the issue of whether procreation is a right or a privilege, or whether there is a necessary linkage between rights and responsibilities, or privilege and duty. Such questions involve the society's larger value system, from which new truths may emerge if resource scarcity impinges critically on national awareness. It may be necessary eventually to consider seriously the implications of our experience with five of the first eight patients seen by one family planning counselor:

A 34-year-old white manic depressive who had twelve pregnancies, the most recent of which was aborted within the year. She had oral contraceptives available but stopped taking them because she was not presently having sexual relations, although she had a "lover."

A 25-year-old white chronic schizophrenic who had three unwanted pregnancies, one terminated by miscarriage and the other two given up for adoption. She would not consider any contraceptive but diaphragm or foam because she had no boyfriend at the time.

An 18-year-old white girl who had an abortion following an out-of-wedlock pregnancy. She married within the year but the marriage was very unstable and her husband was out of work at the time of her being seen by our counselor. Just discharged from the hospital, she was hoping to get pregnant and refused contraception.

A 21-year-old white chronic schizophrenic who had given up an out-of-wedlock baby within less than a year of being seen. She started 28-day pills but discontinued after discharge because she had no boyfriend. Her goal for herself was to find a boyfriend, get married, and have a baby.

A 23-year-old white retarded, chronic schizophrenic who had un-protected intercourse within six month of being seen. She said she would never have sex again until she married. Her goal for herself was to get married and have a baby. She refused contraception.

It is questionable whether the refusal of these women to use contraception is an informed decision, in the individual's best interests. In the latter two cases, the desire for a husband and a baby combined with these women's impaired capacity for reality testing make them extremely vulnerable to sexual exploitation, and the need for effective contraception could arise in a matter of hours. Thus, it is felt that the issue of informed consent or refusal has special ramifications with this population.

Benefits

While this experience suggests that the community may eventually need to consider the problem of "uninformed refusal" to accept contraception, this subsample is in fact not representative of patients seen in any of the three state hospitals in our sample. It is a truism that any innovative program is initially "tested" by referral of the most intransigent, chronic patients, and subsequent cases have supported independent research findings[1,9] which suggest that women seen in psychiatric facilities do *not* differ from the population at large in their desire to have birth control assistance available to them.

Thus, within the framework delineated by contemporary ethical currents, it has been possible to be of assistance to the large proportion of reproductive-age patients who have been admitted to the psychiatric facilities in which we have worked.

In addition to reducing risk for unwanted pregnancy, clinic utilization data suggest that the program is making a significant contribution in terms of increasing the total of health services available to women who are unable to afford private medical care. From the first year's records for three hospitals, it appears that 81% of the women seen in our clinic had received general public assistance before hospitalization or had been registered for Medicaid. Moreover, a large majority of the remaining nineteen percent consisted of patients who had been chronically institutionalized and therefore were not eligible to register for other public welfare assistance (under Public Law 89–97, otherwise known as Title 19 of the Social Security Act, as interpreted by Massachusetts officials).

Age and reproductive histories are additional important factors in evaluating quality of service in a family planning program: nearly half of all women seen were between 16 and 25 years of age, with even more of the contraceptive acceptors in this bracket. About 75% of contraceptive acceptors were single and had been sexually active. Of 61 women in our sample who had ever been pregnant, 31 reported at least one fetal death; patient histories not only suggest that children born to these women would be a financial liability to the society, but also that they would be unwanted by their mothers and liable not to receive adequate care.

Initiating a Program: Objectives and Strategy

Family planning pilot programs have been developed in three state mental hospitals of Massachusetts with the objective of reaching all women patients of reproductive age during their psychiatric hospitalization, in order to: 1) provide sex education and information about the various methods available to prevent unwanted conception; 2) offer gynecological and family planning services before discharge to those patients desiring them; and 3) follow up contraceptive acceptors after discharge, in order to continue providing services and contraceptive supplies directly or in cooperation with an established community-based family planning network.

The target population are the women of reproductive age who are expected to be discharged from inpatient status. or those who are at risk because of sexual contacts during hospitalization.

To encourage a positive reception for an innovative program such as family planning in the psychiatric hospital, care was taken to introduce the idea to hospital staff members in order of their administrative responsibility: below the highest administration level of each hospital, medical, nursing, and social work departments are treated as parallel hierarchies. In a further effort to create a cooperative alliance with the administration, the program offered to be responsible for the gynecological examination which in these hospitals is supposed to be associated with the admission physical.

In the context of integrating our program into an ongoing system, we have developed not one model, but two or three, predicated on the constraints imposed by very different kinds of hospital organizations, objectives, and patient populations.

One model emerged in a major public psychiatric facility that now serves a compact urban catchment area, but that originally was, and still retains important functions as, a teaching and research hospital. There is a high doctor-patient ratio, and first-year residents have front-line responsibility for inpatient services including the day hospital. Second-year residents staff an outpatient walk-in service.

The second family planning intervention model emerged in a hospital that has historic functions as a treatment and custodial center. This hospital's teaching functions are new and for the time being remain secondary. The doctor-patient ratio is relatively low, and until recently many physicians spoke English only as a second language. Acutely ill patients are quickly discharged, but there are considerable numbers who are unable to care for themselves outside of the hospital for more than a brief period and often are functionally, if not congenitally, mentally retarded.

Procedure

Services provided by the family planning program are divided into counseling and gynecology/birth control components. A full-time counselor is responsible for initiating contacts, providing education for patients, assisting in the clinic, and maintaining contact with discharged contraceptive acceptors. The clinic is held weekly at each site for about two hours.

The counselor routinely describes the program to each patient of re-productive age, and appointments for further counseling are made with interested patients. Hospital staff is informed of impending appointments and has the option of advising the counselor and patient that the meeting should, in the patient's interest, be postponed. Clinic referrals are made either for a routine gynecological examination or at the patient's instiga-tion so that she can obtain contraception for herself. Even in the latter case, established procedures at the teaching hospital require a written consultation request before the patient actually attends clinic. The coun-selor dispenses foam, jelly, condoms, and thermometers on her own initiative, but always suggests regular clinic check-ups.

Serology, a GC test, and Papanicolau smear are routine procedures. Pregnancy, monilia, and trichomonas tests are optional. The clinic is further equipped for cautery, but in more serious gynecological condi-tions the hospital staff is informed of the diagnosis, and responsibility for treatment is then assigned to the appropriate medical consultant, as with other physical conditions discovered during a psychiatric hospitalization.

If a contraceptive acceptor has a family physician and consents to his being contacted, the counselor informs the physician of the patient's contraceptive plans, offering to discuss relevant features of the psychiatric history and probable response to the contraceptive method. It seems to us essential to thus enlist the support of the private medical community, alerting them to the special needs of the mentally ill in order that the patient shall not receive conflicting medical directives which might result in discontinuation of contraceptive use.

Inception of contraceptive use is usually delayed until close to the date of discharge or a time when the patient is ready for day care or home visits. However, with IUD acceptors it occasionally has seemed prefera-ble for the initial discomfort following insertion to be experienced in the supportive hospital environment. When a women is allowed to retain her own contraceptive pills during hospitalization, one month's supply is given. At discharge she receives enough pills to take her up to the three-month clinic check-up, and thereafter a supply to last for a three or six month interval, depending on the individual.

Follow-up by the counselor is often patient-initiated as they return for contraceptive supplies, but at other times discharged patients drop out of sight despite regular efforts to reach them. The frequency of *medical* follow-up depends on the contraceptive method chosen and on the practice of the gynecologist attending at a given site: thus, pill acceptors will usually be scheduled for a first return clinic visit in three months and subsequently on a six month basis; IUD acceptors return two to four weeks after insertion (or after the next menstrual period) and again in six months. The physician on duty at the hospital acts as a back-up resource if a woman has difficulty with a method when the counselor is not available. Notes on possible side effects and directions for contraceptive use are on hand for the OD, and at each nurses' station. If medical care is indicated, a woman is referred to the emergency service of a local hospital. Emergencies have not been a major problem and typically have been efforts to gain emotional support from the counselor, for instance, trying to involve her by threats to pull out an IUD.

Resistances

Depending upon the site, initial resistance to the program apparently reflected apathy, religious scruples, or residents' and supervisors' anxiety about counselors preempting their patients' attention in the realm of contraceptive planning and providing an alternate channel for discussion of sexuality. In the latter case, contradictory feelings expressed were that 1) residents are doing all that is needed to be done for patients with respect to sexuality and birth control, and 2) residents have come to learn. Particularly in the wake of criticism that physicians are slow to initiate sexual and contraceptive counseling with patients,[11] they are anxious to develop competence and facility in this area. A resistance specific to one very psychoanalytically oriented ward was that "splitting" discussion of sexual problems damages the therapeutic relationship, especially the transference dimension.

At sites with a former custodial orientation, staff resistance to the program stems from other sources. For example, there is failure to see the patient as sexually active, which may be related both to a denial of sexuality generally and also to strong feelings that patients should *not* have sexual lives. In part, there may be the sometimes punitive view that pregnancy is the natural outcome of intercourse and, particularly among foreign-born physicians, some assumptions about woman's role that conflict with birth control practices.

A procedural arrangement which neutralizes much staff resistance can and should be negotiated prior to beginning services: rather than being made to await referrals, the counselor should be free to introduce herself and describe the program to any patient. Staff still retain control, in that they may specifically recommend that a patient not be seen for further sexual or reproductive counseling, but under this system both inertia and normative expectations favor the program.

It appears that experience with both the counseling and clinic aspects of the service gradually allays most concerns. Contrary to residents' apprehension, the counselor's role does not obviate the need for patients to discuss sexual anxiety and ambivalence over their reproductive functions with their therapists. On the contrary, sex and contraception may become more salient; and without betraying confidentiality, project counselors see it as their responsibility to ask the patient, "Have you brought this up with your doctor?" Depending upon the counselor's training, she may, if necessary, go on to the question, "Why haven't you?" and help the patient deal with her resistance. At other times counseling is even more clearly the catalyst for therapeutic discussion of sex: recently, a sex education session immediately preceded an adolescent's excitedly going to her doctor with whom she had hardly spoken in a week. She now remembered, she said, that her grandfather had practiced "putting it in and out" with her. A possible inference from this event is that at least part of the "forgetting" of early sexual encounters occurs because a child has not the linguistic categories to encode sexual events at the time that they are experienced.

Contraceptive of Choice

The suitability of specific contraceptive methods for the mentally ill is an area of ongoing interest. For example, what is anticipated and what must be evaluated with regard to contraception via the pill?

Our psychopharmacological consultant* advises that depressed patients should begin oral contraception *only* under close supervision because a depressive condition may be either considerably improved or worsened by added hormones, depending upon the etiology of the emotional problem. In some instances hormones can interact with antidepressants to enhance their side effects. An increment in depression can also occur when a deficiency in vitamin B_6 is related to oral contraceptive use; patients being treated for this condition are thus a principal category for whom the birth control pill should be recommended only after careful review. Follow-up attention to mood, behavior, and side affects is essential. As a cautionary measure, an inpatient's prescription for oral contraception is always entered into the order book.

The patients most suited to oral contraception, we are finding, fall into extreme categories. The first consists of young women, often adolescents, who have been admitted to the hospital as a crisis intervention and have a

---

*Richard Shader, Associate Professor of Psychiatry, Harvard Medical School.

good prognosis. Pill use for them is often not only valuable as a birth control method, but also helpful symbolically as an issue through which they can assume effective control over their own lives. It is usually appropriate for these women to keep their own contraceptive pills even while hospitalized, and from routine follow-ups we are encouraged to believe that reliability after discharge is very good. The second category consists of chronic and often retarded patients who are accepting of contraception but cannot be relied upon as effective users. Some in this category have had sexual experiences while hospitalized in which they clearly were passive, if not victimized. So long as hospitalization continues, oral contraceptives administered by the nurse are satisfactory. However, an IUD might be preferable for these women because of events during "escapes" or authorized weekends, and some do make this choice.

The IUD also presents special problems for the mental patient. Although it may look like the contraceptive of choice for this population because of its relative invulnerability to user error, special care must be taken with patients choosing it because of the occasional sequelae of pain, bleeding, and unnoticed expulsion after insertion. It is an elementary precaution, therefore, to educate the hospital staff, as well as the patient, so that they do not ascribe complaints to neurosis or psychotic decompensation.

Coitus dependent methods such as the diaphragm, condom, foam, or rhythm have the obvious flaw of depending upon responsible self-disciplined behavior for their effectiveness. These demands can be managed by some women or couples who are functioning at less than an optimal emotional level, but their chances for success with these methods are thought to be less good than for the population at large.

Conclusion

The sum of our experience is both to reinforce suggestive research data that have pointed to the need for family planning services among mentally handicapped sectors of the population, and to sensitize us to the issues likely to be raised during attempts to introduce a program. This paper has addressed itself to both problems, and will have achieved its purpose if it either stimulates or guides the introduction of such services into community or institutional facilities for care of the psychiatric patient.

Bibliography

Abernethy, V. 1974. Sexual knowledge, attitudes, and practices of young female psychiatric patients. Arch. Gen. Psychiat. 30:180–182.

Abernethy, V. and Grunebaum, H. 1972. Toward a family planning program in psychiatric hospitals. Amer. J. Pub. Hlth. 62:1638.

Angrist, S. et al. 1968. Women After Treatment. Appleton-Century-Crofts, New York.

David, H. 1970. Behavioral research in population planning. Prof. Psychol. 1:208.

Dunham, H. 1965. Community and Schizophrenia. Wayne State University Press, Detroit.

Erlenmeyer—Kimling, L., Rainer, J. and Kallman, F. 1966. Current reproductive trends in schizophrenia. *In* Psychopathology of Schizophrenia, P. Hock and J. Zubin, eds. Grune and Stratton, New York.

Garmezy, N. 1971. Vulnerability research and the issue of primary prevention. Amer. J. Orthopsychiat. 41(1):101–116.

Grunebaum, H. and Abernethy, V. Ethical issues in family planning for hospitalized psychiatric patients. Amer. J. Psychiat. (in press)

Grunebaum, H. et al. 1971. Bases of contraceptive practice in mental patients. Amer. J. Psychiat. 218:6.

Hollingshead, A. and Redlich, F. 1958. Social Class and Mental Illness. John Wiley, New York.

Lief, H. 1965. Sex education of medical students and doctors. Pacific Med. and Surgery 73:52–58.

Odegard, O. 1960. Marriage rate and fertility in pscyotic patients before hospital admission and after discharge. Inter. J. Sbc. Psychiat. 6:25.

Pugh, T. et al. 1963. Rates of mental disease related to child-bearing. New Eng. J. Med. 268:1224–1228.

Schwartz, R. 1969. The role of family planning in the primary prevention of mental illness. Amer. J. Psychiat. 125:1711.

Shearer, M. et al. 1968. Unexpected effects of an open door policy on birth rates of women in state hospitals. Amer. J. Orthopsychiat. 38(3):413–417.

Stevens, B. 1969. Marriage and Fertility of Women Suffering from Schizophrenia or Affective Disorders. Maudsley Monograph Series, Oxford University Press, New York.

Yarden, P., Max, D. and Eisenback, Z. 1966. The effect of childbirth on the prognosis of married schizophrenic women. Brit. J. Psyciat. 112:491–499.

41 TRANSACTIONAL ANALYSIS

Dorothy E. Babcock, M.S., R.N.

A WOMAN WHO HAS BEEN FOLLOWED IN THE OB-GYN clinic is brought to the hospital in labor. She has no idea when she started labor, she has not timed her contractions, and she did not bring the instruction list you went over with her *just yesterday* during her clinic appointment. You know you spoke clearly and slowly, asking her if she understood. You distinctly remember her saying yes and nodding her head. What happened?

Your supervisor questions the number of home visits you made. You get defensive inside, outwardly keeping your cool. What happened?

We usually take communication for granted until we experience difficulty. One way of figuring out what happened in our communication and looking for alternatives is called transactional analysis.

Transactional analysis, or TA, is a system of social psychology which can be used to understand, predict, and change human behavior. It can be used as a treatment method by the psychiatric-mental health nurse and as a communication tool by every nurse in any human encounter. Nurses who are skilled in relating to other human beings find TA concepts familiar. Transactional analysis has much in common with communication, psychophysiological, growth and development, and learning theories.

Each of us has three ways of experiencing ourselves and of relating to others which are called *ego states*; Berne labels these Parent, Adult, and Child(1). These ego states are psychological realities with distinctive feeling tones, ways of thinking, and ways of behaving.

The Parent is that aspect of you and me which has recorded what we perceived our own parenting figures to be, say, and do. Most Parent ego states are nurturing (Nurturing Parent), critical (Critical Parent), and judgmental. This parental part of us defines reality. Parental phrases include words like *always, never, should, good,* and *bad.*

The Adult aspect of us is our computer. The Adult sounds like a news analyst, collecting and giving information on how, when, where, what, and predicting probabilities. This part of us thinks and solves problems.

Our Child aspect feels, wants, and needs. It includes the way we learned to be when we were very young (Adapted Child), as well as all that is spontaneous and gutsy (Natural Child). Phrases such as "Yes, Sir," and "You can't make me!" usually represent the Adapted Child, whereas words like "Yuk!" and "Wow!" characterize the Natural Child.

A clue to detecting ego states at any given moment is one's tone of voice, for instance, demanding (Parent) or squeaking (Child). Body language, such as posture and gestures, also gives us clues: note the characteristic pointing index finger of the Critical Parent or the tilted head of the inquisitive Natural Child.

Transactions

When we relate to each other, a symphony of transactions occurs as energy flows from one ego state to another, back and forth between us. We can analyze each transaction, one at a time, to follow precisely what is going on.

One transaction consists of one stimulus and one response. A part of me—Parent, Adult, or Child—offers you a stimulus, and a part of you responds to that stimulus. For instance, my Child ego state says, "I'm starved!" Your Child ego state responds, "Me too!" Your response is also the stimulus to our next transaction.

Transactions are complementary when the ego state addressed is the ego state that responds. For example, Parent offers the stimulus. "These young nurses don't know what hard work is." Parent responds, "Yes, when I was a student, we worked a 12-hour shift and then went to class." The Child to Child transaction about hunger is also complementary.

Many complementary Adult to Adult transactions take place at a typical change of shift report: "Mr. Jones started fibrillating this afternoon. We got it under control. His vital signs have been stable since 10:00 P.M." Response: "What's the reading on his central venous pressure now?"

Complementary transactions can also occur between different ego states. For instance, a staff nurse is coughing and looks ill. Stimulus

(Child): "Cough, cough, cough!" Response (Parent): "You belong in bed with that cough. Go on home. We'll find someone else to cover for you."

Communication breaks down, however, when a transaction is crossed; that is, when a stimulus evokes a response from an ego state other than the one addressed. For instance, "Will you wait outside while we do this procedure?" is an Adult to Adult request for space to work. The Parent to Child answer, "Well, don't take too long!" changes the tone from an Adult dialogue to a Parental criticism.

Ulterior, or hidden, transactions also cause communication difficulty. They take place on two levels at once: an overt level which is usually Adult to Adult, and a covert level which involves the Child ego state. For instance, the supervisor makes what is an ostensibly Adult request for information: "While reviewing your records, I noticed you made only three home visits last Tuesday. What happened? ("Lazy, do more work.") The public health nurse replies with an Adult-sounding answer: "Yes, if you will notice, I recorded that of the ten patients I visited, seven were not at home." ("Dummy, can't you read?")

When a transaction is ulterior, its outcome is apt to be determined at the covert level. In the example given, the transaction is both ulterior and crossed. It would probably lead to a game and create bad feelings(2).

Strokes

Why would nurses and other care givers take potshots at each other instead of communicating clearly and sticking to business? The answer, according to TA theory, is that they are experiencing stroke deprivation. A stroke is a unit of recognition: a hug, a pat, a smile, a frown, a punch in the jaw. Research has showed that mammals, including humans, cannot survive without adequate stroking or stimulation(3). It has also been demonstrated that painful strokes have as much survival value as pleasant ones. For instance, a jab with a pin is just as much a stroke as a caress with a feather; in fact it is more intense.

Negative strokes are often more predictable than positive ones. If a young boy breaks a lamp, he's much more sure of a parental response to breaking the lamp than if he asks to be held or read to. So, if one is feeling stroke hungry, one can more readily guarantee himself a stroke by setting up a negative situation.

Some nurses are taught to be efficient (Adult) and to care for others (Parent), but not to pay attention to their own needs (Child). This leads to stroke hunger and tempts us to get strokes in crooked, painful ways. Strokes felt in the Child ego state have the most impact; that is, we feel more stroked when our Child ego state has been involved in the transaction. We are better able to stay in our Adult ego state, therefore, when our Child need for strokes is satisfied.

One way of improving communications is to establish a policy of positive stroking. Verbal strokes include, "Hi," "That intubation was smooth." "You smell good, what kind of perfume is that?" and so forth. Nonverbal strokes include smiles, winks, hugs, arm pats, and nudging. None of these strokes takes much time and we can give them without slowing our daily work pace.

It is also important to ask for strokes and notice that we get them. "I'm so tense, will you give me a 40-second neck rub?" "I'm scared. Tell me I can do it!" "Hey, that stroke (nudge, compliment) felt good."

To be meaningful, strokes must be suited to the recipient. None of us is responsible for reading each others' minds. We *are* responsible for letting those around us know what we need. I enjoy hearing I'm a good teacher; another nurse likes people to notice that he persuaded the industrial plant manager to banish contact lenses.

Nothing Ventured, Nothing Gained

Habits serve us well when they free us from thinking about routine procedures so that we can devote our energies to more complex tasks. Habits bind us, however, when we continue to transact in habitual ways that do not work, and they can interfere with effective nursing.

To solve habitual communication problems, we can respond to each other differently, and experiment with new ways to approach our patients. We can analyze the transactions going on, and see what happens if we use another ego state, as in the following example:

A police officer was admitted in serious condition to an intensive care unit. He was accompanied by several fellow officers who were upset, wanted to watch over him, and kept getting in the nurses' way. They asked Critical Parent questions of the nurses, and one added, "He put his life on the line for you!" The nurses were frustrated by the crowd, furious at the accusations, and had no time to vent their feelings (Child). One of their teammates solved the problem.

First, she crossed the officers' critical remarks with a Nurturing Parent invitation that the officers accompany her to the coffee pot and tell her how the accident had happened. She listened sympathetically to their concerns for their friend, and suspected that they had ulterior fears for their own safety which they did not voice. She then appealed to their Adult ego states by requesting two officers to act as liaison between the wounded officer's bedside and the rest of his buddies. Her approach worked.

In the situation where the public health nurse and her supervisor exchanged nasty undercover strokes, the public health nurse actually had several other choices: (1) Critical Parent—"Can't your read? It says very clearly I made 10 visits." (2) Nurturing Parent—"You poor dear, you must get tired of trying to keep the statistics up." (3) Adult—"Although I made 10 visits, I saw only three families in that particular neighborhood. Few residents have phones. I frequently make calls and find no one home. That seems an inefficient use of my time. Have you some alternative suggestions?" (4) Adapted Child—(compliant): "Yes, ma'am." (rebellious): "You're always finding fault!" (5) Natural Child—"But I went to 10 houses! My feet are killing me!"

Any new response helps free us from our usual habit and releases some creative energy. In general, Adult to Adult transactions are most likely to solve problems or at least lead to more effective nursing.

Some nurses object to selecting a stimulus or response on the grounds that it is not natural or honest. By now there are enough data about human learning to know that what feels natural is a well-established habit, and what feels honest is what our Parent ego state believes is right and good(4).

We have the choice of sticking to what we believe and what feels comfortable. We also have the choice of looking further than our current repertoire, and tolerating the risk and discomfort of trying out new beliefs and behaviors.

Transactional analysis can be used for effective patient teaching. One nurse finds TA concepts helpful in structuring lesson plans for diabetics. He finds he is apt to succeed when he first pays attention to the Child ego state of his patients. He invites them to get in touch with their feelings of denial, recognizing both positive and negative feelings as important.

When offering patients Adult information and instruction, this nurse makes a point of clarifying who is in control of the diabetes—the patient, not the physician or any other person. He clearly acknowledges the patient's right to decide how much responsibility to assume. Interventions from the nurse's Adult ego state usually reach the Adult ego state of his patients.

The nurse can also use TA to assess transactions during the teaching process itself. During the prior transaction, the woman who had come to the delivery room unprepared apparently had stopped listening after she heard the nurse's opening remark, "Now, when you go into labor. . . ." When the patient heard the word "labor" she switched into the Child ego state. She nodded her head (Adapted Child) and said yes to the nurse's questions. Her Natural Child was scared: "Labor! Who, me?" No part of her listened.

To solve such a problem, the nurse needs to observe a patient carefully while giving instructions. When we shift ego states, we also change body posture and facial expression. When a patient shifts out of the Adult ego state, eye movements and blink rate change. The nurse can validate her observations by speaking from different ego states: Nurturing Parent— "Your eyes got really wide when I said the word 'labor'. I bet you're feeling a bit scared. That's only natural." Adult—"What are you thinking about right now?" Child—"When I went into labor I. . . ."

Inviting a client to share Child to Child transactions may work particularly well with a patient from another culture. Women of other cultures have told me that professionals are easier to understand and relate to when we talk about our own feelings (share our Child ego state). Evidently we distance ourselves by asking only Adult questions. As one client put it, we "talk like machines with no feelings."

In sum, as we analyze communication problems and plan nursing interventions, asking ourselves the following questions can help us figure out what happened and what to do about it:

• Was that last transaction that I had crossed?
• What ego state am I in right now? My colleague? My patient?
• What ego state shall I use—Critical Parent, Nurturing Parent, Adult, Adapted Child, Natural Child?
• Which choice is most likely to get the job done under the circumstances?
• What am I doing about my need for strokes?

References

1. Berne, Eric. *Principles of Group Treatment*. New York, Oxford University Press, 1966.
2. Levin, Pamela, and Berne, Eric. Games nurses play. *Am.J.Nurs.* 72:483-487, Mar. 1972.
3. Spitz, Rene, and Wolf, K. M. Anaclitic depression. In *Psychoanalytic Study of the Child* New York, International Universities Press, 1946, Vol. 2, pp. 313-342.
4. Babcock, Dorothy, and Keepers, Terry. *Raising Kids OK*. New York, Grove Press, 1975.

42

GESTALT THERAPY, THE HOT SEAT OF PERSONAL RESPONSIBILITY

Stella Resnick

SHE WALKS QUICKLY ACROSS THE ROOM AND PLUNKS herself down on the pillow beside me. Her head flicks back and she smiles excitedly. "May I sit down?" she asks in a thick British accent, even though she's already seated. Big though she is, her mannerisms seem like those of a little girl. Suddenly, she puts her hand over her mouth and her eyes widen. "Oh, sorry about that," she giggles, suggesting that she's asking permission for something she's already done. She doesn't look sorry; she looks delighted.

Florie had sat down on the "hot seat." This was a Gestalt workshop and around the room 12 other people were sitting on big, brightly colored pillows, watching and participating with Florie.

The hot seat is an empty seat next to the therapist which people occupy when they want to focus on themselves with the assistance of the therapist. Although Gestalt therapy is often done in weekly groups or short workshops, most Gestalt therapists also do individual Gestalt therapy.

I ask Florie to repeat her last sentence. Repeating words or actions while paying close attention to one's self often reveals important clues about those words or actions. Florie's words and body language don't match, and I want her to pay attention to the split between what she's saying and doing. She has been saying "Oh, sorry about that" all morning.

Something about that expression is important for her.

Still smiling, but this time with her back noticeably straighter and her head slightly cocked, she repeats, "Oh, sorry about that." Her smile now seems plastered on. She still doesn't look sorry; she's beginning to look haughty. Suddenly her smile widens and a giggle rushes through. Florie is out of touch with her own feelings and actions.

Gestalt therapy has two major aims: assisting the individual to become more 1) self aware and 2) self-responsible.

Self-awareness means knowing yourself, being tuned in to what is happening within you at any moment. With awareness people can recognize their natural, healthy tendencies. They can better distinguish between needs and wants, what feels good or bad, what old programs, old attitudes and habitual ways of doing things are no longer appropriate, and what new learning needs to take place.

Self-responsibility means recognizing that you choose what you do and whom you are. When individuals take responsibility for their lives, they enlarge their alternatives and learn to make choices that enhance and nourish them rather than deplete them. Blaming other people or the situation or fate are ways in which people do not take responsibility for themselves. In Gestalt therapy we talk about the therapy process as one in which individuals learn to mobilize their own resources rather than manipulate others to achieve or insure their well-being.

A MOURNFUL WAIL   I ask Florie to go around the room to repeat her sentence to each person, and pay attention to herself as she makes contact. In Gestalt therapy, people are encouraged to put their words and feelings into action, and to pay attention to themselves as they do so.

Florie walks up to the first person. "I'm sorry," she giggles. "I'm sorry about that." She barely gets the last two words out as her giggle becomes uncontrollable, giddy. She puts her hand over her mouth but she can't stop the laughter.

With the next person, "I'm sorry" just barely squeaks through under the laughter. Florie is getting flushed and her eyes become moist.

She moves on, but this time her words trail off in a mournful wail. She turns quickly away and suddenly shouts angrily, "I'm sorry about that, I'm sorry about that!" "Whom are you talking to?" I ask. She stops for a moment, considers my question then tearfully responds, "My mother."

Florie had found that her seemingly innocuous expression had real meaning for her and was not just a manner of speaking. When Florie started to take responsibility for her words, as well as the behavior that went along with them, she started to become aware of herself, of the anger and pain her words and laughter were covering.

In Gestalt therapy, we don't interpret or analyze the past. Rather, people are encouraged to reexperience the past in the present. Expression is what counts, not the presence or absence of the people from the original situation.

I ask Florie to sit down and imagine that her mother is on a pillow in front of her. "Talk to your mother, Florie," I suggest. "Tell her what you're feeling."

UNEXPRESSED GUILT.   In the course of her work that morning, Florie revealed that her mother was an invalid living in a small town in England. She had asked Florie to stay home and take care of her, and Florie had refused and gone to America. Florie felt guilty and had dragged around the unexpressed guilt in her daily life.

Guilt is often *retroflected* anger, that is, anger that the person directs against oneself, because he or she cannot, will not, express it toward the person who is the source of it. When Florie expressed her guilt to her mother it became obvious that the guilt was indeed anger at her mother. But anger was so unacceptable to Florie that she blocked its expression. She preferred to be angry with herself—guilty—rather than to be angry at her "poor, sick mother." At one point Florie shouted, "I'm not sorry, I'm not sorry. I want to lead my own life. I don't want to live in a small town taking care of a sick mother."

At the end of her session, Florie was smiling softly. She said that for the first time in a long time she felt love for her mother, that she could appreciate both her mother's wanting her to stay and her own eagerness to leave.

Gestalt therapy was developed by Frederick S. (Fritz) Perls and Laura Perls in Europe, South Africa and America, and is a continually developing philosophy, psychology and psychotherapeutic technique. In 1947 Fritz Perls published the first account of the new therapy in his book, *Ego, Hunger and Aggression.* In it he applied the basic principles of Gestalt psychology and of Eastern and existential philosophies to understanding personality and developing a new psychotherapy.

Gestalt is a German word meaning the whole, the entity formed by the particular order of its various parts. Gestalt psychology, which was a well developed theoretical and research oriented school of psychology before Gestalt therapy was developed, proposed that the basic nature of human experience is that it is organized into these patterns or gestalts.

A favorite slogan of the Gestalt school is that *the whole is more than the sum of its parts.* Gestalt psychologists are fond of using optical illusions to demonstrate that the different elements in a pattern combine to form a gestalt that could not have been predicted by knowing what the elements were. The lights on movie marquees that flick on and off and give the illusion of a moving band of lights is a good example of how the gestalt of the moving lights is more than its individual elements.

All experience, not just visual experience, is organized into gestalts. We experience our total environment, both outside and within, not as discontinuous stimuli but as a meaningful whole, in which everything we are and do is related to everything else we are and do.

FINISHING A GESTALT.   Each gestalt is a figure that stands out from some background. The background is the ever-changing whirl of energy or events that takes place every moment of our existence. Even when we're alone, we hear, see, think, feel, act, smell, touch, and so on, down to the molecular level of the constant change going on inside the organism. Out of this constant flow of energy, some gestalt—some experience that is the combination of many individual elements—begins to develop and captures our interest. Interest persists until some action brings this emerging gestalt to some finish. When the emerging gestalt is experienced and attended to, it can melt into the background and leave the foreground free for the next relevant gestalt.

For example, I am sitting here writing and suddenly remember that I promised to telephone a friend about this time. I may decide that it is more important to maintain my train of thought than to call my friend, but now my attention is split. I have two gestalts vying for my interest, and as long as I don't attend to this new gestalt and finish it, I have to use energy to suppress it. I choose instead to telephone my friend, say hello, and tell her I'm too busy to talk. I can now return to my writing with full interest and energy.

Finishing unfinished business is a major task of Gestalt therapy. When Florie started to become more aware of herself, she got in touch with how much energy she had tied up in an unfinished situation with her mother. Rather than express her anger to her mother and come to some closure, she maintained her discomfort by avoiding the issue and suppressing her natural feelings.

Most often, unfinished business interferes with how we relate to the present; it becomes a filter through which all present experience passes. Rather than experience each new situation freshly and creatively, the person with a lot of unfinished business relates to new situations with old responses. A man may be angry and distrustful toward women because he never expressed and finished his feelings of anger toward his mother. A woman may feel perpetually anxious because she never confronted the real source of her fear, perhaps a childhood belief that she is unlovable.

ORGANISMIC SELF-REGULATION.   Finishing unfinished business is one important way that the organism maintains *balance*. When people drag along old feelings, the accumulation throws their systems off balance. Imbalance is always experienced somewhere within the organism as tension.

The natural, physiological tendency of the organism to maintain balance is called homeostasis or *organismic self-regulation*. For example, when the level of sugar in the blood drops, we become hungry, fantasize food, and move toward eating to restore the balance. Part of the self-regulating process is feeling discomfort in our bodies and doing what is necessary to relieve it, whether the tension is physically generated by having too little sugar in the blood or psychologically by fears, need for contact or whatever.

In our culture people learn to be more concerned with what they should do and be than to pay attention to what feels right; they ignore *the wisdom of the organism*, the natural intuitive ability of the body to "know" what's good for it. If we block our feelings of our needs, then we cannot do what it takes to satisfy ourselves and maintain ourselves optimally.

Fritz Perls liked to say that Gestalt therapy was a way of "losing your mind and coming to your senses." Actually, in Gestalt therapy, we don't see the mind and body as separate-but-parallel functions of the human organism, as many of the older psychologies do. Gestalt therapy is *holistic:* the mind *is* the body and body *is* mind. The human being is a gestalt, a unified organism, and his or her mental and physical activities are manifestations of the same thing, his or her total existence.

Gestalt therapy, then, is a process of self-discovery whereby an individual becomes more self-aware and learns to take responsibility for his life by paying attention to himself as a whole person, finishing unfinished business, and developing the various senses, particularly the intuitive ones, in order to be more tuned in to the wisdom of the organism.

DIRECT EXPERIENCE.   Experience is the data of awareness. All experiences take place in the present. An experience of the past is a memory, a mental picture and a feeling occurring in the present. An experience of the future is a present anticipation of what the future might bring. We live in the present. If I am unhappy, I am unhappy right now. If I want to be happy, I first have to be aware of how I am maintaining my unhappiness here and now, and then recognize and choose the alternatives that will make me feel happier.

The only thing any of us can be sure of is what we know through direct experience. Paying attention to yourself means paying attention to the ongoing process of your mental activity and physical responsivity. What and how you are perceiving, sensing, feeling, the kinesthetic cues, gestures, postures of your body and the visualizations, fantasies, dreams, judgments, thoughts, of your mental activity—these are the clues to self-understanding.

SPOKEN MEDITATION.   Gestalt therapists are phenomenological. We deal with what is obvious, with what is going on now without any attempt to explain it or analyze it. We don't ask *why* a person does or feels something because that invites rationalization and defense. Instead we are concerned with *what* they do and *how* they do it.

The Gestalt awareness process is like a spoken and performed meditation. The individual who is on the hot seat, paying attention to him- or herself, starts by reporting out loud what he or she is aware of here and now. The therapist assists the person to be honest—tuned in to the truth of the organism; expressive—finishing old business; and experimental—trying out new ways of being. The therapist guides the person's attention and suggests ways to get more in touch with oneself; the relationship between them is one of mutual respect and equality.

I encourage the person to become an impartial witness while paying attention—that is, to imagine that he or she is not only the one who is speaking and acting, but also an observer, one who watches without evaluating—as a way of developing the ability to more objectively see oneself.

The *awareness continuum* is one of the most basic exercises of Gestalt therapy. Here we ask the individual to pay attention to him- or herself and to report every detail of his or her awareness out loud. The person, say a man, is encouraged to focus his awareness on what he is feeling, sensing, imagining. As he practices the awareness continuum, he finds his focus might shift from an awareness of what's happening outside him to a movement he makes, to an image, to a feeling, to a thought, or whatever. Practicing the awareness continuum is a way of practicing being aware as well as developing the skill of focusing inward as a method of self-observation. As the awareness shifts to different experiences, something emerges as having the most energy, catches the interest and is pursued.

"IT FEELS TERRIBLE."   Once I was doing a demonstration of Gestalt therapy before a group of about a hundred people. A woman—let's call her Mary—who had never done any Gestalt work before sat down beside me. After giving a demonstration of the awareness continuum I asked Mary to do the exercise herself. With her eyes closed, Mary began to report her experience. At one point a big smile flashed across her face, she laughed and said in a loud voice, "I imagine that everyone is looking at me and it feels terrible."

Precise language facilitates awareness. I asked Mary to be more direct with her language. Now, when she repeated her modified statement as "I feel terrible," she recognized that her statement was inaccurate, that she didn't really feel terrible. "But," she said questioningly, "my hands are shaking and my voice is trembling," as though this were some indication that she should be feeling terrible.

In Gestalt therapy we ask people to *make the implicit explicit* by exaggerating their behavior as a way of doing with awareness what was previously unconsciously and automatically done. I asked Mary to stand up and shake on purpose. At first she refused, but I coaxed her a bit, and when she got up and started to shake her hands and body, she began to laugh and she exclaimed loudly, "Hey, this is fun!" When she sat back down on the chair, she looked vibrant and happy, and said in a strong, clear voice, "You know, I don't often let myself have a good time. God, that was more fun than I've had in a long while."

When people pay attention to themselves, they are attending to three different but interrelated varieties of their experience: their mental activity, their feelings and bodily sensations, and their actions. All of these different experiences are important for individuals to be tuned in to if they are to increase their self-awareness and self-responsibility.

FIXED IDEAS.   *Mental activity includes thinking and image-making,* such as deliberating, visualizing and dreaming. In the process of growing up people develop habits of thought; fixed attitudes and ways of interpreting the world. Much of the time these fixed attitudes are introjected from the parents—swallowed whole without evaluation—and never assimilated or integrated with the rest of the personality.

As people pay attention to themselves they begin to recognize how their habitual ways of thinking color their experience, limit their alternatives, and restrict their positive, nourishing, creative ways of being. Becoming conscious of these fixed ideas and thought patterns often leads to giving them up in favor of a more open, less judgmental view of the world.

The other part of mental activity is the internal pictures that flash before the "mind's eye." Most, if not all, needs are represented mentally first before they are acted on. When we're hungry we picture the food we want. When we're cold we may picture a sweater. We rehearse before we act. By paying attention to these inner pictures, individuals can get a better sense of their needs and desires, and their behavior can then be more congruent with what is going on inside them.

Sometimes people don't take responsibility for their inner pictures but project them onto other people instead, much like a movie projector projects an image onto a screen. We often project parts of ourselves that we don't like and see our own unfriendliness or criticalness or hate as outside of ourselves, not as our own but as the other's.

A PROJECTION EXERCISE.   In Gestalt therapy we try out different experiments as ways of understanding our internal process. To see how projection works you might try the following. Sit close to and directly opposite another person who is interested in doing the exercise with you.

Without talking, both of you close your eyes and each pictures a face of anyone not present—someone you feel something about. Really examine the face you are visualizing, and when you feel that you have the image firmly fixed, open your eyes and project the image onto the face of the person sitting opposite you. Maintain the image for about a minute, looking at the person you're with and "seeing" the other face. Pay attention to how you feel. Then close your eyes again and rest for a few seconds. When you're ready open your eyes again, and this time simply look at the face of the person you're with. You will notice when you open your eyes to really look at the other person how your feelings change and how much more clearly you see him or her. In order to maintain a projected image we have to let our eyes go slightly out of focus and not see the real person as clearly.

In Gestalt therapy people "own" their projections by play-acting how they imagine other people are seeing them, evaluating them or judging them. When they play out their fantasies in this way, they can see and experience that it is their own self-judgments and self-criticism with which they are torturing themselves.

CAR, COUNTRY ROAD, FRIEND, SELF.   Dreams are seen as projections in Gestalt therapy, so rather than engage in the intellectual exercise of analyzing dreams, we experience them by acting them out. All the parts of the dream are seen as parts of the dreamer projected into story form. The individual plays out all parts of the dream. If a woman dreams about driving with a friend in a car down a country road, she plays not only herself and the friend but the car and the country road as well. She may have a dialogue between herself as the car and herself as the country road to discover and re-own whatever parts of herself were projected as a car, a country road, her friend and her dreamed self.

One of the most frequent questions a Gestalt therapist asks of the person paying attention to him or herself is "What are you feeling now?" *Feelings* are energy, a sense of excitement having a location somewhere on or within the body, extending over a certain area and having a certain intensity. We can ask about feelings then, not only what do you feel, but also where do you feel it, how much of an area does it cover, how much do you feel it? If we are out of touch with what we are feeling, we can't use these signals adequately to satisfy our needs, enhance our pleasures or reduce pain. Pain is an important signal that something is not right within and needs attending to. Unfortunately, some people are so out of touch with their feelings that they think it is natural to be in pain, to be unhappy, and don't do what it takes to reduce their pain/unhappiness. They may adapt to their pain so that they are mostly unconscious of it, but it is always present, influencing their behavior and experience.

People sometimes confuse feelings and thoughts. Since feelings are facts and thoughts can be fictions, it is important to be able to distinguish between the two. For example, "I'm feeling that you don't care about me," is a thought, not a feeling. I tell myself that you don't care about me and it may or may not be true. "I'm feeling sad, or tense, or cold," is a reporting of feeling. With feelings you can point to the place you're feeling something, where in your body you feel sad or tense or cold.

DISCHARGING EMOTION.   Feelings include emotions like anger or joy; sensations like pain or shakiness; and occasionally the tension of certain need states like feeling hungry or sexy. Experience takes place at many different levels at once, and emotion is a good example of that. We don't feel angry only in the gut but all over the body. There is a tendency to bare the teeth as shoulders and arms tense; hands naturally form into fists, hostile pictures flash before the mind's eye. There is a sense of energy and we want to stomp and yell.

Every emotion is associated with its characteristic expression, like stomping and yelling in anger or crying in sadness. When emotion is not discharged through its expression, tension builds up. It is as though blocking the expression of a given emotion freezes it and locks it into the body where it stays. Unfinished business stays unfinished. People who don't express their anger stay angry; they may retroflect their anger and become guilty and depressed, or their anger may ooze out in small subtle ways as in sarcasm or irritability. In either case their anger stays in their system, influencing their health and well-being and their relationships with other people.

When people learn to hold back their feelings all their lives, their bodies build up tension and take on the physical structure of the emotions they are not allowing themselves to feel and express. People who are angry and don't express it look angry all the time. The same is true for fear, or sadness, or guilt.

In Gestalt therapy people get in touch with their resistance to expressing their feelings. For example, people often learn to deny their feelings in early childhood in order to become more acceptable to their parents; consequently they tend lose touch with their authentic selves.

Recently I worked with a man who had been in a weekly group with me. Jack is tall, rugged looking and has led an adventurous life; yet his shoulders always seemed tense, his chest bloated, and he seemed restless and suspicious.

FREE TO FEEL AFRAID.   At one point in his work, Jack started to get concerned about how people in the group felt about him, what they were thinking. I asked Jack to own his projections, to play-act being the group and act out what he imagined they were thinking about him. As the group, Jack became sneering and angry at the empty pillow where "Jack" was sitting. When Jack sat down on the pillow to experience how he related to his portrayal of the group, he felt afraid, and for one of the first times in his life, he admitted to being afraid. I encouraged him to let himself feel his fear, to be afraid.

At first Jack simply sat on his pillow looking afraid, not knowing what to do. He seemed stuck. He knew how to be sneering and angry but didn't know how to be afraid. Finally Jack put his hands up to his face and started to make soft, gutteral, moaning sounds. Suddenly he began to scream. His eyes were wide, and his shoulders were way up almost sucking his head in. Soon Jack was crying softly and repeating, "I *am* afraid. I *am* afraid."

Later in the session, Jack revealed that he saw his father as continually putting him down for showing signs of fear. He had denied his fear to please his father and gain his approval. "Be a man. Be a man," Jack kept shouting when he was playing his father. When Jack played himself he became aware of the pain he had chosen to live with in covering up his nature.

Actions reflect the inner process of mental activity and feelings. What we do reflects whom we are. In fact, sometimes when we cut off feelings, or when feelings and images are vague and unidentifiable and we don't know what we need or want, the best clue to what's going on is to watch what we do or else try out different behaviors and see which "feels right."

DOUBLE MESSAGES.   In Gestalt therapy we ask people to pay attention to their actions as clues to awareness. How they are standing, sitting or breathing is information to them about themselves. Small gestures often reveal something going on that the individual may not be aware of. I've seen people making an affirmative statement while their heads were shaking "no." When they became aware of this "double message" they often became aware of some conflict: part of the person felt "yes" while another part felt "no."

In Gestalt awareness process, just as people act out their projections or dreams or unfinished business, they also get in touch with their inner conflicts by acting them out. If an individual became aware that part of him or her were saying "yes" to something and another part "no," he or she would act out the conflict by playing both roles—the part that feels "yes" and the part that feels "no." Each part would have a voice and the person would enter into a dialogue with these different voices.

Where the two voices begin to repeat themselves and no resolution is immediately apparent, we say that the individual is at an impasse—he or she is stuck. In Gestalt therapy people play out their conflicts until they get to their impasse and then they are encouraged to stay stuck—to stay at that creative zero point where both sides of themselves seem balanced in conflict. If the person stays with the empty space and the feeling of discomfort often accompanying it, some sudden insight or some explosive expression of feeling eventually breaks through the stalemate and the person discovers some creative solution uniting the two parts. Then the individual begins to move from fragmentation of the self toward awareness and integration of the different parts.

Jack had experienced this impasse when the sneering angry part of himself, which he had projected at the group, confronted the frightened resisting part of himself. When he allowed himself to stay stuck, not knowing what he would do, but maintaining himself in the situation, he broke through his resistance to express his authentic self. Scared, he became freer to be whom he really is once he expressed his fear.

Not only do people notice what they are doing as clues to understanding themselves and act out their conflicts as a way of integrating their fragmented parts, but people are also encouraged to do something new, to try out new and different ways of expressing themselves. As Laura Perls puts it Gestalt therapy is existential, experiential and experimental. In Gestalt therapy groups, people experiment in a safe environment with expressing their feelings, revealing their fantasies, being authentic with other people, as well as experimenting with how it feels to play the village idiot or tell a story in gibberish or dance a feeling.

Gestalt therapy is not only a clearing of the unfinished business, the projections, the introjections and the fixed ways of being that prevent spontaneity and choice, but it is also a training in the skills by which people can continue to grow on their own, outside of the therapy situation. Even when they are not involved in any on-going therapy experience, people continue to practice and develop the ability to learn from themselves through noncritical self-observation, to trust their bodies and the natural expression of their feelings, to risk exploring new and different ways of being in the world.

Gestalt therapy is not oriented toward adjustment. The values of Western society encourage people to suppress the feelings of their bodies and to live in their heads instead. Through various influences like the growth movement and the women's liberation movement these deadening values along with others like self-denial and living for the future are beginning to break down. We are developing a new philosophy of life that is evolving from the old. Gestalt therapy as a philosophy—a way of life—as well as a psychology of human behavior and a psychotherapy, contributes to this developing new consciousness. In its emphasis on awareness, balance, organismic self-regulation, being in tune with the body, expressing feelings, and taking responsibility for one's own life and experience, Gestalt therapy articulates a healthy orientation to life through which people can be allowing and comfortable with themselves and accepting and loving with others.

43 BEHAVIOR MODIFICATION: TWO NURSES TELL IT LIKE IT IS

Edith J. Burley, R.N.

Thelma B. Steiger, B.S.N.

THE CONCEPT OF SYSTEMATIC REINFORCEMENT, WHICH HAS ALSO been referred to as operant conditioning, experimental analysis of behavior, or behavior therapy is a powerful tool in the modification of aberrant behavior. One of the findings of the psychology laboratory is that behavior is influenced by the immediate consequences of that behavior, and symptoms ranging from tantrums to severe autism can be modified by conditioning.

A behavior modification program has been in effect at Haverford State Hospital for two years. With the approval, support and continued interest of the hospital administration, two psychologists undertook a project in behavior therapy. The goal of the project was twofold: (1) to give dignity and independence to the chronic patient, and (2) to attempt to prevent an accumulation of a chronic psychotic population in the hospital. The basic mechanism underlying this program is the premise that people tend to behave in ways that "pay off." They avoid behavior associated with bad effects (negative reinforcers) and they repeat behavior associated with rewards (positive reinforcers).

Basic assumptions underlying a behavior therapy program are: (1) maladaptive behavior is learned in the same way that adaptive behavior is

Reprinted with permission from *Journal of Psychiatric Nursing and Mental Health Services*, January-February 1972.

learned. No special mental or physical disease process is assumed. (2) The task of psychotherapy is not assumed to be an effort aimed at the removal of intrapsychic conflicts via insights or changes in the personality structure. Psychological treatment involves the utilization of a variety of methods to devise programs which control the patient's environment, behavior and the consequences of behavior in such a way that presenting problems are resolved. (3) Because maladaptive behavior is learned, the techniques employed in the program can be drawn from the whole fund of experimental data in the field of human and animal learning.

Evolution of the Program

The head nurse and psychiatric aides on the behavior modification unit are a "hand picked" team. They were given minimal orientation to their functions within the program by the psychologists who initiated the program. For the most part, they learned by doing and by trial and error, with much patience and dedication. They spent a great deal of time with patients.

The ward was equipped to house fifty patients. The floor plan included a large, pleasantly accommodated living room situated close to the nursing office and doctor's office. This unit has its own dining area and a beauty parlor. Adequate sleeping quarters are provided by dormitories, private and semi-private rooms. One room was transformed into a "general store" and another area was labeled "skid row." This latter area will be described later.

There were fifty women assigned to this unit, ranging in age from seventeen to seventy, all of whom had been hospitalized from ten to twenty years. Seventy percent of these patients were diagnosed as schizophrenic. The rest were placed in diagnostic categories of mental retardation and organic brain damage. Because of the long period of hospitalization and the apparent resistance to many treatment modalities, any change would have to be for the better when one considered a typical day on 14 East, before the program began. Through the program the staff was able to rise to the challenge of a very difficult group of patients.

At 6:00 A.M. the night personnel turned on lights and asked the patients to "please get up." By 6:30 A.M. personnel finally assisted everyone out of bed; in many cases this would mean lifting patients out of bed and getting them on their feet. Many patients had to be dressed by the staff.

Between 7:00 and 7:30 A.M. the patients were called for medication. When they did not respond, they had to be located.

At 8:00 A.M. all patients were corralled into the dining area for breakfast. Many times this meant getting them out of bed again.

Between 8:30 and 10:30 A.M. personnel tried to coax patients to make beds, and finally made the beds for them. One-fifth of the patients were bathed each day. There was a bath book and personnel decided when each patient should take a bath. If patients did not bathe themselves, staff lifted them into the tub and bathed them.

By 10:30 A.M. all patients were sitting in the living room staring at a blaring television. Staff then started the housekeeping for the day.

Eleven thirty A.M. was round-up time again. Many patients were asleep in their chairs in the living room. Medicine was brought to them, and we helped them to the dining room to eat lunch. Many patients had to be spoon fed all meals.

At 1:30 P.M. patients were due at either recreational or occupational therapy. This again was planned by personnel; patients had no choice. Staff herded patients into a group, dressed them in outdoor clothes and plodded off to the activity of the day. When they arrived at the occupational and recreational therapy area, patients sat and stared while personnel engaged in activities meant for patients, trying to kindle a spark of participation, but to little avail.

About 3:00 P.M. the group trudged down the hill to their building. Staff removed the patients' coats and put them away while the patients dropped back into the chairs in the living room, perhaps to doze until taken to supper. As one nurse put it, "Our working day is now over. We are not encouraged about tomorrow; it will be the same. Our work is monotonous. We all lack enthusiasm. We have the feeling of not accomplishing a thing. We are glad to turn the unit over to the next shift." No wonder the nursing staff welcomed a chance to try something new.

Before the behavior modification program could start, the staff realized it would be profitable to have patients' families involved. The relatives of all patients were invited to attend an orientation session on a given evening. A film provided by Smith, Kline and French was shown; the program and its goals were explained. There was a question and answer period; the psychologists and head nurse participated in responding. At this time staff tried to interview each family to find out what kind of behavior preceded the patient's admission to the hospital. This was most difficult. Many families merely said "she was not acting right." Doctors would translate this at the time of admission as "bizarre behavior." What was needed, however, were specific behavior traits. The interviews required time and patience before families could recall behavior in descriptive terms (i.e., she would not get out of bed in the morning, she would not take a bath, did not care for the house, neglected the children). During these interviews staff also tried to learn what the family expected of this patient when she was discharged. Would she live at home? What would her duties be? Must she support herself?

Perhaps selected diary notes of the head nurse will most clearly show how the program got underway.

AUGUST 18:   This is the "big day" for 14 East, the first day of the modification program. We went around to each patient with a token and said: "This token is for lunch." As we were met with many questioning looks, there were some who did not want to take the token, but they finally accepted it to please us. At lunch all of the patients turned in the token at the dining room door.

AUGUST 21:   We have continued this procedure for three days, adding the other meals. The patients are used to "paying" a token for meals. Today we put a notice on the bulletin board (this board is in a very prominent place, next to the television). This notice stated that tokens would be given out at a card table next to the nursing station door, just before the doors to the dining room opened. We stayed at the table about five minutes after the dining room was opened. At this point some of the patients had not read the notice and they missed the first meal. All showed up for the next token.

AUGUST 23:   Some patients are too lethargic to get up out of their chairs twice, once for the token, then again to go to the dining room. They wait until the very last minute to pick up their token just before going to the dining room. One little lady who could hardly care for herself, took it upon herself to help another very confused patient. We overheard conversations exchanged between patients such as, "Did you get your token yet?" and "Don't lose that, you'll miss your meal!" This is very heartwarming to us because up to this time these patients rarely verbalized and walked around quite unaware of their surroundings.

AUGUST 25:   We posted another notice stating that tokens would now be given only between certain times. We made these times one-half to one-quarter hour before the dining room doors opened. Now when the patients forgot to read the notice, they have no chance of coming back to the table and getting that token. Again, some of the patients missed the first meal, however, they were bright and early for the next meal token.

AUGUST 27:   Today was a little hard on personnel. We now wait for the patient to state what she wants when she comes to the table.

The reason it was hard on personnel was that in all our previous training we are taught to anticipate the patient's needs and to fulfill those needs. Now we have to act as though we do not see the needs.

SEPTEMBER 12:   Lunch tokens are now given out at 9:15 A.M. and patients take care of them until lunch time which is 12:15 P.M.

SEPTEMBER 21:   When the patients' nails were checked at 9:15 A.M., many were told they had dirty nails, to go clean them, and we would give them a lunch token. Ten patients had dirty nails; they all made an attempt to clean them; they all received a token for lunch.

SEPTEMBER 22:   Today when we checked patients' nails, we had nail brushes and files ready for use. Those with dirty nails were told, "Today you are allowed to go clean your nails, and then we will give you a lunch token. In the future you will have to have clean nails the first time you come for your token." Only one patient would not accept either brush or file to clean her nails. She did not receive a lunch token. As we oberved the patients in line, we can see life awakening in them. One patient got out of line and tried to borrow a nail file from another patient. This required an exchange of words, an awareness of "the other." Two other patients were standing quietly in line. When it seemed to dawn on them that we were going to check nails, they immediately looked at their nails. One left the line and went to wash her hands, the other started to clean the nails of one hand with the nail of the other. Later today we posted notices on the bulletin board:
— Nail brushes and nail files may be borrowed any time. Just ask at the nursing station.
— Between 9:00 and 9:15 A.M. lunch tokens will only be given to those with clean nails.

SEPTEMBER 24:   Despite the improved response of patients to the token given for clean nails, five patients missed lunch today. Most of the others who have been caring for their nails now have not only cleaner but better shaped nails. They notice this change and have big smiles on their faces when they show us their hands.

SEPTEMBER 30:   It was decided in team meeting today that from now on we would make another modification:
For clean nails say: "Here is another white token, you will need one token for the day room and one token for lunch."

For dirty nails say: "I cannot give you two tokens because your nails are dirty. Here is one white token. You can use it to get into the day room, or you can use it for lunch. It is up to you."

OCTOBER 1:   Today we started giving two tokens for clean nails and only one for dirty nails. With this one token the patient is forced to make a choice. Will she use it for lunch or for the privilege of sitting in the day room? If she used it for the day room, she will miss lunch. If she uses it for lunch, she has to wait in the hallway, standing or sitting on the floor, and there is no smoking permitted.

OCTOBER 3:   Today we started giving patients two free tokens at 4:15 P.M. They may use one for dinner and one for going to bed. If they refuse or won't pay for the bed, they must sleep in the day room all night. Three patients preferred to hoard their tokens; they spent the night in the day room.

OCTOBER 4:   Now, between 8:45 A.M. and 9:15 A.M. patients may receive one token for clean nails, and one token for beds made. They have 30 minutes to return and make their bed. No free tokens are given now. One patient slept in the day room tonight, however, none of the patients who spent last night in the day room did a repeat performance.

OCTOBER 17:   Automatic ground privileges were cancelled for everyone today. Occupational and Industrial therapies were also cancelled. Today patients were given one token for each of the following:

clean nails
acceptable grooming
bed made
cleaning chores done

These tokens can be used for breakfast, lunch, and supper, entrance to the day room, or to pay to get off the ward to go out on the grounds. Ward cleaning chores are worth one token if done satisfactorily. Some patients have more than one job, thus earn more than one token. Patients who had seemed very lazy work quite well at ward cleaning now.

OCTOBER 27:   Employment agency started. Hours 10:30 A.M. to 11:00 A.M. Any patient desiring a job whereby they can earn tokens may apply. *Notice posted:* Starting tomorrow one token will be given when morning medication is taken on time (7:30 A.M.).

NOVEMBER 1:   Dance therapy started at 4:00 P.M. 14 patients participated. Now that the patients respond more like living beings, volunteers and activities personnel are more encouraged to try to work with them. *Notice posted:* Trips off grounds are available for two or more persons at a cost of five tokens. Inquire at the nursing stations.

NOVEMBER 2:   Two patients made arrangements to go to the opera with the chaplain. Two patients went on a shopping trip with the psychologist.

NOVEMBER 11:   Many articles have been donated for the patients' "general store" (cigarettes, candy, costume jewelry, some articles of clothing, grooming articles, etc.). *Notice posted:* The store will be opened on Monday at 9:00 A.M. Articles are priced as marked.

NOVEMBER 14:   Store opened. Ten articles sold.

NOVEMBER 18:   *Notice posted:* One token charged for a visitor on the unit. Two tokens charged for visitors off the unit. A juke box has been donated to the unit. Three records played for one token.

DECEMBER 1:   *Notice posted:* **MOVIE PASS** on sale for five tokens. Four patients signed up to go, each paid ten tokens, five for the pass, and five for the trip off the grounds.

DECEMBER 29:   *Notice posted:* **ROOMS FOR RENT** Private room—three tokens, Semi-private room— three tokens and Dormitory—one token. If too many want private or semi-private rooms for us to accommodate them, then the room goes to the highest bidder. . . .and that is how it all began.

Each patient's program is tailor-fitted to her individual needs. Before behavior can be modified, it is necessary to find out what is reinforcing to the patient. Each patient is different. One may work to have a private room. For another, meals are very important. To another, a cigarette is most important. After the best reinforcer is found, a goal for the patient is planned and small steps taken in that direction. Pushing for results too fast can lose the patient. A procedure that is not working after 10 to 14 days is dropped, and another procedure is initiated with the same goal in mind. What works for one patient may not work for another. Before any procedure is started, it is imperative to have a base line. Behavior must be measured and recorded again for 10 to 14 days. This enables staff to determine if the tokens change behavior.

While tokens are paid for all desired behavior (reinforcing the positive), unacceptable behavior is ignored. If ignoring the undesirable behavior does not extinguish it, then tokens are charged for the undesirable behavior. It is up to the patient to decide if she wants to stop the unacceptable behavior or pay tokens. A patient can do anything she wants on this unit as long as she pays for it. For example, if a patient wants to go into the day room and cause a disturbance by shouting, throwing chairs and cursing, the charge for disturbing the peace is four tokens. Hitting another patient is also expensive, five tokens.

Patients are paid for "good behavior" according to each one's capabilities. One patient only had to comb her hair to earn enough tokens to live comfortably for the day. However, as soon as this response was established for three or four days, the requirements were increased. Requirements were added gradually until she was on a par with the rest of the patients.

Every patient is paid differently for every job. There are two patients who dislike going out, so they are paid to go to the canteen and have a card signed. This means they have to leave the unit, walk to the canteen (one block of fresh air) ask someone to sign their card, return to the unit, and come to the pay line with their signed card at the scheduled time. All other patients pay tokens for going to the canteen. After the patients are going to the canteen and perhaps starting to enjoy it, the payment is cut in half and continues to diminish until after a short time patient is paying for the right to go to the canteen just as the other patients do. A similar procedure has been used with patients who will not go on day passes or weekends. Large sums are paid for the first times until they have sampled the privilege. Then the sum is gradually decreased until the economy is turned around and they are paying for the privilege.

There are patients who do not socialize with either personnel or other patients. These patients are given jobs in which talking is a necessity. Telephone answering service on the unit is one such job. The patient is trained to answer the phone: "14 East, with whom would you like to speak?" After they are comfortable with the assignment, they will be moved to a job like storekeeper, or receptionist in the lobby, which involves greeting the visitors to the building and calling the proper information into the unit.

Again, from the head nurses' diary:

"We have one patient who spends most of her waking hours peeking out of the locker or bathroom door. She never ventures out to mingle with other patients. This behavior was completely acceptable to personnel; she never broke a rule. She was so easy to care for, but we really were not doing anything to help her. We accepted her as she was, and did not expect her to do anything else. She missed a meal because she was in one of her favorite spots. An attendant who walked past her in the afternoon of the day of this new notice overheard a remark which really set us back on our heels; "I sure won't miss the next token, I'm hungry!"

We have a young retarded girl in the program. For months before the program started we had been unwittingly reinforcing undesirable behavior. We thought we were making things easier for ourselves. Whenever medicines or meals were called, she always pushed in first. It seemed much easier to let her have her way! Now she is learning to wait her turn and, although she is still putting up a small "fuss," her behavior is much better than two and one-half weeks ago. One token-time she was escorted to the end of the line when she tried to push in ahead of the others. She was angry, but did not know how to handle the situation. She tried to get rid of the psychologist by saying, "Bye-Bye man," but this didn't work, so she cooperated until she arrived at the gate of the dining room at which time she looked around at the psychologist and broke the token in half. She was allowed to use the broken token this time, but was told we did not accept broken tokens. She has only broken one other token. She got angry when she could not push ahead at the dining room door and threw the token to the floor, breaking it. At this point she missed a meal. (We all had to support each other since we all wanted to giver her another chance. This was a very hard lesson for all of us.) Since then we have not had another broken token from Linda.

One little lady who just sat around all day was placed on the program. She had to be coaxed to go to any assignment or activity. She never showed any emotion, and she also never missed a meal or broke a rule. However, she missed one of the notices and she did not get her token in time to eat one night. At this point we saw her show emotion for the first time. She really was very "spunky," she spoke up about no meal, and asked to report us to the doctor. This was granted. When she reported us, the doctor listened to her complaint and then explained to her that he knew all about the program and that he was the one who put her name on the list and that she was expected to cooperate. She, at this point, was so angry at herself, the doctor, and the personnel, that she acted more alive. She speaks more and openly states that she does not like the program. However, she is cooperating completely.

A new patient came to the ward and was added to the program after it had been in progress about two weeks. The patient only had "walking sight" and was very confused; it was decided we would give her a token just before each meal for a day, before she would have to ask for her token. This plan worked for just one meal. Another patient took it upon herself to get her and take her to the table and tell her to ask for her token the same as all the other patients.

Personnel feelings no longer have as much effect on patient care. For example, on a day when the staff was feeling happy and all the world was bright, all patients were allowed ground privileges, extra television hours and other "goodies." The next day, if personnel were tired and cranky, no patients were allowed out until all housekeeping was done, and there might be no television. This cannot happen with our program. If a patient has the agreed upon number of tokens, then she can leave the unit no matter how personnel feel. The patient decides what she wants, pays for it and gets it.

The difference in the atmosphere in our unit is dramatically shown by the present daily schedule.

At 7:00 A.M. lights are turned on. Within the next half hour it is each patient's responsibility to come to the staff. She receives a white chip if she takes her medicine in this half hour, a red chip if she shows she is wearing clean underwear and a blue chip for taking a bath or shower.

By 8:00 A.M. the day room is swept and mopped, furniture and window sills are dusted. Six patients are paid to do these chores, if one does not show up for work by 7:30 A.M., volunteers are solicited. A patient can only be a volunteer if she has already done her own assigned work.

Tokens are collected for breakfast as the patients go to the dining room at 8:15 A.M. During breakfast, beds and rooms are checked by staff.

At 8:45 A.M. workers with early assignments off the unit have their grooming checked (hair, dress, nails and lipstick). They are paid in the measure agreed upon. Some of these patients go to make beds on the geriatric units. Two patients go to school.

From 9:00 A.M. to 9:30 A.M. all other patients are due at grooming line. They are no longer called. It is their responsibility to come.

At 9:15 A.M. the door opens for workers who are due at work off the unit by 9:30 A.M. These include: two patients who work in the patients' library; two patients who make cancer dressings; two patients who go to the tailor shop; one patient who is attending a nurses' aide course, and one patient who bathes, feeds, dresses and walks two retarded patients.

At this time patients may pay for where they wish to spend the morning, in the living room or on the grounds. Also during this time staff not engaged in the pay line inspect work assignments on the unit. Each assignment is checked once. If it is incomplete, then a volunteer may finish it for extra tokens.

One patient carries the key to the front door. She opens the door for early workers and each half hour after that. This is like having another member of the team. She saves personnel so much time and enjoys being paid for her "very responsible job."

At 9:30 A.M. the store is opened. Here patients can purchase small variety articles with tokens; no money is used. The store opens every time the patients are paid, thus they can immediately see the reward of their good grooming and work. The storekeeper is a patient who gets a token for taking care of customers.

At 9:30 A.M. another patient makes and serves coffee to patients and personnel. A coffee ticket, which may be exchanged for a cup of coffee, is purchased at the store or the office. The coffee maker and server earns one token for each cup of coffee she serves.

A clean-up girl washes the cups and pot so that it is ready for next coffee time. One patient is paid for doing her personal laundry. She must bring her clothes to personnel by 10:30 A.M. If they are clean, her card is signed so that she will be paid at the next pay period.

Second pay period begins at 11:30 A.M. Those patients who have worked off the unit return with their signed papers. All jobs are treated as real employment. Patients are docked for being late, not completing a job, leaving before the job is complete, refusing an assignment, or inappropriate behavior. The store is open for shopping.

Tokens are collected as patients enter the cafeteria for lunch. After lunch patients pay for where they want to spend the afternoon. They may also purchase the right to take a one hour nap. The penalty for being found in bed napping without prior arrangement is double the cost for naps.

Three patients go to feed patients in geriatrics.

At 1:00 P.M. the door opens for workers who leave for the serving room, school, clerical pool and the library. Several are assigned to Occupational Therapy.

Payment for afternoon work is made at 3:30 P.M. and the store is again opened for immediate reward.

Supper tokens are collected and at 5:00 P.M. patients pay for the room where they want to spend the evening and for a private single bedroom, if desired.

During the evening a cup of juice or milk is served by a patient for the price of one token.

As patients progress toward dealing with the "real world" outside the hospital, living becomes more complex. The work assignments become more meaningful rather than being merely "busy work." The concept of unemployment insurance has been introduced to the token system economy. The patient may pay two tokens per week to the unemployment insurance. If she becomes ill and cannot work for a few days, or in the event that staff in charge of a given work area have no work for the patient on certain days, then the patient may be paid for the job from her unemployment insurance fund.

Banking privileges are also made available now. The "lead slugs" used as tokens may become heavy and cumbersome to carry around, so the patient may "deposit" any surplus in "the bank." The amount of her deposit is recorded on a bank card which is then issued to her. The principle of banked tokens earning "interest" when deposited over a period of time is also applied.

If a patient becomes "indigent" because she chooses not to work for tokens, she may miss meals and have to live in an area called "skid row" by the patients. This is a short hallway and stark room devoid of furnishings. Patients rarely choose to spend longer than a twenty-four hour period in the "skid row" area. Staff is careful not to let patients become so low in token funds that this endangers health or safety.

Medical orders for the physically ill may be tied right into the program. There is one patient who receives token payment for doing her postural drainage exercises. Small comforts and securities can also be purchased; for example, a patient may rent a soft chair in the living room, locker key, and television room privileges weekly.

Assessment and Benefits of the Program

Social awareness and caring for others has been fostered by the program which initially paid patients to care for the physically sick patients (i.e. carry meal trays, read to patients, etc.). Now, patients often give these small attentions to others spontaneously, without thought of remuneration. In every instance this program gives the patient the dignity of making her own decisions.

Many newly assigned psychiatric aides are upset about the way the ward 14 East is organized. It usually takes between two days to a week before the newcomers are praising the program. Many come with the idea that it is cruel to make a patient pay for meals and bed. This attitude fades very quickly when they see what the patients are able to do just because they are expected to succeed and are shown that we believe in their potential for better health.

Here are some reflections of the head nurse of the unit after two years of work on this program. "If administration is not supportive and even enthusiastic about the program, don't start it. It will fail without the backing of administration. Team work is essential. As soon as possible involve all personnel on all shifts in the program. You will see the members of a shift become more enthusiastic as their responsibility for the program is increased. All shifts should overlap by at least an hour; this improves communications between shifts and keeps the program consistent. As personnel become involved in the program they contribute more ideas. Use everyone's idea. Even though you think some ideas may not work, try them as soon as possible. This is so reinforcing to personnel that they will come up with more and more ideas, and some of them will be very, very good.

Personnel do not become discouraged on this unit. Patients' records clearly show trends of improvement, and this acts as a catalyst to the staff's enthusiasm.

This program has some overall financial benefit also. The patients on the behavior modification program take less medication. A recent study conducted by hospital staff has shown that there is $1,000 saving on medication bills per twenty-five patients a year. A group of twenty-five patients off the program received 120 pills (22c per patient) per day. A group of twenty-five patients on the program received only 60 pills (11c per patient) per day.

Although individual patient's progress is meticulously charted, perhaps the best measurement of the effectiveness of this program is evident in the patient's own words:

"This token business is O.K. but I want to earn the real kind of spending money now so I need a real kind of job". . .

"This program is helping me plan ahead for the day when I am earning and budgeting my own money" . . .

"I think its terrible to have to pay for my meals with those slugs, but it makes my day more interesting because I have to do different things to earn them" . . .

"This is the fairest and squarest way I've ever been treated, and I been in many a hospital. Here I can earn anything I wants or needs" . . .

We have observed that there is less "crazy" talk. The patients are now talking more about realities, i.e., the wages are too low (tokens), the prices are too high, or the work expected is too hard. There are fewer physical complaints. There has been a decrease in inappropriate behaviors, and disturbing the peace on the unit is practically extinct. Grooming and personal hygiene have marvelously improved. There is less fighting and friction among patients, more socialization between patients and between patients and personnel. Patients help one another both in earning tokens and giving advice as to how they should be spent or saved. More letters are being mailed to families, more phone calls are being made to families and there are more weekend passes to go home. Patients are asking for more privileges (and are receiving them) such as shopping trips, passes to go out to eat or to go out to a show.

Satisfaction for nursing staff comes with being able to truly help their patients toward better health. The nursing personnel at Haverford State Hospital are so pleased with what they have been doing on Unit 14 East that they welcome interested visitors who come to observe the program and return to their home hospitals to start similar programs.

44 BURNED OUT

Christina Maslach, Ph.D.,

JUST BEFORE CHRISTMAS, A WOMAN WENT TO A poverty lawyer to get help. While discussing her problems, she complained about the fact that she was so poor that she was not going to be able to get any Christmas presents for her children. The lawyer, who was a young mother herself, might have been expected to be sympathetic to the woman's plight. Instead, she found herself yelling at the woman, telling her, "So go rob Macy's if you want presents for your kids! And don't come back to see me unless you get caught and need to be defended in court!" Afterward, in thinking about the incident, the lawyer realized that she had "burned out."

Hour after hour, day after day, health and social service professionals are intimately involved with troubled human beings. What happens to people who work intensely with others, learning about their psychological, social or physical problems? Ideally, the helpers retain objectivity and distance from the situation without losing their concern for the person they are working with. Instead, our research indicates, they are often unable to cope with this continual emotional stress and burnout occurs. They lose all concern, all emotional feeling, for the persons they work with and come to treat them in detached or even dehumanized ways.

For the past few years, I have been studying the dynamics of burnout in collaboration with co-workers at the University of California in Berkeley. We have observed 200 professionals at work, conducted personal interviews and collected extensive questionnaire data. Our sample

Reprinted with permission from *Department of Health and Social Services Quarterly* Winter 1976, Vol. 34.

includes poverty lawyers, physicians, prison personnel, social welfare workers, clinical psychologists and psychiatrists in a mental hospital, child-care workers and psychiatric nurses. Our findings to date show that all of these professional groups (and perhaps others that you can think of in your own experience) tend to cope with stress by a form of distancing that not only hurts themselves but is damaging to all of us as their human clients.

For one thing, the worker's feelings about people often show a shift toward the cynical or negative. According to one social worker, "I began to despise everyone and could not conceal my contempt," while another reports, "I find myself caring less and possessing an extremely negative attitude." In many cases, professionals who have burned out from stress and can no longer cope begin to defend themselves not only by thinking of clients in more derogatory terms but even by believing that the clients somehow deserve any problems they have. As one psychiatric nurse reported to us, "Sometimes you can't help but feel, 'Damn it, they want to be there, and they're fuckers, so let them stay there.' You really put them down."

There is little doubt that burnout plays a major role in the poor delivery of health and welfare services to people in need of them. They wait longer to receive less attention and less care. It is also a key factor in low worker morale, absenteeism, and high job turnover (for a common response to burnout is to quit and get out).

Further, we found that burnout correlates with other damaging indexes of human stress, such as alchoholism, mental illness, marital conflict and suicide. The suicide rate of police officers, for example, is 6½ times higher than that of people in non-law enforcement occupations, and psychiatrists contribute more than their share of numbers to the suicide toll.

If stress cannot be resolved while on the job, then it is often resurrected at home. Sometimes the professional is unaware of the causes and wrongly attributes the increased fighting to something that has gone wrong in the family relationship. As one correctional officer put it, when talking about the pressures of working in prison, "None of my three wives understood."

Burnout varies in severity among different professions and is called by different names (some law enforcement groups refer to this suppression as the "John Wayne syndrome"), but the same basic phenomenon seems to be occurring across a wide variety of work settings.

In our project, we are uncovering the interpersonal stresses that plague these workers, learning what (if any) preparation they receive to cope and isolating the techniques that they use to "detach" themselves

from clients or patients. Also, we seek to identify the human consequences for American society that result from use of such distancing techniques, and we are addressing ourselves to solutions. What can be done
to prevent the destructive process of burnout?

The verbal and nonverbal techniques used to achieve detachment
were remarkably similar among all the many professional groups we
studied. By reducing the worker's emotional involvement, these techniques make a client seem less human, more like an object or a number.

We found that a change in the terms used to describe people was one
way of making them appear more objectlike and less human. Some of
these terms are derogatory labels ("They're all just animals" or "They
come out from under the rocks"). Others are more abstract terms referring to large, undifferentiated units, such as "the poor," "my caseload" or
"my docket."

Another way of divorcing one's feelings from some stressful event is to
describe things as precisely and scientifically as possible. In several
professions, the use of jargon (e.g., "a positive GI series," "reaction
formation") typically serves the purpose of distancing the person from a
client who is emotionally upsetting in some way.

Patients are often labeled by their immediate medical problem, such as
"He's a coronary." While this aspect of the patient is the most important
one that a physician should be attending to, the fact that it is often the
only one means that the patient's complex humanness—his or her accomplishments, hopes and feelings and beliefs—is disregarded or ignored.

A related technique that we discovered involves recasting a volatile
situation in more intellectual and less personal terms. For example, in
dealing with a mental patient who is being verbally or physically abusive,
a psychiatric nurse may try to stand back and look at the patient
analytically so as not to get personally upset. "I think that if someone on
the outside were to hit me, I would get really angry and hit them back," a
nurse told us. "But I don't get angry if a patient hits me, because it's a different situation. The patients who strike out are not really angry at you—
they're striking out in fear, or they're so out of it that they don't even
know what they're doing. Sometimes a patient is striking out at the devil.
So, at the moment, you happen to look like the devil, but it's not you personally that he's striking out at—so I don't get angry at that."

Another way of distancing is to make a sharp distinction between job
and personal life. Many professionals whom we studied do not discuss
their family or personal affairs with their co-workers, and they often re-
frain from discussing their experiences on the job with their spouses and
friends. "My husband and I have an explicit agreement that neither of us
will 'talk shop' at home. I'm in social work, and he's in clinical practice.

Neither of us wants to burden the other with more emotion-arousing anecdotes from the day, as we each have had enough of our own to cope with," explained one of our subjects.

Some of the prison personnel even refused to tell people what their job was. In response to questions, they would only say, "I'm a civil servant" or "I work for the state." By leaving their work at the office and not reliving it once again at home, the emotional stress is confined to a smaller part of the professional's life.

One social worker in child welfare stated that if he did not leave his work at the office, he could hardly stand to face his own children. Likewise, when he was at work, he could not think of his family because he would then overemphathize with his clients, leading to unbearable emotional stress. As one might expect, he doesn't have the usual family photos on the office desk. Rules forbidding staff to socialize with their patients or clients outside the job setting can help to bring about this clear distinction.

For many psychiatrists, a drawback of going into private practice is that job and private life can merge in disturbing ways. As one of our respondents put it, "Everytime you hear your telephone ring at night, you think, 'Oh, no—I hope it's not a patient.' At times it seems as if you can't ever get away from your patients' problems for some peace and quiet for yourself. When I worked at the hospital, there wasn't the same problem because when I went home for the day, another shift came on—and so I could relax in the evenings because I knew that if any of the patients needed help, there was someone else there to provide it."

Another technique for cooling emotion is to minimize physical involvement in a tense encounter. How does it happen? We observed a number of ways. Some people physically distanced themselves from others (by standing farther away, avoiding eye contact or keeping their hand on the doorknob) even while continuing a minimal conversation. Withdrawal was also achieved by communicating with the patient or client in impersonal ways—superficial generalities, stereotyped responses and form letters.

In some cases, professionals simply spend less time with their patient or client, either by deliberately cutting down the length of the formal interview or therapy sessions, or by spending more of their time talking and socializing with other staff members. Many of the psychiatric staff were able to point to specific patients with whom they limited their interaction. "There was one woman who was very suicidal. She had injured herself in some bizarre ways and had set herself on fire several times on the ward. She was extremely depressed, and I did a lot of work with her. One day I had to spend my entire eight-hour shift with her, and I was so down by the time I left that I knew that I had to limit my time with her. I wouldn't spend more than two hours with her because she really got to me after a while," a psychiatric nurse told us. Or, in another case: "There's a 13-year-old schizophrenic boy that I'm working with now who thinks he's a machine, or a 'mutant.' I like him, but he frustrates me tremendously. Sometimes all I can handle is a 30-minute conversation with him because he's very nongiving. Sometimes I deal with the frustration by separating myself from the patient. I won't spend as much time with him; instead, I'll spend more time with other patients whom we're achieving a little more with."

Related to withdrawal is the technique of "going by the book" rather than unique factors of a situation. It's another way of short-circuiting any personal involvement with a client or patient. By applying a formula, the professional can avoid having to think about the nature of the problems. Also, the emotional stress triggered by taking responsibility for unpopular or painful decisions can be eluded if a worker says, "I'm, sorry, but its not my fault those are the rules around here, and I have to follow them."

For the social welfare workers, one of the major signs of burnout was the transformation of a person with original thought and creativity on the job into a mechanical, petty bureaucrat.

For many of the people whom we observed, social outlets proved to be a more gratifying, if ironic, route to detachment. They solicited advice and comfort from other staff members after withdrawal from a difficult situation. Such social support eased the stress and pain, fostered a sense of distance from the situation and tended to neutralize the emotions. Reported one of the profession, "When we get together, we bitch a lot to each other. We hash things out. We laugh at it sometimes. We talk about it a lot and try new ways. It helps to talk about it, and if you can't see it another way, then somebody else might be able to."

Social support also led to a perception of diffused responsibility among staff members, which helped the individual worker to feel even more remote from troublesome clients. Another social technique was the use of humor. Joking and laughing about a stressful event reduced personal anxiety by making the situation seem less serious, less frightening and less overwhelming. The battlefield surgeons in M*A*S*H*, who made "sick" jokes and flirted with the nurses while they performed grave operations, are a particularly apt example of this technique at work. As one of our respondents put it, "Sometimes things are so awful and so frustrating that in order to keep from crying, you laugh at a situation that may not even be funny. You laugh but you know in your heart what's really happening. Nevertheless, you do it because your own needs are important—we're all human beings, and we have to be ourselves."

Many of these detachment techniques can be used by professionals either to reduce the amount of personal stress or to cope with it successfully while still maintaining concern for the people they must work with. However, because some forms of these techniques preclude any continued caring, we found that they often degenerated into the total detachment and dehumanization of burnout. In these cases, the worker's attempts at emotional self-protection came at the expense of the client, patient, child, prisoner, etc. The professionals donned such thick armor that nobody could get through.

At the moment, we cannot present a total solution to the problem of burnout. However, our work thus far has pointed to a number of factors that could reduce the harm done by burnout or prevent its occurrence altogether.

Burnout often leads to a deterioration of physical well-being. The professional becomes exhausted, is frequently sick and may be beset by insomnia, ulcers and migraine headaches, as well as more serious illnesses. Some of the prison guards reported physical problems with their back and neck, although only a few seemed to realize the psychosomatic nature of these ailments. "On the way home from my first day on the job," says one guard, "I realized that my neck hurt. The muscles were tight, and that caused me to have a headache. Perspiration was heavier than normal. Later on, I realized that my neck and back would begin to get stiff and sore and painful just before I went to the prison—and it would last until I got home again."

In order to cope with these physical problems, the worker may turn to tranquilizers, drugs or alcohol—"solutions" that have the potential for being abused. Better measures include regular vacations (where one can rest completely and "recharge one's batteries") and physical exercise. In a booklet on burnout, put out by the Drug Abuse Council, Dr. Herbert Freudenberger suggests, "Encourage your staff and yourself to exercise physically. If you want to run, do it. Play tennis, dance, swim, bicycle, exhaust yourself on the drums. Engage in any activity that will make you physically tired. Many times the exhaustion of burnout is an emotional and mental one that will not let you sleep."

Burnout often becomes inevitable when the professional is forced to provide care for too many people. As the ratio increases, the result is higher and higher emotional overload until, like a wire that has too much electricity flowing through it, the worker just burns out and emotionally disconnects. The importance of this ratio for understanding burnout is vividly demonstrated in the research on child-care workers that I recently conducted with Ayala Pines. We studied the staff members of eight child-care centers where staff-to-children ratios ranged from 1 to 4 to as high as 1 to 12.

The staff from the high-ratio centers worked a greater number of hours on the floor in direct contact with the children and had fewer opportunities to take a break from work. They were more approving of supplementary techniques to make children quiet, such as compulsory naps and the use of tranquilizers for hyperactive children. They did not feel that they had much control over what they did on the job, and overall they liked their job much less than did the staff from low-ratio centers.

Social welfare workers said that a high ratio of clients to staff was one of the major factors forcing a dehumanized view of clients. "There are just so many, you cannot afford to sympathize with them all," explained a social worker. "If I only had 50 clients, I might be able to help them individually. But with 300 clients in my caseload, I'm lucky if I can see that they all get their checks."

When staff ratios are low, then the individual staff member has fewer people to worry about and can give more attention to each of them. Also, there is more time to focus on the positive, nonproblem aspects of the person's life, rather than concentrating just on his or her problems. For example, in psychiatric wards with low staff-patient ratios, the nurses were more likely to see their patients in both good times and bad. Even though there were upsetting days, there were also times when the nurses could laugh and joke with the patients, play Ping-Pong or cards with them, talk with their families and so on. In a sense, these nurses had a more complete, more human, view of each patient.

Opportunities for withdrawing from a stressful situation are critically important for these professionals. However, the type of withdrawal that is available may spell the difference between burnout and successful coping. The most positive form of withdrawal that we observed is what we have called a "time-out." Time-outs are not merely short breaks from work such as rest periods or coffee breaks. Rather, they are opportunities for the professional to voluntarily choose to do some other, less stressful, work while other staff take over client/patient responsibilities. For example, in one of the psychiatric wards we studied, the nurses knew that if they were having a rough day, they could arrange to do something else besides work directly with patients. "There are times on the ward when I know that I'm not as capable of giving that much of myself, so I'll sit in the office and do a lot of paperwork. The way our schedule is, it gives you the opportunity to do that. You can withdraw and choose to attend meetings for a while. Or you can ask to get assigned to medications, so that you spend the entire day in the medicine room. Then, the only time you see patients is when you're calling on them for medicines." In this system, when one nurse took a time-out, the other nurses would cover for her and continue to provide adequate patient care.

In contrast to sanctioned time-outs were the negative withdrawals of "escapes." Here, the professional's decision to take a break from work always came at the expense of clients or patients, since there were no other staff people to take over. If the professional was not there to provide treatment or service, then people in need simply had to wait, come back another day or give up. The professionals were more likely to feel trapped by their total responsibility for these people; so they couldn't temporarily withdraw without feeling some guilt. When guilt was heaped upon the already heavy emotional burden they tenuously carried, the load often became too much to bear.

The use of sanctioned time-outs versus guilt-arousing escapes seemed to be primarily determined by the structure of the work setting. Time-outs were possible in well-staffed agencies that had shared work responsibilities, flexible work policies and, most importantly, a variety of job tasks for each professional, rather than just a single one. When institutional policies prevented the use of voluntary time-outs, we found lower staff morale, greater emotional stress and the inevitable consequence of more dissatisfied citizens, frustrated at not getting the care they needed.

The number of hours that a person works at a job is very likely to be related to that person's sense of fatigue, boredom, stress, etc. So one might suspect that longer working hours would lead to a higher burnout rate. However, our data reveal a somewhat different pattern of behavior. Longer hours are correlated with more stress and negative staff attitudes only when they involve continuous direct contact with patients or clients.

Our study of child-care centers provides a good illustration of this point. Longer working hours were related to signs of burnout when the longer hours involved more work on the floor with children. They were more approving of institutional restraints on the children's behavior, and when they were not at work, they wanted to get as far away as possible from children and child-related activities. Staffers who worked just as many hours but spent a smaller proportion of time in direct contact with children did not develop such negative attitudes toward young people. Instead, they felt positively about them and about the child-care center in general. Perhaps the quality of caring, if not mercy, may have to be time-shared.

In many of the institutions we studied, there was a clear split in job responsibilities—either the professionals worked directly with clients or patients, or they worked in administration. As an example, most of the child-care workers spent all their time on the floor with the children, while the directors only had a few (if any) hours with the children and spent the rest of their time in administrative work and meetings. Burnout was more likely to occur for the workers. Often, they would then escape into administrative work.

We were initially surprised to discover how many social workers were returning to school to get advanced training for this kind of higher level, "nonclient" work (and we found it bitterly ironic that clients should be such outcasts in a profession that would not exist without them). As one social worker said, "We can all point to people who have burned out—who are cold, unsympathetic, callous and detached. And each of us knows that we have the potential to fit that role as well, if we haven't already. And that's why we're going back to school to become administrators or teachers or whatever—so that our client contact will be limited and we won't be forced to become callous in order to stay sane.'

Our findings on the effect of prolonged direct contact suggest some job changes that would modify the amount of such direct contact. Possible work alternatives include shorter work shifts, greater opportunities for time-outs, or jobs that involve varied work responsibilities so that an individual staff person is not constantly required to be working directly with other people.

The availability of formal or informal programs in which professionals can get together to discuss problems and get advice and support is another way of helping them to cope with job stress more successfully. Contrary to the beliefs of some skeptics (one physician stated that such a system would only provide the nurses with another opportunity to chit-chat rather than work), such support groups serve a very valuable function for their professional members. Burnout rates seem to be lower for those professionals who have access to such a system, especially if they are well-developed and supported by the larger agency.

Some of the psychiatrists reported being part of a social-professional support group when they were doing their residency. They would meet regularly to discuss problems that they were having in treating their patients, to vent frustrations or to report their successes. After leaving the hospital and entering private practice, some of these psychiatrists found that the lack of such a group was a serious, unanticipated loss to them. "I felt cut off, isolated—I didn't feel I had people whom I could turn to when problems arose, and whose opinions I could trust," one therapist told us. Some psychiatrists even made efforts to rejoin the hospital meetings of the residents, although not always successfully.

Since health and social service workers often experience strong emotional reactions, efforts must be made to constructively deal with these feelings and prevent them from being extinguished, as in burnout. We were surprised to find that many of our subjects did not know that other people were experiencing the same feelings they were; each of them thought their personal reaction was unique. And it was easy to keep this illusion, because they rarely shared feelings with colleagues. In many cases, workers felt that something was wrong with them—they were "bad persons" to have such feelings—and several had sought psychiatric help to deal with what they thought was personal failing.

Even though many of these professionals keep their feelings to themselves, it is painfully clear that they have a strong need to talk to someone about them. Throughout our work, we have been struck by the outpouring of emotional responses to our research from health and social service professionals. They are extremely eager to talk with us about the problems of detached concern and burnout. In fact, we often receive calls from other professional people who have heard about our research. For example, while we were collecting information from the staff of the psychiatric ward at a county hospital, several of the nurses from the alcoholism treatment ward contacted us and asked to be interviewed as well. All too often, their reason for volunteering for the research was "I know that I have burned out—but I want to understand why."

Our findings show that burnout rates are lower for those professionals who actively express, analyze and share their personal feelings with their colleagues. Not only do they consciously get things off their chest, but they have an opportunity to receive constructive feedback from other people and to develop new perspectives and understanding of their relationship with their patients/clients. This process is greatly enhanced if the institution sets up some social outlets such as support groups, special staff meetings or workshops. In general, we found that those professionals who are trained to treat psychological problems were better able to recognize and deal with their own feelings.

In contrast, prison guards who experienced great fear were constrained from expressing, or even acknowleding, it by an institutional macho code, one consequence of which was the channeling of this emotion into psychosomatic illnesses. According to one former prison guard, "Male identity is a killing factor within the all-male prison society. Concern of any kind is all too often translated as weakness. All new correctional officers must learn to control their emotions, especially the incredible fear. Each of us reacted to the fear in his own way, but we had no way to release tensions."

It seems clear from the research findings to date that health and social service professionals need to have special training and preparation for working closely with other people. While they are well trained in certain healing and service skills, they are often not well equipped to handle repeated, intense, emotional interactions with people. As one poverty lawyer put it, "I was trained in law, but not in how to work with the people who would be my clients. And it was that difficulty in dealing with people and their personal problems, hour after hour, that became the problem for me, not the legal matters per se."

In recommending that these professionals receive training in interpersonal skills, I do not mean to suggest that somehow these people are antisocial types who are personally unable to relate to other people. Rather, I believe that their occupations require them to operate in situations of unique stress, for which their previous life experiences have not adequately prepared them. Any of us, facing such a stressful set of circumstances, would probably burn out fairly quickly, but we expect these professionals not to do so. Such an expectation, however, is unwarranted unless they have careful training.

Such training should focus on the personal stress involved in the work—what its sources are, what the constructive and ineffective techniques for dealing with it are, what the possible changes in attitude and emotions are (and why they occur). In other words, professionals need to be made aware of the importance and relevance of their psychological state to their work with other people.

In addition, it is important that they understand their own motivations for entering their particular career and recognize the expectations they have for their work. As Freudenberger points out in his booklet, staff members can be on a variety of "trips," a self-fullfilling ego trip; a self-aggrandizement ego trip; a self-sacrificing, dedication-to-others ego trip; or a trip to deny their own personal problems.

Although many of our subjects stated that they wished they had had prior preparation in interpersonal skills, some reported that there was no time for it in their already packed curriculum. Others felt that such preparation was just "icing on the cake" and not an essential part of professional training. The view of several physicians was that the competent practice of medicine was all that they need to know to be successful in their career, and that any psychological training simply amounted to knowing how to make "small talk" with their patients. Such a skill was viewed as pleasant but unimportant. In my opinion, this viewpoint is sadly in error, for it trivializes an essential aspect of the doctor-patient relationship and fails to recognize that both the doctor and the patient are human beings whose personal attitudes and emotions can affect not only the delivery of health care, but also how and even whether it is accepted.

Is burnout inevitable? Some professionals seem to think so and assume that it is only a matter of time before they will burn out and have to change their job. The period of time most often cited in one psychiatric ward was 1½ years, in free clinics it was usually one year and some poverty lawyers spoke of a reduction of the former four-year-stint down to two. I would like to think that burnout is not inevitable and that steps can be taken to reduce and modify its occurrence. My feeling is that many of the causes of burnout are located not in permanent traits of the people involved, but in certain specific social and situational factors that can be influenced in ways suggested by our research.